T0332001

*Shariah and the Halal Industry*

# SHARIAH AND THE HALAL INDUSTRY

MOHAMMAD HASHIM KAMALI

OXFORD
UNIVERSITY PRESS

# OXFORD
UNIVERSITY PRESS

Oxford University Press is a department of the University of Oxford. It furthers
the University's objective of excellence in research, scholarship, and education
by publishing worldwide. Oxford is a registered trade mark of Oxford University
Press in the UK and certain other countries.

Published in the United States of America by Oxford University Press
198 Madison Avenue, New York, NY 10016, United States of America.

Library of Congress Cataloging-in-Publication Data
Names: Kamali, Mohammad Hashim, author.
Title: Shariah and the halal industry / Mohammad Hashim Kamali.
Description: New York : Oxford University Press, 2021. |
Includes bibliographical references and index.
Identifiers: LCCN 2020056049 (print) | LCCN 2020056050 (ebook) |
ISBN 9780197538616 (hardback) | ISBN 9780197538630 (epub) |
ISBN 9780197538647 (Digital-Online) | ISBN 9780197538623 (updf)
Subjects: LCSH: Muslims—Dietary laws. | Halal food industry—Law and legislation. |
Halal food industry—Law and legislation—Malaysia.
Classification: LCC BP184.9.D5 K36 2021 (print) |
LCC BP184.9.D5 (ebook) | DDC 297.5/76—dc23
LC record available at https://lccn.loc.gov/2020056049
LC ebook record available at https://lccn.loc.gov/2020056050

DOI: 10.1093/oso/9780197538616.001.0001

1 3 5 7 9 8 6 4 2

Printed by Integrated Books International, United States of America

# Contents

# Introduction

THIS INTRODUCTION DISCUSSES five themes, beginning with a summary and overview of the book, followed by a similar overview of the halal industry and its market presence. Then follows a brief discussion of the sources of shariah and the need for continuous research and *ijtihad* (independent reasoning) to respond to newly arising issues on halal and *haram*. The chapter ends by touching on a rather difficult aspect of the subject, namely the negative impacts of meat eating on the environment, and also looks at meat eating in Islamic history and its religious overtones.

## Summary and Overview

The volume at hand is composed of three parts. Part I, titled "Shariah Perspectives," provides a detailed review of the data of shariah over twenty chapters devoted to a variety of interrelated subjects. Thus, it expounds the permissible (halal, *mubah, ja'iz*), the prohibited (*haram, mahzur, mamnu'*), and that which may fall in between, including the gray areas (*al-mashbuhat*) that are not clearly evaluated in the existing data of shariah, and are therefore open to fresh research and *ijtihad*, such as issues concerning food additives, preservatives, genetically modified organisms, and chemical enhancers.

Chapter 6, on *haram*, is the most detailed in Part I, mainly due to its centrality to the whole of this book. This chapter provides a detailed review of the shariah rules and guidelines on *haram*, beginning with the definition of *haram* and its classification into several types, all of which have a bearing on the degree of severity of the transgression involved. Then follows a section on the grounds of *haram*, which leads, in turn, to another section on the mixing of halal and *haram* in the same subject matter and how the shariah may deal

*Shariah and The Halal Industry*. Mohammad Hashim Kamali, Oxford University Press. © Oxford University Press 2021. DOI: 10.1093/oso/9780197538616.003.0001

with it. The succeeding three chapters (Chapters 7–9) examine *istihalah, istihlak,* and necessity and forgetfulness, respectively—subjects that may be seen as extensions of *haram,* but are presented in separate chapters for reasons of reader convenience.

Our review of the shariah principles in Part I serves two main purposes, one of which is to introduce the halal market and its factual presence. It thus expounds the theoretical underpinnings of the market realities of the halal industry, enabling the average reader to better understand what has always been practiced by Muslims with a degree of devotion, even enthusiasm, and is now finding new avenues of expression. The second purpose is to take the more advanced reader of the subject a step further to acquire knowledge of the tools of research into shariah and enabled to engage in the reconstruction and reform of some of the applied aspects thereof. The reader will also find in many places references to where the applied shariah rules may need to be adjusted in order to respond more effectively to contemporary changes and issues of concern to the halal industry. The first group of readers is thus presented with an examination and review of the rules of halal and *haram* and the renowned scale of Five Values (*al-ahkam al-khamsah*) that explain the underlying concepts and values of the halal industry. This explanatory section is then taken a step further through a presentation of a set of other shariah principles that enable the reader to understand how and where to do research in order to revise and reconstruct the existing rules in line with new market developments.

In addition to the introductory review of the sources of shariah, the reader also finds chapters on *fatwa* issuance, and *fatwas* that the Malaysian and other *fatwa* issuing authorities may have validated on matters of concern to the halal industry. Chapter 1 provides a broad outline of shariah, followed by two separate chapters expounding the principles of permissibility (*ibahah*), and of cleanliness (*taharah*), respectively. There is also a chapter (Chapter 17) on the principle of selection (*takhayyur*) that shows the researcher how to exercise selection, or preference, among the available interpretations of shariah offered by the various schools of Islamic jurisprudence in favor of that interpretation which may best relate to contemporary conditions. A chapter then follows on the subject of "piecing together" (*talfiq*), which in many ways resembles *takhayyur* but also differs from it in other respects.

Part I also presents, toward the end, a chapter on "Islam and Science," which looks into the ways scientific research can be integrated into shariah, as part of modern research on issues of concern to the halal industry. This chapter thus looks into four halal-related issues of contemporary concern, namely the use of electric stunning in halal slaughtering, halal vaccines, genetically modified organisms in the food chain, and the environmental impacts of meat eating. But even in its earlier sections, Part I familiarizes the reader with a number of doubtful matters (*al-mashbuhat*), such as gelatin, insulin, and chemical additives, that are open to fresh responses and research into the sources of shariah. In sum, the twenty chapters in Part I provide a number of explanatory sections that are then supplemented by additional readings into the *ijtihad*-related aspects of the shariah of concern to the halal industry. The chapter examines to what extent the shariah may be said to have the resources to accommodate new changes and move abreast with the challenges of modernity and science. A full response to this question would really fall beyond our scope, but what is presented here in connection with the subject matter of this book is hopefully sufficient to engage the interested reader in preliminary responses to the question raised. That said, in terms of the language flow and the progression of chapters, the entire book is written with an average reader in mind.

Part II, titled "Halal Industry in Malaysia," reviews milestones of development that include four main areas: the issuance of halal standards, halal certification procedures, the development of halal parks, and that of the halal pharmaceuticals sector. Sixteen halal standards have been issued since 2004 by the Department of Standards Malaysia, all presented in separate booklets of about ten to twenty pages each, dealing with the shariah and regulatory aspects of the various segments of the halal industry. Some are thus concerned with an exposition of basic shariah principles of general application on the subject of halal and *haram*, whereas others relate to food and beverage, halal slaughtering, *halalan-tayyiban*, halal cosmetics, halal pharmaceuticals, medicine and supplements, halal management, packaging, transportation, and so forth. The other three "milestones of development" discussed in Part II basically supplement the "halal standards" in that companies and individuals who fulfill all the halal standards qualify for the issuance of halal certificates and logos they can then exhibit on their premises and products. The establishment of halal parks in the various states and strategic locations of Malaysia also seeks to facilitate a more efficient development of halal standards. Halal parks are based on the concepts of facilitation, easy access, and better control of the scientific research aspects of halal standards, although they tend to offer a microcosm of the larger spread of the halal industry generally. Finally, halal pharmaceuticals represent a salient segment of the halal industry and its rapid progress into in a new area in line with the applied Halal Standards of Malaysia.

Part III of the volume reviews regional and international developments of the halal industry in the ASEAN region and elsewhere, including China, Japan, South Korea, and a number of European countries. Also featured in this part is a section on "imported meats" from non-Muslim-majority countries by Muslim countries and consumers. This is followed by a chapter on halal tourism, with a brief review of its history, development, and diversification in Malaysia, Indonesia, and Turkey. A discussion then follows on some of the negative reactions to halal, "halal phobia,"[1] and halal reputational issues. The book ends with a conclusion and a number of actionable recommendations.

## World Halal Market

Our review of halal market trends in the various parts of this volume reflects on its size and potential growth directions. There are approximately 1.84 billion Muslims in the world today, making up around 24.4 percent of the world population, or just under one-quarter of the human inhabitants of the earth. Muslims the world over are showing, especially in recent decades, a greater awareness of halal and *haram* in their choices and lifestyles. Their number is also expected to rise to 2.2 billion by 2030. The growing Muslim population worldwide translates into a rising international demand for halal products and services. Halal is now a global industry and agenda at a time of ever-increasing globalization, which also bodes well for the growth of the world economy as a whole. The young and fast-growing Muslim demographic, a substantial and fast-growing Islamic economy, and the greater affluence of some Muslim countries in the Middle East and Asia are among the leading market indicators of demand for halal products today. However, rapid growth also presents challenges surrounding halal compliance issues and reputational risks. International attitudes and rapid technological changes also entail important

---

1. "Halal phobia" echoes a parallel but larger phenomenon, namely that of Islamophobia. Whereas Islamophobia means the fear of Islam, real or imaginary, halal phobia similarly means fear and apprehension, justified or otherwise, of halal. This involves the skeptical, negative, and sometimes hostile reception of the halal brand and concept by individuals, organizations, and even markets. More particularly, it refers to the culture-cum-religious resistance that certain sectors of society in Western countries such as France, the United States, and even Singapore have voiced, rightly or wrongly, against halal. Many tend to see it as another manifestation of radical Islam. It thus appears that halal phobia is a subset of Islamophobia, and the two often go hand-in-hand.

responsibilities concerning ethical governance of the halal industry and its proper regulation worldwide.[2]

According to Kuwait Finance House research, the value of the global halal economy is expected to be US$6.4 trillion in 2018. Of this grand total Islamic finance and halal food sectors are expected to contribute US$3.9 trillion and US$1.6 trillion, respectively. Also, according to the Global Islamic Economic Indicator (GIEI), Malaysia and the United Arab Emirates are two of the fifty-seven member countries of the Organisation of Islamic Cooperation (OIC) and sixteen non-OIC countries that have the best halal ecosystems. The halal ecosystem signifies a dynamic system that consists not of an isolated development, but rather a complex network of businesses, institutions, government agencies, and nongovernmental organizations (NGOs). It is equipped with the means to detect instances of noncompliance according to an established set of criteria. The halal park concept mentioned earlier is driven by building a halal ecosystem that is internally self-contained and able to facilitate well-planned and controlled development. Singapore, the only non-OIC state listed among the top fifteen GIEI countries also has one of the best halal ecosystems. Based on reports by the Islamic Development Bank and Thompson Reuters, the rapid growth of the halal economy worldwide is driven by strong demand from both Muslim and non-Muslim consumers.[3]

As for the question of why are countries like Italy, Spain, Thailand, Japan, China, Brazil, and South Korea are keen to invest in the halal industry, and why Brazil's BRF and other multinationals like Nestle, Carrefour, Walmart, MasterCard, and Marriot have engaged in the provision of halal products and services, the answer is surely profitability for the most part, but also perhaps their interest in halal values such as purity, integrity, and caring. It has been widely reported that the British, French, and Dutch, rightly or wrongly, tend to associate Islam with violence, yet at the same time these same countries are keen to participate and be active players in the world halal market.[4]

The emergence of the halal industry as a market reality and commercially lucrative sector of the Islamic economy is relatively recent, developed mainly in the last few decades, as part of the Islamic revivalism of the latter half of the twentieth century. The halal industry emerged even after the Islamic banking

---

2. Cf. Shah, "Fostering a True Halal Economy," 12. See also Tieman, "Safeguarding Halal Reputation," 14.

3. As reported in Mohamad, "Halal Economy," 18.

4. Mohamad, "Halal Economy," 18.

and finance phenomenon, but gained momentum with the onset of globalization (or perhaps resistance to it) that addressed and began to penetrate markets and media, but also to influence lifestyle and culture. Although the industry is still in its early stages of development, it has experienced remarkably rapid growth, especially since the first decade of twenty-first century. Its rapid progress is partly due to its stringent rules on food safety, cleanliness, and economic fair play that appeal to the consumer public, both Muslim and non-Muslim. As with the Islamic banking and finance industry that preceded it, the halal industry is also seen as market-driven more than it is knowledge-driven. Market players and industry specialists now stress the need to enrich past achievements and rapid market advances with a better understanding of their underlying Islamic principles, as well as scientific knowledge relevant to its current and future growth.

## Religion and Culture

Religiosity is the main cause, of course, of why Muslims observe the lawful and unlawful in their dietary choices. Yet it is interesting to note that Muslims who are not so pious in other respects still tend to observe these rules, partly because dietary laws are usually observed from early childhood as part of religious and family traditions. They are deeply entrenched in the customs and culture of societies, and for many they become a part of their identity. To illustrate this, one may refer to the story of Nariman, who was born in Egypt, lived in Britain for more than ten years, and is now back in her homeland:

> Years after I stopped practicing all other aspects of Islam, I was still fasting during Ramadan. . . . Although I mostly don't know, nostalgia still makes me fast the odd few days every Ramadan. It makes me feel part of an event that links me with other human beings, family and friends but also millions that I don't know: we all feel hunger together, we all sit down to eat at sunset.[5]

Nariman says she found it easier to break other dietary restrictions, but fasting was "the last to go." "Perhaps because as a child, it was a sign of being grown-up," she explains, "it made you proud to be allowed to fast with the

---

5. Consiglio, "Food: the Last Bastion of Faith."

adults. . . . So that will always be linked for me to a sense of achievement, of proving that I can." She says that going against the restrictions of what to eat and when not to eat is like "breaking deeply ingrained taboos": "It can be liberating but can also feel like you've cut yourself loose, which is potentially scary."[6]

The impact of religion on food consumption depends on the nature of its teachings and the manner in which they seek to regulate a certain area or subject, people's customary practices, and how they understand and interpret the teachings of their religion. Most leading religions forbid certain foods, such as pork in Judaism and Islam, or pork and beef in Hinduism and Buddhism (Christianity, which has no major food taboos, is an exception). Consumption of animal products, and more specifically meat and meat products, is often addressed in scriptural sources and regulated by rules concerning the slaughter of animals.

Besides the two basic sources of Islamic law, the Qur'an and the Sunnah, other sources and proofs are also used in determining the permissibility of food and beverage. Whereas the Qur'an is the most authoritative source, the Prophet Muhammad's sayings and exemplary conduct, or his Sunnah, though for the most part explanatory to the Qur'an, also provide original rulings on a variety of issues, including halal and *haram* in animals, birds, and marine life that are not addressed in the Qur'an. Halal products are often defined as ones that are shariah-compliant, meaning they are clear of *haram* elements, exploitation, and injustice, and are neither harmful nor intended to advance harmful purposes. Halal products and services must also be free of alcohol, pork, blood shed forth, carrion, and meat that has not been slaughtered according to Islamic rituals.

As already mentioned, halal and *haram* are an entrenched part of the Muslim faith, which is why they have been traditionally observed without any statutory or executive orders. This is partly because of the Qur'anic directives on halal and *haram* and how they address the believers. To quote the Qur'an:

> O ye who believe! Eat of the good things We have provided you with and be grateful to God if it is Him you worship. (al-Baqarah, 2:172)

The believers are reminded time and again to eat what is halal and also *tayyib* (pure and wholesome):

---

6. Consiglio, "Food: the Last Bastion of Faith."

O you people! Eat of that which is in the earth, lawful and wholesome (*halalan tayyiban*). (2:168)

Eat of the good things We have provided for your sustenance, but commit no excess therein. (Taha, 20:81)

In addition, the faithful must invoke God's name when eating meat. This is understood to mean that an invocation must be made at the time an animal is being slaughtered:

So eat (meat) on which God's name has been mentioned, if you are believers. (al-An'am, 6:118)

And eat not (of meat) on which God's name has not been pronounced. For that would be an abomination. (6:121)

The majority of Muslim scholars have held that this last verse refers to the proper slaughtering of only the permitted animals. Since Muslim dietary laws relate to divine permissions and prohibitions, those who observe them earn a reward in the hereafter and those who violate them may be penalized. Meats and other substances of animal origin that are specifically prohibited are spelled out in the Qur'an as follows:

Forbidden to you (for food) are: carrion, blood, the flesh of swine, and that on which has been invoked the name of other than God; that which has been killed by strangling, or by a violent blow, or by a headlong fall, or by being gored to death; that which has been partly eaten by a wild animal, unless you are able to slaughter it (in due form); that which is sacrificed on stone (altars); and meat that is divided by raffling with arrows. (al-Ma'idah, 5:3)

Although clear textual prohibitions are enough to establish religious obligations, it is believed that many of them are also based on health reasons, and what is prohibited is largely due to their impurity and harm.

## *Harm (Darar) and Repulsiveness (Khubth)*

Two of the salient shariah principles that have influenced juristic opinion are manifest harm (*darar*), and natural repulsiveness (*khubth*). There are a number of rulings in the scriptural sources that permit destruction of harmful or dangerous creatures such as snakes, scorpions, rats, and predatory animals, which have consequently been classified as non-halal on grounds of *darar*. So also are animals and substances that are naturally repulsive and thus classified under *khaba'ith*, such as rotten food and decayed carcass, even of halal animals.[7]

Animals that are halal for human consumption need to be ritually slaughtered according to specified methods, as already mentioned, with only two exceptions, based on the authority of hadith: fish and locusts. As for animals that are non-halal for human consumption, their slaughter and death from natural causes are about the same. Slaughter will not make them halal for eating, but regardless of the manner of their death, many of their body parts, such as their hair, bone, skin, and fat may be used for other beneficial purposes. The one exception to this is the swine, which is unlawful altogether, including their skin, bone, and hair, according to the Hanafi school of law, though other leading schools have recorded disagreement on this, and many have allowed the use of porcine derivatives for beneficial purposes other than eating, especially when they have undergone the process, for instance, of substance transformation (*istihalah*) as in the case of gelatin and insulin. These are elaborated in the following pages.

Muslim jurists of the past have discussed the source evidence on halal and *haram* and formulated guidelines to regulate their applications to animal slaughter and dietary subjects. Whereas the shariah identifies *haram* substances in food from animal sources in clear detail, it takes a different approach to the identification of halal/permissible in foodstuffs and beverages, as these are not always identified by name but rather by indicators that are not entirely free of doubt. Gray areas of doubt have consequently existed and often called for fresh juristic inquiry and *ijtihad* as to their permissibility. The existing *fiqh* manuals provide details concerning most of the familiar varieties of animals, birds, insects, seafood, etc., either by name or by their general characteristics, but these are still not exhaustive. Yet the incessant diversity in our times of food varieties and market products, as well as new developments in science and technology, continuously impact the *fiqh* positions on dietary substances, which necessitate, in turn, continuous research and review of the content and composition of food products from the shariah perspectives. This is not even confined to new products, but could involve revision and substitution of some of the existing *fiqh* rules in light of new scientific evidence and market developments.

---

7. Cf. Wizarat, *al-Mawsū'ah al-Fiqhiyyah*, vol. 18, 336.

Current issues of GMOs (genetically modified organisms) in foods, animal feed, and hormones are often discussed in the light of these concepts, and in several other sources and principles of Islamic jurisprudence. Biotechnology, unconventional sources of ingredients, synthetic materials, and innovations in animal slaughter and meat processing are also among the issues that Muslim scholars, government regulatory bodies, and institutions of specialized research are dealing with to help consumers make better informed choices.

## Meat Eating Then and Now: Environmental Impacts of Meat Eating

With regard to the enormously damaging impacts of meat eating on the natural environment, this is expected to be difficult to change for various reasons. Meat is historically known to be humanity's earliest food, and it was taken raw at first until roasting became known. Islam basically confirmed the importance of meat both as a nutritional food and for its good taste. Reports further confirm meat eating as a preferable food type among the Arabs, who habitually regarded meat as the best food, which may arguably be reflective to some extent of their desert lifestyle and a certain shortage of other food varieties. It also remains true that meat eating has dominated the history of food almost everywhere, not least in the Muslim countries and communities, with the exception perhaps of the followers of Hinduism, who are mainly vegetarian. A meal is hardly seen to be complete, to this day, without meat, and for larger occasions, not just one but many meat varieties and dishes are required. That said, some of this fascination with meat might also be changing due to changeable market conditions and the wider selections of food availability in the marketplace, and also greater awareness of health hazards associated with excessive meat consumption, especially red meat.

The Qur'an mentions meat in about a dozen places, nearly all in a positive light. In one place, in a reference to the sea as a source of sustenance, it is mentioned that the sea is "for you to eat thereof flesh that is fresh and tender" (al-Nahl, 16:14; Fatir, 35:12). This is, by implication, understood to be a reference mainly to fish. In another place, poultry is mentioned as food of the "People of Paradise": "and the flesh of fowl—any that they may desire." (al-Waqi'ah, 56:21). In yet another reference to the dwellers of Paradise, God Most High promises, "and We shall bestow on them of fruit and meat any they may desire" (al-Tur, 52:22). Elsewhere in a reference to the people of

Moses (the Jews), when they asked for varieties of food other than Manna,[8] and for quails, to be sent to them from On High, they asked for produce of the earth such as cucumber, garlic, lentils, and onion, but were asked then, "Will you exchange the better for that which is lesser?" (al-Baqarah, 2:61). This is indicative perhaps of a certain preference for the flesh of quails over these other food varieties just mentioned.[9]

In an elevated (*marfu'*) hadith on the authority of the Companion Abu Darda', it is also stated that "meat is the best food of the people of this world and those of the Paradise."[10] In addition, the Qur'an in various places mentions certain other food items, such as milk, honey, figs, grapes, olives, and pomegranates, mostly in a positive light, which tends to confer a certain sanctity on them. Muslims do pay attention to all of this, as many believe that the mere mention of these food varieties in the Qur'an is indicative of encouragement for reasons not only of natural purity and appeal, but also their health benefits.

Reports from the leading Companions also confirm their preference for meat. 'Ali ibn Abu Talib is thus quoted to have recommended meat consumption: "for it improves the skin color, lightens the stomach, and improves one's manners." In another report attributed to Nafi', he speaks of his fellow Companion 'Abd Allah ibn 'Umar, who would not miss out on meat during Ramadan and also during travel. Nafi' reported what 'Ali b. Abu Talib had said, that "one who abandoned meat for forty nights, his manners are adversely affected." Similar statements have been recorded from the Successors (the generation immediately following the Companions), some of whom praised meat as helping one's eyesight, and others as an energy booster. A few other personalities are quoted to have spoken similarly on the good effects of meat consumption, with the proviso, however, that it is taken in moderation.[11]

When one confines one's food intake to meat sources alone, however, it is likely to be greatly harmful. For meat, although good in itself, does not include many of the necessary nutrients. The second caliph, 'Umar b. al-Khattab, is quoted in this connection to have said, "Beware of meat, as its

---

8. *Manna*, which is found to this day in the Sinai region, is a gummy saccharine secretion found on a species of tamarisk. See Ali, *Meaning of the Holy Qur'an*, 29, fn. 71.

9. Cf. al-Harithi, *Al-Nawazil fi'l-At'imah*, vol. 2, 497–498.

10. Ibn Majah, *Sunan Ibn Majah*, hadith no. 3305, 785, "*sayyidu ta'am ahl al-dunya wa ahl al-jannati al-lahm*." The hadith is said to be a weak hadith.

11. al-Jawziyyah, *Zaad al-Ma'ad fi Huda Khayr al-'Ibad*, vol. 4, 303–304; al-Harithi, *Al-Nawazil fi'l-At'imah*, vol. 2, 499.

harm to one's health can be no less than that of alcohol."[12] One observer named 'Abqirat, who apparently had knowledge of nutrition, is quoted by the renowned Hanbali scholar Ibn Qayyim al-Jawziyyah (d.751/1350) to have given the following advice: "[D]o not make your bellies into the graveyard of animals."[13] Excessive meat eating is also noted to cause, or play a role, in developing diseases such as gall bladder and kidney malfunction, as it increases urine acidity, or urea. A nutrition specialist, Dr al-'Alami, has further added to this that excessive meat consumption can cause sciatica, rheumatism, diabetes, the narrowing down of arteries, and high blood pressure.[14]

Livestock farming and meat consumption, especially red meat, have severe impacts, not only on human health and well-being, but also on the earth's environment and sustainability. The vast and still increasing meat consumption causes forest destruction, wildlife extinction, excessive greenhouse gas (GHG) emission, and global climate change.[15] As a protein source for the world's rapidly expanding middle-class populations, increased meat consumption will likely put excessive strain on the earth's well-being, exceeding planetary boundaries of safety.

Domestically raised ruminant meat has a much higher carbon footprint in producing protein than other meats, and especially greater than vegetarian sources, based on a global meta-analysis of life-cycle assessment studies.[16] Scientific research further shows that ruminant animal production is the largest source of anthropogenic methane emissions, and also accounts for more than any other land use, covering 26 percent of Earth's terrestrial surface.[17]

In the chapter on "Islam and Science" we juxtapose traditional Islamic perspectives on meat consumption with these new findings, bringing to light indisputable evidence that calls for urgent attention. Drastic changes have clearly taken place due to persistent abuse and neglect of the environment, with environmental degradation reaching a crisis level. Recommendations

---

12. Recorded in Imam Malik, *al-Muwatta': Kitab Siffat al-Nabiy: Bab ma ja'a fi akl al-Lahm*, hadith no. 1742, 569; al-Zurqani, Muhammad bin Abd al-Baqi. *Sharh al-Zurqani 'ala Muwatta' al-Imam Malik*. Cairo: Maktabah al-Thaqafah al-Diniyah, 2003.

13. Ibn Qayyim, *Zaad al-Ma'ad*, vol. 4, 313.

14. Dar al-'Alami Hushar, as quoted in al-Harithi, *al-Nawazil fi'l At'imah*, 499–500.

15. The present author acknowledges with thanks that much of the data discussed here is derived from an IAIS Malaysia research paper by its visiting fellow Daud Abdul Fattah Bachelor, titled "Islamic Perspectives on Reducing Meat Consumption to Promote Earth's Sustainability" (2018).

16. Ripple et al., "Ruminants, Climate Change and Climate Policy," 2–5.

17. Bland, "Is the Livestock Industry Destroying the Planet?"

are given for shariah researchers to absorb and integrate these new realities into their work agenda on environmental protection efforts, in addition to reviewing at a glance some of the shariah positions and principles that could be utilized as aids to new research on environmental issues.

Lastly, the reader will note that the Arabic versions of the quotations from the Qur'an, hadith, and Islamic legal maxims appear under three separate appendices at the end of this volume. The English translation of all of these appear in the running text, and the addition of their Arabic originals is for purposes of added accuracy and the benefit of Arabic-conversant readers.

# PART I

## Shariah Perspectives

### Introductory Remarks

One of the main concerns of the various chapters in this part of the book is to beef up the shariah input within the rapidly developing global halal industry. This is partly in response to a groundswell of opinion that obtains among industry practitioners and others that the halal industry in Malaysia and elsewhere is fashioned by rapid market developments, and the shariah input therein has therefore not been receiving due attention—not dissimilar perhaps, to developments in Islamic banking and finance that preceded the emergence of the halal industry. Both are important in that they bring into the global arena Islamic tenets and principles that touch people's lives, both Muslims and non-Muslims, on an increasingly widening scale. Yet barring those with specialized knowledge, the general public is poorly informed on the principles that underline actual developments in the halal industry. This awareness needs to be conveyed in ways that present a blend of theoretical knowledge side by side with its practical developments, and that show clearly how the one relates to the other. This too has been a motivating factor of this book and its thematic arrangement, especially of Part I, which is devoted to an exposition and review of shariah principles.

The twenty chapters of various lengths in Part I are broadly devoted to a review of important shariah principles of relevance to the understanding of halal and *haram* in Islam. The selection presented here includes an introductory chapter on the shariah (meaning, history, and sources), followed by chapters on the principle of original permissibility (*ibahah*), the principle of original cleanliness (*taharah*), the principle of substance transformation (*istihalah*), and that of extreme dilution (*istihlak*), as well as a chapter also on *fatwa* issuance in shariah. Another major chunk of Part I deals with an exposition of the renowned shariah scale of Five Values, namely the prohibited (*haram*), reprehensible (*makruh*), the obligatory (*wajib*), the commendable (*mandub*), and the permissible (halal, *mubah*, and *ja'iz*). A chapter is also devoted to doubtful matters (*mashbuhat*) that may fall in between halal and *haram*, such as food additives, genetically modified organisms, chemical enhancers, and so forth. The chapter on the requirements of a valid slaughter (*al-dhabh*) describes the shariah rules on the subject and the manner of their application in Malaysia. Chapters are also devoted to the roles of necessity (*darurah*) and forgetfulness (*nisyan*) in the understanding of *haram*, followed by a review of the role of general custom ('*urf*), in the determination of halal and *haram*, and finally a chapter on Islam and science. We also present a selection of salient legal maxims of Islamic law (*qawa'id kulliyyah fiqhiyyah*) of particular relevance to the understanding of halal and *haram* in shariah.

The exposition here of the classifications of *haram* into various types also helps to provide a degree of insight into this exceedingly important aspect of the shariah. We examine the grounds of *haram*, which include, in addition to filth and manifest harm, intoxication, poisonous substances, and unlawful acquisition of food that belongs to others. What follows next is a general introduction to shariah, which is followed, in turn, by chapters on the principles of original permissibility (*ibahah*), cleanliness (*taharah*), and others.

# *I*

# *Shariah*

## MEANING, DEFINITION, HISTORY, AND SOURCES

THIS OPENING CHAPTER will examine the following aspects of shariah:

- The meaning and definition of shariah.
- The distinction between shariah and *fiqh*.
- The higher purposes (*maqasid*) of shariah.

## *Meaning and Definition*

Shariah literally means "the way to the watering place," or "the path to correct guidance, salvation, and relief." Shariah is defined as the totality of guidance that God Most High has revealed to His Prophet Muhammad pertaining to the dogma of Islam, its moral values, and its practical legal rules. Shariah is thus a broad concept that is not confined to legal rules, but rather comprises the totality of guidance that God Most High has revealed to humankind.[1]

Shariah has often been described as a diversity within unity—diversity in detail and unity over essentials. The basic Islamic belief in the finality of divine revelation (*wahy*) contained in the Qur'an and its timeless validity has had a unifying effect, ensuring continuity in the understanding of fundamentals. Shariah originates in the Qur'an and Sunnah, and it consists of both specific rules and broad principles of legal and moral import. The clear and specific

---

1. al-Tahanawi, *Kashshaf Istilahat al-Funun*, 835. In a modern work, the Islamic Council of Europe defines the shariah as "the totality of ordinances derived from the Qur'an and Sunnah and any other laws that are deduced from these two sources by methods considered valid in Islamic jurisprudence." Azzam, *Universal Islamic Declaration of Human Rights*, 16.

*Shariah and The Halal Industry.* Mohammad Hashim Kamali, Oxford University Press. © Oxford University Press 2021. DOI: 10.1093/oso/9780197538616.003.0002

injunctions of the Qur'an and Sunnah constitute the core of the shariah, and the understanding that they impart is expected to be self-evident. However, in view of the fact that a much larger portion of the Qur'an is open to interpretation and *ijtihad*, unanimity and consensus in the *ijtihadi* part of shariah has been difficult to obtain. But even so, the jurists of different ages were able to identify a broad line of agreement over interpretations on which they could find supportive evidence in the precedent of the Prophet's Companions or the *ijtihad* of leading ulema. Unity over some interpretational aspects of the shariah is thus reflected in the idea of general consensus, or *ijma'*, whereas diversity over detail is the subject matter of *ikhtilaf* (juristic disagreement).

The rules of shariah are concerned with three major themes: dogmatic theology, which is the subject of *'ilm al-kalam*; the moral teachings of Islam, which fall under *'ilm al-akhlaq*; and practical legal rules pertaining to *'ibadat* (devotional matters) and *mu'amalat*, (civil transactions), which constitute the subject matter of *fiqh*. Shariah is thus primarily concerned with regulating relationships among individuals and those of the individuals with their Creator. It does this by expounding the limits of proper conduct, by defining the essentials of the faith, and by delineating the rituals of worship. The rules of shariah are thus concerned with establishing a basic order of values and measures that protect the integrity of its five higher objectives (*maqasid*), namely life, faith, intellect, property, and lineage.

Dogmatic theology is mainly concerned with liberating humanity from belief in superstition and inculcating faith in God Most High, belief in the fundamentals of Islam, and a sense of enlightened conviction in its values. The moral teachings of Islam (*'ilm al-akhlaq*) are basically concerned with educating the individual by encouraging him or her to exercise self-discipline and restraint in the fulfilment of natural desires, and also a sense of commitment to moral virtue. The ulema are generally in agreement on the primacy of faith and morality (*'aqidah* and *akhlaq*). By comparison to these, *fiqh* is a mere superstructure and a practical manifestation of the dogma and morality of Islam.

## Shariah and Fiqh

Shariah is often used synonymously with *fiqh*, but it is, as already noted, wider than *fiqh* and comprises, in addition to the legal rules of *fiqh*, instruction on morality and dogma. *Fiqh*, which literally means "understanding," is defined as the knowledge of the practical rules (*ahkam 'amaliyyah*) of shariah, which are deduced from their detailed evidence in the sources. *Fiqh* thus consists of the practical rules of shariah that are mainly derived from divine revelation as contained in the Qur'an and Sunnah, and not from the pure application of human reason ('*aql*).[2]

A ruling (*hukm*) of shariah may convey a command or a prohibition, in which case it is known as *hukm taklifi* (defining law), or it may not contain an injunction as such but expound the necessary conditions and requirements for the proper implementation of the *hukm taklifi*. This type of ruling is technically known as *hukm wad'i* (declaratory law), which basically supplements the *hukm taklifi*. To fulfill a contractual obligation is a *hukm taklifi*, but the textual ruling that the parties to a valid contract must be adult and sane is a *hukm wad'i*, which imposes no obligation as such but specifies the valid application of the original ruling.

*Fiqh* is knowledge of the practical rules of shariah concerning the daily activities and conduct of the individual in such areas as civil and commercial transactions, crimes and penalties, matrimonial law, taxation, or devotional matters such as prayer and fasting. The practicalities of conduct are evaluated on a scale of five values of obligatory, recommended, permissible, reprehensible, and forbidden. To say that *fiqh* is concerned with practical rules of conduct would preclude dogmatic theology from the purview of *fiqh*. The last point in the definition of *fiqh* provides that these practical rules are deduced from the detailed evidence that is available in the sources of shariah; that is, the Qur'an and Sunnah and a number of other proofs which are expounded in the science of the sources of law, the *usul al-fiqh*. The rules of *fiqh* may not, in other words, be obtained from a source, such as international treaties, that is not a recognized proof.

Both *fiqh* and shariah originate in the same sources, but shariah is more closely associated with divine revelation (*wahy*). *Fiqh* is a product largely of juristic opinion—that is, *ra'y* (personal opinion) and *ijtihad*, which do not command the same authority as *wahy*. Juristic opinion is also more susceptible to differences of interpretation and disagreement in accordance with the change of time and circumstances. It thus appears that knowledge of halal and *haram*, the clear injunctions as well as the broad and general principles of the Qur'an and Sunnah, constitute the common denominator of both the shariah and *fiqh*. But *fiqh* extends the general guidance of shariah in regard to matters that are not fully regulated in the source materials of shariah. With regard to the need for continuous research and *ijtihad*, it will be noted that

---

2. al-Jurjani, *Kitab al-Ta'rifat*, 222; Al-Amidi, 'Ali bin Muhammad. *Al-Ihkam fi Usul al-Ahkam*. Beirut: al-Maktab al-Islami, 1982, 5.

the source data of shariah are not expected to provide clear rulings or exhaustive details on all varieties of animals and plants and all newly arising issues. The source data of shariah provide some guidelines that may help researchers in their quest for answers to new issues.

The rules, or the *ahkam*, of *fiqh* mainly occur in two varieties. First, there are *ahkam* that are founded in a clear text (*nass*), such as the essentials of *'ibadat* (worship matters), prohibition of adultery and of marriage between close relatives, and so forth. These are self-evident and therefore independent of interpretation or *ijtihad*. This part of *fiqh* is simultaneously a part of the sacred and permanent shariah. Second, there are rules that are formulated through the exercise of juristic deduction and *ijtihad*. Because of the possibility of error in this exercise, the rules that are so derived do not command finality. They may be based on interpretation of a particular text or on sound legal reasoning. The conclusion in either case is not in conflict with any textual ruling, and it secures in the meantime a benefit (*maslahah*). This is not necessarily a part of the permanent shariah, and the *mujtahid* (scholar competent to exercise *ijtihad*) who has reason to depart from it in favor of an alternative conclusion may do so without incurring a transgression.[3]

*Fiqh* develops the shariah in light of the changing conditions of society through the modality of *ijtihad*. But the harmony of *fiqh* and *ijtihad* with the principles of shariah is not always certain. Only when the ruling of *ijtihad* is supported by a conclusive consensus, or *ijma'*, does that ruling acquire the binding force of a *hukm shar'i*. The edifice of *fiqh* is thus built by the cumulative rulings of *ijtihad* that the jurists have formulated in response to particular issues.

The *fiqh* (applied Islamic law) is thus concerned mainly with extracting practical legal rules from the data of the primary sources. Muslim jurists of the various schools (*madhhabs*) of Islamic law have provided additional details on numerous aspects of the scriptural directives on halal and *haram*. Yet when a new situation arises that is not covered in the scriptural sources, or in the existing *fiqh* interpretations, it may be addressed through independent reasoning (*ijtihad*), which is when a qualified scholar or group of scholars exert themselves fully to derive the needed solution. This could be attempted by recourse to one or more of the subvarieties of *ijtihad*, as are also expounded in the science of the sources of law, the *usul al-fiqh*, or through original and independent interpretation that does not violate the basic principles.

---

3. Cf. al-Shatibi, *Al-Muwaqat fi Usul al-Shari'ah*, I, 31; Zaydan, *al-Wajiz fi Sharh al-Qawa'id*, 66; al-Nabhan, 11.

The sources of Islamic law that are expounded in *usul al-fiqh* are of two kinds: the revealed sourced, or the Qur'an, and the authentic sayings and exemplary conduct of the Prophet Muhammad, or his Sunnah/hadith. The latter sources are the rational or nonrevealed sources that are many, including, for instance, analogical reasoning (*qiyas*), which is to construct a new ruling of Islamic law by drawing an analogy with an existing ruling or *hukm* in the Qur'an or Sunnah. Another rational source is consideration of public interest (*istislah*, also known as *maslahah*), which consists of a rational ruling that proceeds over a lawful subject matter and meets the public interest while also not violating any of the principles of shariah. Juristic preference (*istihsan*) is another formula for extracting new rules, and it applies when an existing ruling of the law is applied to a case but somehow fails to deliver justice or seems unfair under the circumstance. By recourse to *istihsan* the qualified jurist/judge constructs a ruling that is preferable and just. *Istihsan* as such may be seen as an equivalent in Islamic law of the Western law doctrine of equity/fairness.

These are all the subvarieties of *ijtihad*, albeit offering different formulas for the application of *ijtihad*, which has now also acquired a collective dimension in that it is undertaken not only by individual scholars, or *mujtahids*, as used to be the case, but also by the *fiqh* academies and learned institutions with significant insight into the shariah as well as contemporary disciplines. In our coverage of scholastic positions on various issues of concern to halal and *haram* in animals and other substances, we have looked into the resources of both the Sunni and Shii jurisprudence for comparative purposes, but also in our quest to explore the prospects of greater standardization of the increasingly globalized halal market.

As already noted, *ijtihad* is in the nature of a juristic opinion that does not establish a binding rule of shariah. *Qiyas*, or reasoning by analogy, is a subvariety of *ijtihad*, and it consists of drawing an analogy to that which is already regulated in the Qur'an or Sunnah. As will be noted below, Muslim scholars have often determined the ruling of an unknown animal or bird, one that is not mentioned in the existing sources or precedents, by its resemblance, or analogy, to that which is familiar and known—such as the giraffe, which is not mentioned in the Qur'an or Sunnah, but is held to be halal due to its striking resemblance to the camel, on which there is a ruling. The *usul al-fiqh* sources also mention a variety of other proofs and formulas that could be employed as the tools of *ijtihad*.[4]

---

4. Fuller details on *ijtihad* and all its subvarieties are found in Kamali, *Principles of Islamic Jurisprudence*.

Halal is a broad shariah value and concept that is not confined to food and beverage, but also extends to medicine, cosmetics, pharmaceuticals, hotels, and resorts, and the scope seems to be expanding, especially in its contemporary understanding, which takes a holistic approach to halal.

Food and beverage varieties are evaluated by the renowned scale of five values (*al-ahkam al-khamsah*) which consist of the obligatory, recommendable, permissible, reprehensible, and forbidden (*wajib, mandub, mubah, makruh*, and *haram*, respectively). Food and beverage that are regulated by a decisive ruling of the Qur'an and Sunnah mostly fall under either the obligatory (*wajib*) or the prohibited (*haram*) categories, and Muslims are obliged to observe them. In addition, Muslims are encouraged under the concept of recommendable (*mandub/mustahab*) to pay attention to guidelines on how the halal and *haram* may best be practiced, and how to attain refinement in safety and purity in food, the treatment of animals, and so forth. The opposite of recommendable (*mandub*) is reprehensible (*makruh*), which often consists of neglecting that which is recommended (*mandub*), or it may consist of doubtful practices that bend the rules, or clumsy and objectionable conduct. Whereas halal and *haram* are mandatory, the *mandub* and the *makruh* are in the nature of moral advice and do not impose strict obligations. It is due to a much larger space that is occupied by the recommended, the reprehensible, and the permissible (*mubah,* halal, *ja'iz*) that Islam is often said to be a "way of life" not strictly confined to dos and don'ts, but that also guides the faithful in so many other ways in the conduct of their daily lives in family and society, business transactions, morality, and culture.

## *Higher Purposes (*Maqasid*) of Shariah and Custom (*'Urf*)*

An aspect of the shariah guidelines that has historically been neglected but has been the focus of renewed interest in recent decades is the higher objectives, or *maqasid*, of shariah, which can also be utilized, side by side with the existing data of *fiqh* and *usul al-fiqh*, as a basis of independent reasoning (*ijtihad*) in the formulation of new rules. The *maqasid* are divided into different types. The essential purposes (*maqasid daruri*, or *daruriyyat*) are five: the protection of religion (*hifz al-din*), protection of life (*hifz al-nafs*), protection of rationality and intellect (*hifz al-'aql*), protection of property (*hifz al-maal*), and protection of lineage (*hifz al-nasab*—also known as *hifz al-nasl*). These are all values that must be protected and prioritized as far as possible in lawmaking, *fatwa*, and *ijtihad*. These values often bring into the picture the macro aspects of shariah and the end results of its detailed rulings—in contrast, one might say, to the more literalist preoccupations of *fiqh* and *usul al-fiqh*. This also partly explains why the *maqasid* have become the focus of renewed attention in recent decades.[5] The essential *maqasid* can thus be the basis of *ijtihad* conducted by qualified shariah scholars.

How do *fiqh* and shariah differ from the *maqasid al-shariah*? The main difference is that *fiqh* consists of detailed rules, whereas the *maqasid* refer to the purposes of those rules. The *fiqh* rules makes provisions, for instance, on the right of maintenance between close relatives, but the purposes/*maqasid* of those rules are protection of the family unit (*hifz al-nasab*) and preservation of the ties of kinship among its members. Similarly, the *fiqh* rules require that at least one of the two countervalues in exchange contracts (*'uqud al-mu'awadat*), such as sale and purchase, must be present at the time of contract. The purpose of this ruling is protection of property (*hifz al-mal*) against excessive uncertainty (*gharar*), destruction, and loss. Whereas the *fiqh* rules on halal articulate the rule-based jurisprudence, the *maqasid* perspective also looks at the broader picture that the smooth flow, for instance, of the marketplace and production of the safe, clean, and lawful varieties of food substances should be encouraged and made available to the people. In this way the *maqasid* look at the rules of *fiqh* and shariah from a different angle: whereas the *fiqh* is rule-based, the *maqasid* are purpose-oriented more than they are rule-based. *Maqasid al-shariah* also protect the *fiqh*/shariah against distortion, manipulation, and abuse. For it is possible to follow the rules of *fiqh* but distort and even violate their purposes, especially in financial transactions that ostensibly comply with the *fiqh* requirements but which are often constructed in ways that seek to secure the prohibited usury/*riba*.

Yet it should be added that shariah, *fiqh*, and *maqasid* all expound different dimensions of the same reality: *fiqh* and *maqasid* arise, as indeed they must, from the shariah itself, such that there can be no substantive disconnect between them. This is in view of a certain tendency nowadays toward the excessive use of "*maqasid shariah*," such that it is fast becoming a catchphrase, especially in the discourse of the uninitiated—meaning anyone who likes an idea and then claims it to be one of the *maqasid*! One should also avoid seeing the *maqasid* as a first reference when there is a clear text on the subject. The present writer recently read an unpublished article he was sent for a review, wherein the writer, with an evidently skin-deep knowledge of shariah, used

---

5. See for more details on the *maqasid*, see Kamali, *Shariah Law: An Introduction*, 123–141. See also Kamali, "Actualisation (*Taf'il*) of the Higher Purposes of Shariah." .

the *maqasid* as the authority for *zakah* (obligatory alms). This totally ignores the fact that the obligation of *zakah*, which is one of the five pillars of Islam, is based on the clear text (*nass*), being the first authority on the subject. One is naturally appreciative of the fact that *maqasid* are the focus of renewed attention, but one may also have reason to be wary that this desirable development does not lead to careless applications and abuse.

Another source of law and judgment that is recognized in *usul al-fiqh* is the general custom (*'urf*) of society that can be the basis of *ijtihad* when it is free of harm and corruption. Many rulings of *fiqh* on the varieties of foods and beverages are influenced by the prevailing customs of people. The position is also similar with regard to scholastic differences between *lawful* and *unlawful* in food varieties.

The leading schools of Islamic law have on the whole recorded differential rulings on a variety of animals, birds, sea creatures, etc., some of which are exceedingly liberal, whereas others are more restrictive. One of the reasons for these wide-ranging differences is the customary practices of the various communities in which they emerged, such as geographical and climatic conditions of the early scholastic centers, but also the fact that, barring a few exceptions, the Qur'an hardly specifies animals by name, as they are understandably too numerous, and juristic opinion thus tends to rely mainly on interpretation, people's sound customary practices, and other methods mentioned earlier. Yet juristic opinion often remains at the level of *ijtihad* that stops short of general consensus, and may therefore be liable to change with the change of circumstances and living conditions of the people.

In order to be valid, an *'urf* must fulfill three conditions:[6]

1. It is the collective practice of a large number of people; hence the habits of a few or even a substantial minority within a society are not valid *'urf.*
2. That it is sound and reasonable; hence recurring practices among some people in which there is no benefit or which partake in prejudice and corruption are excluded from the purview of valid *'urf.*
3. That *'urf* does not violate a definitive text or principle of shariah.

A controversial practice in Malay traditional healing methods that illustrates a corrupt/invalid *'urf* is that of *berjamu*, a highly elaborate ritual for the purpose of appeasing spirits and other invisible beings. The ritual is performed

---

6. Kamali, *Principles of Islamic Jurisprudence*, 95.

either to cure illnesses or even to appease the sea spirits. Apart from mere incantations and standard offerings, *berjamu* is sometimes extended to the sacrifice of animals such as cows, buffaloes, and goats, as a form of gift to the unseen entities. The act of slaughtering animals for the sake of anyone other than God Most High is a grave issue in Islam and totally unacceptable in the name of *'urf.*[7]

---

7. For details, see Abdullah, and Kamali, "Malay Traditional Customs."

## 2

# The Principle of Original Permissibility (Ibahah)

THE NORM OF shariah with regard to food and beverage, the choice of clothes one wears, and the sale and purchase of all these, as well as conclusion of other contractual transactions over them, is that they are all permissible based on the original principle of permissibility (*ibahah*). Permissibility thus becomes a basic presumption that is only abandoned when there is evidence to suggest abandonment. A legal maxim on permissibility simply reads that "[t]he norm [of shariah] in all things is permissibility unless there be evidence to establish a prohibition." (*al-aslu fi'l-ashya' al-ibahah hatta yadullu al-dalil ʿala al-tahrim.*)[1] The main purpose of permissibility in this maxim involves utilization, including consumption and all other appropriate uses of the available resources of the earth for human benefit. That said, the maxim under review applies to matters on which there is no clear ruling in the sources of shariah, and it does not, as such, apply to matters that have been regulated and determined by a clear text. Quoted in authority for this maxim are the following Qur'anic passages:

- He [God] has created for you (*khalaqa lakum*) all that is in the earth. (al-Baqarah, 2:29)
- Say: who has forbidden the beautiful (gifts) of God, which He has produced for His servants, and the clean and pure sustenance (He has provided)? (al-Aʿraf, 7:32)

---

1. Cf. Zaydan, *al-Wajiz*, 181.

*Shariah and The Halal Industry.* Mohammad Hashim Kamali, Oxford University Press. © Oxford University Press 2021.
DOI: 10.1093/oso/9780197538616.003.0003

The first of these verses is explicit on the subjugation by divine authority of the earth and all its resources for the benefit of humankind, a benefit that includes consumption for sustenance of animal and plant resources.

The reference to clean and pure sustenance derived from wholesome produce and resources of God's creation is again clear evidence on the permissibility of food and beverage, as well as clothing and transport, that humankind may enjoy in all reasonable ways. This verse is couched in a question format, which is meant to draw attention to and emphasize the divine grant of permissibility it conveys.[2] Also quoted in support of the maxim is the hadith on the authority of Abu Darda' (quoted below), wherein the Prophet has reportedly said that the halal and the *haram* have been determined in the Book of God, and in regard to what has not been so determined and on which God Most High has remained silent, it is exonerated.

Instances where *fiqh* scholars have illustrated the correct understanding and application of the maxim of original permissibility include the following:

- With regard to an animal on which no ruling is found in the sources and it is difficult to determine whether it is permissible or not, it is considered to be permissible. With regard to a plant or tree that is not known by name but also no one has said anything about its harm, then it is presumed to be permissible based on this maxim.
- The permissibility of a great variety of clothes, household items, and new inventions on which no shariah ruling had existed has also been determined by reference to this maxim. This is also said with regard to trades, transactions, and contracts on which the shariah sources are silent but they are clear of usury and harm, they are also presumed to be permissible.[3]

*Ibahah*, in the language of *fiqh* scholars, is often an equivalent expression for freedom. The principle of original permissibility means, in other words, that freedom is the normative position of shariah with regard to foodstuffs, animals on land and in the sea, customary matters, commercial transactions and contracts, and other matters. All are permissible and the shariah grants basic freedom of action with regard to them and indeed all other matters that fall under the purview of *ibahah*. That said, the renowned Andalusian Maliki scholar al-Shatibi (d.790/1388) makes a point that to some people *ibahah* may

---

2. Zaydan, *al-Wajiz*, 181.

3. Zaydan, *al-Wajiz*, 182–183.

appear differently than to others, and that people are entitled to follow their own best judgments. A learned person may see something that others may not, and his or her specialized knowledge and understanding may point to a certain doubt or difficulty in the object of the observation. Al-Shatibi then comments that when doubt or difficulty proves persistent and the observer cannot see a way out of it, abandonment would seem advisable. When there is the apprehension, in other words, that what is deemed permissible may in some ways lead to what is reprehensible (*makruh*) or even prohibited (*mamnu'*), then it is best to abandon it.[4] Muslim jurists also maintain that expatiation in pursuit of permissibilities (*al-tawassu' fi'l-mubahat*) that can lead one to indulgence and doubtful practices is not encouraged on grounds of personal piety. This advice is, however, confined to doubtful situations, but does not apply with regard to *mubah* and halal that is clear of doubt. For the shariah does not advise severity and self-denial in the enjoyment of what God Most High has made permissible.[5]

The principle of permissibility is closely related to its allied principle of original nonliability (*bara'ah al-dhimmah al-asliyyah*), which is the nearest Islamic equivalent of the common law principle of presumption of innocence, both of which mean that no one is guilty of an offense unless the contrary is proven through lawful evidence. Article 98 of the Ottoman Mejelle[6] thus proclaims that original nonliability is the basic norm of shariah. This principle is also derived from the data of the Qur'an and hadith, which need not be reviewed here, but the present writer has provided a fuller treatment of them elsewhere in his previous publications.[7] Yet a point of difference between the shariah principle of non-liability, and the presumption of innocence may be that the former is not confined to criminal law matters and applies equally to civil claims and litigations. A claim by itself will not therefore prove anything unless there is evidence that liability exists. Nonliability in shariah simply means that people are free to do what they wish in order to achieve the purposes they pursue in their daily lives, in work, in business, and

---

4. al-Shatibi, *al-Muwafaqat*, vol. 1, 120 as quoted in al-Raysuni, *al-Haram fi'l-Shariah*, 237.

5. al-Raysuni, *al-Haram fi'l-Shariah*, 238–239.

6. The Mejelle was the civil code of the Ottoman Empire in the late nineteenth and early twentieth century. It was the first attempt to codify a part of the shariah-based law of an Islamic state. The code was prepared by a large team of scholars, containing 1,851 articles, from 1869 to 1876, and entered into force in 1877. It is the first codified collection described as the first successful attempt to render the Hanafi *fiqh* into a legal civil code comprehensible to the layperson and not just to scholars.

7. For details, see Kamali, *The Right to Life*, 86–87 and passim.

indeed all other areas, provided they do not violate the law or cause harm and prejudice to others. *Ibahah* is also expressive of this purpose, both within and outside the criminal law context.

According to another legal maxim, "the norm in benefits is permissibility, and it is prohibition in regards to harm." (*al-aslu fi'l-manafi' al-ibahah wa fi'l-madaar al-tahrim.*)[8] When the shariah declares something either *haram* or halal, it is for reasons primarily of their inherent harms or benefits, respectively, but in regard to matters and objects on which the shariah has remained silent, they are all permissible. The principle of permissibility thus extends to all objects, foods and drinks, animals, acts, and transactions that are not considered to be harmful.[9]

In yet another supportive maxim, it is stated: "when there is total silence [in shariah] on the permissibility or prohibition of something, it is exonerated." (*kull ma sukita 'anhu 'an ijabihi aw tahrimihi fa-huwa 'afwun.*)[10] This is an endorsement, again, of the original principle of permissibility, and a manifestation of God's expressed desire to bring ease to the people. In support of this is also quoted the Qur'anic verse that reads, in the relevant part, that "Your Lord is never forgetful" (Maryam, 19:64), which evidently means that His silence is purposeful and can never be attributed to His forgetfulness. It is stated by way of explanation that God Most High and his Messenger have identified the permissible and the prohibited, but when they have chosen to remain silent over something, it is an indication of its permissibility. To this effect, it is provided in an elevated (*marfu'*)[11] hadith on the authority of Abu Darda': "What God has made permissible in His Book, it is halal, and what He has prohibited is *haram*, and what He has remained silent about, it is exonerated. So accept from God what He has exonerated, for He never forgets anything, [and then cited the verse] "and your Lord is never forgetful."[12]

---

8. al-Suyuti, *al-Ashbah wa'l-Naza'ir*, 133; al-Raysuni, *al-Haram fi'l-Shariah*, 143.

9. al-Raysuni, *al-Haram fi'l-Shariah*, 145.

10. This is a statement of Imam al-Shafi'i in his *al-Risalah*, 201. It is also stated as a legal maxim in Ibn Taymiyyah, *al-Qawa'id al-Nuraniyyah al-Fiqhiyyah*, 222. See also al-Raysuni, *al-Haram fi'l-Shariah*, 99. Al-Shafi'i, Muhammad bin Idris. *Al-Risalah*. Edited by Ahmad Shakir. Cairo: Mustafa al-Bab al-Halabi, 1940.

11. A *Marfu'* hadith is one that a Companion says that could not be originated in his own opinion, but only through his observation of the Sunnah of the Prophet.

12. The hadith is recorded in al-Hakim, *al-Mustadrak 'ala Al-Sahihayn*, vol. 2, 406–407, hadith no. 3419, and also al-Bayhaqi, *al-Sunan al-Bayhaqi*, vol. 6, 12. See also al-Raysuni, *al-Haram fi'l-Shariah*, 101.

Original permissibility is also held to be the basic position regarding animals. They are all permissible for human consumption unless there is evidence to the contrary, and this is the majority position of the Maliki, Shafi'i, and Hanbali schools. Imam Abu Hanifah is, on the other hand, inclined toward prohibition unless there be some indication to suggest that the animal in question is permissible. Abu Hamid al-Ghazali (d.505/1111) of the Shafi'i school and Ibn Muflih al-Hanbali (d.763H/1362CE) have also held that the basic norm regarding animals is permissibility unless there is evidence to the contrary. Abu Hanifah's position has thus been marginalized by most other jurists.[13]

To declare something permissible, one is consequently not required to produce supportive evidence for it beyond what may be obvious to the senses. Plant food and animal flesh are thus clean if general practice and reason indicate such and when there is no obvious sign of impurity and harm to suggest prohibition. No further shariah proof is necessary. Yet to overrule the basic presumption of permissibility requires decisive evidence. If this evidence consists of a text, it must be decisive both in meaning and transmission. This is the subject of a legal maxim, which states that "prohibition can only be established by means of definitive evidence." (*la yuqta'u 'ala tahrimi shay'in illa bi-yaqin.*)[14] In connection with this, Yusuf al-Qaradawi (b. 1926) has suggested, rightly perhaps, that it is sufficient that the text in question is authentic and conveys a clear meaning (*nass sahih al-thubut sarih al-dalalah*), because a text of this kind is generally sufficient to establish a practical ruling of shariah outside the sphere of worship (*'ibadat*)—and also sexual intercourse with a member of the opposite sex, for this is only permitted through a valid marriage, as elaborated below.[15] The evidence that overrules *ibahah* may be shariah evidence that suggests prohibition or reprehensibility due to manifest harm (*darar*). But the proof of harm can also be based on rational and scientific evidence. Rational evidence alone cannot establish *haram*, but rational evidence can establish harm.

Juridically, permissibility is a *hukm* (law or value of shariah) as in the renowned scale of Five Values (*al-ahkam al-khamsah*). Permissibility as such is defined as an option (*takhyir*) the Lawgiver has granted to the competent

---

13. Ibn Juzay, *al-Qawanin al-Fiqhiyah*, 298. See also al-Harithi, *al-Nawazil fi'l-At'imah*, vol. 2, 503.

14. al-Raysuni, *al-Haram fi'l-Shariah*, 100.

15. al-Qaradawi, *Bay' al-Murabahah li'l-Amir bi'l- Shira'*, 13.

person to do something or not to do it, with no preference for either side.[16] This option may be granted by the shariah, in which case there would be a ruling on it in the sources, such as the permissibility of eating and drinking in the Qur'an (al-Baqarah, 2:60; al-A'raf, 7:31), and it would as such be a juridical permissibility (*al-ibahah al-shar'iyyah*), or it may be by way of exercising the principle of original permissibility due to the absence of any prohibition, and this would be an instance of original permissibility (*al-ibahah al-asliyyah*). Consuming avocado, for instance, is not mentioned in any text, but it is presumed to be permissible by way of *ibahah asliyyah*. But once there is a shariah ruling on an original permissibility, then it becomes a juridical *ibahah*.

The option in a juridical *ibahah* may sometimes be imbedded into an obligation, but the Lawgiver grants a choice in respect of the manner of its fulfillment. With regard to the atonement of a false oath, for instance, the Qur'an (al-Ma'idah, 5:89) prescribes one of three acts by way of compensation for the wrongdoing of taking a false oath: feeding ten poor persons, providing clothes for them, or freeing a slave (when this was possible), whichever one may choose. This option is in the nature of a juridical permissibility imbedded in an act of atonement (*kaffarah*). Permissibility may also be granted by a human person, such as when the owner permits a hungry person to consume his food, or allows him the use of his animal or car.[17] It thus further appears that permissibility can either involve the usufruct of something but not consumption of the object itself, as in the use of a car, or it may involve consumption of the object itself, as in the case of the owner permitting a hungry man to consume his food. This also signifies a certain difference between *ibahah* and ownership. Whereas the owner can use what belongs to him himself or allow someone else to do so, permissibility is in the nature of freedom, which does not confer upon a person the right to transfer it to someone else. A person is permitted, for instance, to eat food in a wedding feast to which he or she is invited, but not allowed to do anything else with that food, nor to transfer it to a third party. In a similar vein, *ibahah* does not confer on the person the power of representation (*tawkil*). The invited guest in our previous example is not authorized therefore to appoint a representative (*wakil*), unless, of course, this is expressly permitted by the owner. *Ibahah* pertaining to usufruct (*ibahat al-intifa'*) usually incurs liability for compensation.

---

16. Wizarat, *al-Mawsu'ah al-Fiqhiyyah*, vol. 1, 128.

17. Wizarat, *al-Mawsu'ah al-Fiqhiyyah*, vol. 1, 132. See also al-Zuhayli, *al-Fiqh al-Islami wa Adillatuh*, vol. 5, 494.

In the event the user of an object damages or destroys it, that person is liable to compensate the owner. *Ibahah* of the capital objects (*ibahat al-a'yan*) also does not preclude liability for compensation in the absence of prior permission of the owner, such as when a hungry person eats food belonging to another person without permission. But there is no liability if it is with a prior permission—although the jurists have recorded different views on this.[18]

It thus appears that *ibahah* is a limited juridical concept that does not include the privileges of ownership. Juridical *ibahah* can be established, not only by the Qur'an and hadith, but also by general consensus (*ijma'*), people's customary practice (*'urf*), public benefit (*maslahah*), and independent reasoning (*ijtihad*). These are broad juridical concepts that may overlap with, or subsume, one another and also admit evidence from different sources. For instance, the concept of public benefit (*maslahah*) can be the basis of *ibahah*, but this may also utilize scientific evidence that can be given in respect of substances that were either not known or not used as food items before, and then *ijtihad* can also originate in *maslahah*, or indeed in general custom, and so forth. The general acceptance or otherwise of people seem to be playing a crucial role in the acceptance or otherwise of animals and meat varieties for food, which often concurs with the shariah concept of *ibahah*. But, as already noted, *'urf* can establish a juridical *ibahah* as well, as it is a recognized shariah evidence.

It may be mentioned in passing, however, that certain other expressions also occur in the Islamic sources that convey similar juridical meanings to that of *ibahah*, such as exoneration (*al-'afw*), soundness (*al-sihhah*), permissibility (*al-jawaz*), and, of course, also *halal*. These are parallel concepts for the most part, but not identical, as there are technical differences between them, but these need not detain us here, as the discussion would involve a certain linguistic analysis of Arabic words, and subtle juridical differences.[19] They are mentioned in passing to convey awareness, as some of these terms also occur in the scriptural sources of concern.

One may, however, say a word about *mubah* and halal, which are synonymous for the most part, yet halal is said to be a wider concept than *mubah*. Halal is the opposite of *haram*, and it can, as such, include the other four value points in the renowned scale of Five Values, namely the permissible (*mubah*),

---

18. Cf. Wizarat, *al-Mawsu'ah al-Fiqhiyyah*, vol. 1, 134.

19. For a discussion of terminology on *ibahah* and its parallel concept, see Wizarat, *al-Mawsu'ah al-Fiqhiyyah*, vol. 1, 127f.

recommendable, obligatory, and reprehensible, according to the majority. Something may thus be halal but reprehensible at the same time, or halal and recommendable at the same time, or even halal and obligatory at the same time. For instance, the Prophet has said in a hadith that "the worst of all halal before God is divorce." Divorce is thus halal and *makruh* both. Eating less than one's full stomach is halal and recommendable both—as the Prophet has recommended such in another hadith, and some of his Companions, especially 'Umar al-Khattab, have spoken much about the harms of overeating. *Mubah* is a category of its own in the scale of Five Values, and is less inclusive as such than *halal*. Whereas halal can subsume *mubah*, *mandub*, *makruh*, and even *wajib*, *mubah* does not subsume any other value point. This is rather a technical discussion, however, and we do not propose to lengthen it any further.[20]

When the principle of permissibility is applied to something, it becomes permissible, or *mubah*, and it is this term that features most in the juristic discourse on *ibahah*.

---

20. See Wizarat, *al-Mawsu'ah al-Fiqhiyyah*, vol. 1, 127f.

# 3

# The Permissible (Mubah,
# Also Halal, Ja'iz)

MUCH HAS ALREADY been said in the preceding chapter on this subject. Here the focus of the discussion is on the *fiqh* treatment of *mubah* as a value category, including its sources, varieties, and how it is understood by the leading schools of Islamic law. Of the three Arabic words that appear in this heading, halal and its derivatives occur more frequently in the Qur'an and hadith, whereas the *fiqh* literature is more inclined to employ *mubah* and ja'iz.[1] *Mubah*, and also halal, may be defined as an act, object, or conduct over which the individual has freedom of choice, and for which its exercise does not carry either a reward or a punishment. Halal/*mubah* may have been identified by explicit evidence in the shariah or by reference to the presumption of permissibility, as already mentioned.

The scale of Five Values, namely the obligatory, recommended, permissible, reprehensible, and forbidden (*wajib*, *mandub*, *mubah*, *makruh*, and *haram*, respectively) does not occur in the Qur'an or hadith in that order, and they are introduced by the jurists based on their general understanding of shariah. The Qur'an may use the word *halal* or its derivatives directly, or else declare that "there is no sin," "no liability," "no blame" in doing something, or that "God will not take you to task" for such and such, all of which imply permissibility. A variety of expressions are also used in the scriptural sources

---

1. The reason why *fiqh* scholars opt for a different terminology may be due to the sensitivity that the Qur'an attaches to the pronouncement of halal and *haram*. For this is the prerogative only of God, as elaborated below. A slight difference in the meaning of these terms may also be relevant to note: whereas *mubah* and *ja'iz* refer to something about which the *shariah* is totally neutral, halal often implies a degree of purity, particularly in the context of foodstuffs, and may as such imply preference that is not totally neutral.

*Shariah and The Halal Industry.* Mohammad Hashim Kamali, Oxford University Press. © Oxford University Press 2021. DOI: 10.1093/oso/9780197538616.003.0004

to convey the reprehensible and that which is recommended. Thus, when one reads in these sources expressions such as "God does not love" such and such, or when an act is described as "an abomination," "disliked," "misguided," and so forth, it would indicate something is reprehensible (*makruh*), and the opposite of such expressions, or when an act or object is favorably described or praised, may also imply something is recommendable (*mandub*).[2]

The textual guidelines on halal suggest that no unnecessary restrictions should be imposed on the basic freedom of the individual's personal choice in what he or she wishes to consume, and the scope therefore of prohibitions should not go beyond what has been specifically determined by the text. The permissible, or halal/*mubah*, has thus been left as an open category that applies to all that which is not forbidden. The Qur'an thus says in an address to the Prophet: "They ask thee what is lawful to them (as food). Say lawful (*'uhilla*) unto you are (all) things good and pure" (al-Ma'idah, 5:6); and "O people! eat of what is on the earth, lawful and good (*halalan, tayyiban*)" (al-Baqarah, 2:168, 172); and then again: "O ye who believe! Forbid not (*la tuharrimu*) the good things that God has made lawful (*ahalla*) for you" (5:87). To extend the scope of the halal even further, the text declares, "It is He Who has created for you (your benefit) all things that are on earth" (al-Baqarah, 2:29).

The Prophet has said in an open address to the people: "Eat, drink, and give charity, and wear clothes without extravagance, arrogance and self-aggrandizement. For God loves to see His servants exhibiting His bounties on them."[3]

This open outlook on halal/*mubah*, lawful, and pure has enabled the jurists, in turn, to formulate general guidelines, including the legal maxim on *ibahah* discussed in chapter 2, but which may be reiterated: "permissibility (*ibahah*) is the basic norm (of shariah) in all things unless there be evidence to establish a prohibition."[4]

---

2. The Arabic expressions used for *mubah* are: *lā ithma, la junāḥa, lā ba'sa, lā yu'akhidhukum Allāh*, etc.

3. Hadith recorded in *Sunan al-Nasa'i, Sunan Ibn Majah* and *Musnad of Ibn Hanbal*—as also quoted in al-Zuhayli, *al-Fiqh al-Islami*, vol. 3, 505–506.

4. The Arabic version of the maxim is: *al-aṣlu fi'l-ashyā' al-ibāḥah ḥattā yadullu al-dalīl 'alā al-taḥrīm*. Cf. al-Suyuti, *al-Ashbah wa'l-Naza'ir*, 60. A legal maxim normally consists of an abstract and epithetic statement of a *fiqh* position based on the overall reading of available evidence in the Qur'an and hadith. By way of explanation, al-Suyuti raises the question as to the permissibility for human consumption, for instance, of giraffe, saying that the jurists have not taken a position on this and it is therefore halal in the light of the said maxim and also the fact that giraffe is not a predatory animal.

This basic permissibility subsumes the two other shariah values, namely the recommendable and reprehensible. For these two consist of persuasive advice that may or may not be followed, and there is no obligation to comply with them. This is why the prominent Zahiri scholar of Andalus, Ibn Hazm al-Zahiri (d.1064/456) has reduced the Five Values earlier mentioned to only three, namely the obligatory, the prohibited, and the permissible, adding the point that the recommended and the reprehensible are essentially subsumed by the permissible (*mubah*). Muslim jurists have also held, as already mentioned, that any textual evidence that overrules the presumption of permissibility must be decisive, as a *haram* cannot be established by doubtful evidence, such as a weak *hadith*, or a Qur'anic verse that does not convey a clear meaning—in which case the subject would be governed by the presumption of original permissibility.[5]

The Malikis are the most liberal with regard to the permissibility of foodstuffs from animal sources that may have been classified as reprehensible or even forbidden by the other schools. The Shafi'is, Hanafis, and the Ja'fari or Twelver Shia are moderate, whereas the Hanbalis tend to be restrictive. The Malikis permit all varieties of land and sea animals and birds, including the stray animals (*jallalah*) that feed on filth, and also birds of prey, as well as elephants, ants, worms, and beetles, to be permissible for human consumption. Most other schools have declared many of these as reprehensible if not forbidden.[6] The permissive position of the Maliki school refers to the basic norm of permissibility with regard to all animal varieties, birds, insects, and marine animals on which the Qur'an or Sunnah contain no ruling. A similar position has also been held by some early jurists, including 'Abd al-Rahman b. 'Amr al-Awza'i (d.774/157), Yahya b. Sa'id, as well as two leading figures among the Companions, Ibn 'Abbas and Abu Darda'.[7]

There are three types of *mubah*/halal. First, *mubah* that does not entail any harm to the individual, whether he or she acts on it or not, such as traveling, hunting, or walking in the fresh air. Second, *mubah* whose commission is permitted due to necessity, although it is essentially forbidden. This may include

---

5. al-Qaradawi, *al-Halal wa'l-Haram fi'l-Islam*, 23; al-Qaradawi, *Bay' al-Murabahah*, 13. A sound (*sahih*) hadith, as opposed to a weak one, is defined as a hadith with an unbroken *isnad* (chain of transmitters) all the way back to the Prophet or a Companion, consisting of upright persons who possessed retentive memories and whose narration is not outlandish (*shadh*), and it is free of both obvious and subtle defects (*'ilal*). Cf. Kamali, *A Textbook of Hadith Studies*, 139.

6. For details, see al-Zuhayli, *al-Fiqh al-Islami*, vol. 3, 510f.

7. Cf, Wizarat, *al-Mawsu'ah al-Fiqhiyyah*, vol. 18, 336.

the consumption of alcohol or carrion to save one's life.[8] The third variety of *mubah* refers to conduct that Islam has prohibited but which was committed before the advent of Islam, or with reference to converts, before they embraced the religion. For instance, wine-drinking was not prohibited until the Prophet's migration to Medina, hence it fell under *mubah* until the revelation of the Qur'anic verse that finally declared it forbidden (i.e., al-Ma'idah, 5:90).[9] Abu Hamid al-Ghazali has further explained that it is incorrect to apply *mubah* to the acts of a child, an insane person, or an animal, nor would it be correct to call the acts of God Most High *mubah*. Acts and events that took place prior to the advent of Islam are not to be called *mubah* either. *Mubah* has again been subdivided into three types:

1. Acts that are *mubah* for the individual but recommendable for the community as a whole. Eating certain foods, such as vegetarian food, butter and milk, and so on, is *mubah* for the individual, but it is recommendable for the community as a whole to produce them and make them available in the marketplace.
2. Acts that are permissible for the individual but obligatory (*wajib*) for the community as a whole. Under normal circumstances, eating, drinking, and marriage may be permissible for the individual, but to ensure their availability is an obligation for the community and its leadership. Similarly, it is permissible for the individual to choose his or her line of work and profession, but the community as a whole is under obligation to ensure the survival of certain types of industries, trades, and professions.
3. Acts that are permissible on an occasional basis but forbidden if pursued regularly. For example, an occasional use of harsh words on one's child is permissible, but forbidden if practiced all the time, and reprehensible if practiced frequently.

---

8. Cf. Kamali, *Islamic Jurisprudence,* 429.

9. Cf. Kamali, *Islamic Jurisprudence,* 429.

# 4

# *Halal and* Tayyib *Compared*

TAYYIB (LIT. PURE, clean) refers to objects, acts, and conduct that are not only permissible (halal, *mubah*) but also considered to be pure, clean, and wholesome by the people of sound nature. *Tayyib* invokes people's approval, often regardless and independently of customary practice.[1] A somewhat vexed question has arisen, however, as to whether *tayyib* is embedded in the nature of things, or in individual persons' taste and judgment, or indeed in people's custom and culture. With reference to the Qur'an, in particular the verse that expounds the mission of the Prophet on three main points—one of which is that "He declares to them as lawful what is good (and pure), and forbids to them what is evil (and impure)" (al-A'raf, 7:157)—commentators say that the main context of this verse is Arab customary practices. Ibn Qudamah (d. 620/1223) thus wrote that the *tayyibat* and the *khaba'ith* are those that were so practiced by the people of Hijaz (Mecca and Medina), especially the city dwellers among them. For they were the main audience and recipients of the Qur'an and Sunnah of the Prophet. To understand the words of the text, one must therefore refer to their custom ('*urf*), not of any other [people]."[2] This is also representative of the majority of jurists who understand Arab customary practices as the main reference of determination of *tayyib*, or the opposite of it, *khabith*, and say that people's tastes vary so much that it will be too subjective to refer to individual persons' verdicts. Customary practice is thus held to offer a better criterion. The critics say, however, that customary practices of people also vary a great deal: what may be considered as *tayyib* in food and drink by some people, may be viewed differently by others.

---

1. Cf. al-Qaradawi, *al-Halal wa'l-Haram*, 31.

2. Ibn Qudamah, *al-Mughni*, vol. 13, 83.

*Shariah and The Halal Industry.* Mohammad Hashim Kamali, Oxford University Press. © Oxford University Press 2021.
DOI: 10.1093/oso/9780197538616.003.0005

To confine the Qur'an interpretation to Arab custom would also be problematic for those who lived in remote places and times, including twenty-
first-century Muslims. It is generally maintained, nevertheless, that *tayyib*
and *khabith* are what people make of them, and not necessarily ingrained in
the nature of things. The discussion is moved further by other more recent
observers who accept customary practice as the principal criterion of *tayyib*,
but add that it is the custom of the middle class, as it were, not of the far left,
nor the far right, and that it refers mainly to the urban populations, not the
Bedouins.[3] To illustrate the point, non-Arabs (i.e., *al-'ajam*) do not like or
consume locusts, which were, however, liked by the pre-Islamic Arabs. And
yet the Arab taste has also changed, and locusts are not liked by them now.
When reference is made to the eating habits and practices of the Muslim
populations of India, Europe, Turkey, and elsewhere, one often finds them to
differ greatly from one another. So it is difficult to establish clear, universal,
and unchangeable criteria for *tayyib* and *khabith*.[4] That said, most legal traditions and customs tend to provide their own specifications that help to offer
a degree of clarity to the understanding of *tayyibat*, as we too are advancing a
certain context for *tayyibat* with reference to the burgeoning halal industry in
twenty-first-century Malaysia and elsewhere in the Muslim world.

The opposite of *tayyib* (pl. *tayyibat*) is that which is objectionable and unclean and which repels people of good taste and the general public, even if
some people may find it otherwise.[5] As the discussion below on the grounds
of *haram* indicates, the basic relationship of halal and *haram* to *tayyib* and
*khabith*, respectively, is an intrinsic and natural inclination of *tayyib* toward
halal and of *khabith* toward *haram*. *Tayyib* is used in the Qur'an and the pro-
phetic Sunnah to describe something that is good and wholesome. In reference to food, for instance, the Qur'an calls on people to consume food that is
both permissible and wholesome:

> O People, consume from earth [only] what is halal and *tayyib*, and
> follow not the footsteps of the devil. (al-Baqarah, 2:168)

Since God Most High has determined the halal and *haram* for people's
benefit (*maslahah*), this becomes the basic cause and rationale behind all

---

3. For details, see Fadlullah, *Fiqh al-At'imah*, 32.

4. Ibid., 33.

5. al-Qaradawi, *al-Halal wa'l-Haram*, 56.

the laws of shariah on halal, *haram*, and *tayyib*. Most of that which is halal is *tayyib*, and most of that which is *haram* is also *khabith*. When this natural relationship is disturbed, as it has been in some cases in the Qur'anic narrative regarding certain communities and nations, it has been for specific reasons.[6] *Haram* in shariah is thus grounded in either natural repulsiveness (*khubth*) or harm and prejudice (*darar*), or of the two together. Broadly, whatever is purely or predominantly harmful and repulsive is *haram*, and that which is purely or predominantly beneficial and clean is halal.[7]

## Tayyib *in Scholastic Jurisprudence*

*Tayyib* did not, however, represent a juridical category, in that the existing *fiqh* literature did not specify a separate value point by this name next to, one might say, that of the permissible (*mubah*/halal). The renowned scale of Five Values thus speaks only of five value points wherein *tayyib* is not featured as a separate category. But as our review and analysis of the halal industry in Malaysia and elsewhere show, it seems that *tayyib* is now being recognized as an extension of the basic concept of halal. Yet in the conventional *fiqh* terms, Muslims were required to ensure that what they did, ate, or drank was halal/ permissible in shariah, even if it was not pure, *tayyib*, or of best quality. It was seen by the *fiqh* scholars of earlier times as good enough for Muslims to observe the rules of halal without being asked to go a step beyond halal to that of *tayyib*. One was legal and the other basically moral and marked a step beyond on the rank of virtue. If someone chose to aim at what was *tayyib*, that would be better, preferable, and morally virtuous. But placed in the context of the halal industry, and of the standards of cleanliness and hygiene today, it is perfectly valid, in the present writer's view, and even closer to the letter of the Qur'an, to adopt *tayyib* as an extension of halal, and read it as an integral part of the scale of Five Values. In some cases, superior market facilities and supplies may even place Muslims residing in advanced and developed countries in a better position, where it is easier for them to choose only what is of better quality and *tayyib*.

---

6. Certain *tayyibat* were thus prohibited to the Jews as a matter, however, of reprimand and punishment (cf., Q al-An'am, 6:146; al-Nisa', 4:160).

7. In the case of liquor for example, the Qur'an explains its prohibition: "say that it is sinful but also benefits the people in some way, yet its evil is greater than its benefit" (al-Baqarah, 2:219). See also al-Qaradawi, *al-Halal wa'l-Haram*, 31.

In the context of the global halal industry, this means working to supply products "that are sustainable, not damaging to the planet, and pursuing business models that are ethical, responsible and not exploitative."[8] With this holistic understanding of halal and *tayyib*, one would be able to integrate the halal industry with Islamic banking and finance to construct a wholesome or *tayyib* business and supply chain working as extensions of one another.

Imagine, for example, a company that supplied halal chicken. First and foremost, the company should be funded in a fully shariah-compliant way, perhaps through shariah-compliant trade financing contracts, and financed by an Islamic bank. It should pay and treat all its employees fairly, with the kindness and respect (*ihsan*) that are central to the teachings of Islam. Then the chicken should be farmed in a sustainable, environmentally friendly and ethical manner to ensure a good quality of life for it in due fulfilment of humankind's responsibility as *khalifah* (trustees) and stewards of the earth. It should, of course, be slaughtered according to the proper halal rituals, transported with consideration of the damaging carbon emissions generated by certain kinds of fuel, and even packaged in sustainable and recyclable packaging wherever possible. Finally, it should be sold to retailers and consumers at prices that are fair for all involved in the transaction. This would not only be a wholesome and *tayyib* value chain, but would also help realize the full potential of an Islamic economy within the wider global economy, especially where customers are increasingly seeking ethical and sustainable options.[9]

The foregoing would suggest the adoption of *tayyib* as a target and even benchmark for evaluation of the halal industry performance and attainment of excellence in its products and services. To do so would also provide grounds for new developments in *fatwa* and *ijtihad* as to whether Muslims should only accept products and services that combine both halal and *tayyib*, and even make this into a juridical requirement that halal certification authorities and individual consumers should follow as a consolidated category and criterion of best performance.

It is characteristic in many ways, perhaps, of all law in that legal rules tend to aim at the very high or the very low, as the case may be, of value points pertaining to conduct—as compared to what people normally do in their daily lives. One may thus engage in deceitful activities and selfish pursuits, or eat unhealthy food and things which are merely permissible, but the law will not

---

8. Shah, "Fostering a True Halal Economy," 14.

9. Shah, "Fostering a True Halal Economy," 14.

take one to task for it, so long as the conduct in question does not amount to a crime or a clear violation of the law. This does not mean, however, that the shariah is not concerned with the higher reaches and objectives of personal conduct, which is why one also finds in the same scale of Five Values the category of recommendable, as well that as of reprehensible. In the case of permissible/halal food, the law permits Muslims to eat certain things, such as snails, worms, locusts, lizards, and even vultures and crocodiles (according to some interpretations at least), none of which can be said, however, to be *tayyib*. The distinction between halal and *tayyib* pertaining to victuals can relate more widely perhaps to Maliki jurisprudence, which permits the eating of a large variety of animals, birds, mammals, and insects that are merely tolerated but evidently fall short of *tayyib*. Since *tayyib* in the choice of food is all about purity and natural appeal, it belongs, for the most part, to the category of recommendable or *mandub*, and not necessarily to that of merely *mubah* or halal, or could at times signify an overlapping category between *mubah*/halal and *mandub*. *Tayyib* as such should be the optimal in the choice of food and highly recommendable also for the food industry and outlets to provide that which is clean and naturally appealing.

## Tayyib *beyond Victuals*

*Tayyib* is, furthermore, not confined to food, but goes beyond, in the language of the Qur'an and hadith, the strictly legal to an all-embracing value-based outlook on life, from objects to speech, conduct, personal lifestyle, environmental beauty, and personal accomplishments of individuals. *Tayyib* thus extends to aspects of conduct, such as the line of work one does (cf. Q al-Baqarah, 2:267—*min tayyibati ma-kasabtum*), just as it sometimes appears next to right ethical conduct, or *salihat* (Q al-Mu'minun, 23:51—*kulu min al-tayyibati wa'milu salihan*). Pleasant speech also partakes in *tayyib*; as is the clear purport of the Qur'an (al-Hajj, 22:24—*hudu ila'l-tayyibi min al-qawl*), and that of the hadith to the same effect, which declares a pleasant word (*kalimah tayyibah*) as a form of charity. So also are pure and upright individuals, men and women, who may rank as *tayyibun* or *tayyibat*, respectively (cf. Q al-Nur, 24:26)—and even pleasant and comfortable residences (*masakin tayyibah*—Q al-Tawbah, 9:72; al-Saff, 61:12). *Tayyib* is, as already indicated, used in the Qur'an as the antonym of *khabith* (objectionable, unclean, reprehensible), be it in food and drink, or other aspects of personality and conduct. *Tayyib* as such is a major theme of the Qur'an that encapsulates an exceedingly wide range of applications, well beyond food and beverage, and may well be described as an attribute of the Muslim personality, and that of Islamic civilization.

Furthermore, references to *tayyib* that occur in numerous places in the Qur'an and hadith often juxtapose halal and *tayyib* side by side (cf. al-Baqarah, 2:167; al-Ma'idah, 5:4, 5:87; al-A'raf, 7:157; al-Nisa, 4:160). In other places, the Qur'an addresses the Prophet and the believers to "eat the *tayyibat*" or "eat the *tayyibat* from the sustenance We have provided you with" (al-Mu'minun, 42, 51; al-Baqarah, 2:172), thus using the *tayyibat* separately from its litmus halal base. Reading them all together leaves little doubt, however, that halal is also *tayyib* for the most part, but also that *tayyib* can stand alone, in that something can be halal but may not qualify as *tayyib*. It is thus interesting that the Qur'an makes *tayyib* a target for the *halal* itself. This is the clear purport of the verse that reads, in an address to the Prophet, "They ask you what is permissible (*uhilla-* a derivative of halal) for them—say that which are *tayyibat*" (al-Ma'idah, 5:4). It is also typical of the Qur'anic usages of these terms that halal is mentioned first and *tayyib* after, as if the text is conveying the message that *tayyib* is a step beyond halal.

The industry awareness of the scope and potential of *tayyib* in its Malaysian context can be seen in the following interview extract of Jamal Bidin, the former head of the Halal Development Corporation (HDC), who said that the halal industry in Malaysia not only looks at the Islamic or shariah requirements, but also at the hygiene and safety aspects, which have been part and parcel of the halal standards for a long time. He added that, moving forward, halal in Malaysia should also take into account environmental issues, adopt fair trade practices and ward off child labor, to be on a par with European standards. "This is because, in the concept of *halalan tayyiban* (permissible [and desirable] for consumption), the word '*tayyiban*' means good things, so it also means good for the environment and the different segments of society."[10]

There is much scope and potential in Islamic banking and finance (IBF), and in takaful Islamic insurance, to take *tayyib* and *tayyibat* as the next benchmark in their journey for higher achievements. IBF and takaful regulatory authorities may need careful planning for the purpose, as integrating the *tayyib* concept is likely to take time, but it would bring greater credibility and value into their respective sectors. IBF has only in the last few years adopted the halal banking and halal finance concepts as a mark of its realization that halal finance is a broad concept, and integrating it into the fabric of its

10. Ismail, " 'Halal' Is Not Just about Food," interview with Jamal Bidin, 12.

operations will add to customer appeal and bring greater Islamic credibility to its products and services. To the best of the present writer's knowledge, the expressions *tayyib* and *tayyibat* have not yet been adopted by the IBF industry advisors and specialists, let alone the industry operators. Since IBF is fairly well regulated and, in many ways, more controlled than the halal industry, just as the former has also a longer history in terms of market presence and product development compared to the halal industry, it would seem advisable for the IBF to take *tayyib* and integrate it, on a graduated scale to begin with perhaps, develop it into measurable metrics, and then measure excellence in product development and performance by it.

It is perhaps due to a variety of factors that Islamic jurisprudence and the *fiqh* value schemes have, to all intents and purposes, treated the Qur'anic usage of *tayyib* and its plural *tayyibat* as moral categories compared to halal and *mubah*, which are legal. Yet Islamic law and jurisprudence are not meant to be static and do have the resources to develop in line with significant changes in the living conditions of Muslims. The shariah principles of *maslahah* and *ijtihad* can also respond to new opportunities and challenges as they occur. We believe that the gap may be narrowing and that future progress in the halal industry, as well as IBF, may provide grounds for integrating *tayyib* and *tayyibat* into the regulatory and applied aspects of their operations, which would have in effect elevate *tayyib* from a moral, praiseworthy and recommendable category into an applied practical and legal requirement.

To ascertain *tayyib* as a subset of *mandub*, or even a category in its own right, in the context especially of victuals, is even more meaningful in view of the many new developments in food sciences, genetically modified food varieties, and the mixing of additives and ingredients in the mass production of foodstuffs and supply chains. Factory production lines and commercially driven food processing methods also tend to widen the scope of doubt in the natural goodness of food supplies in the marketplace. The halal food industry is thus well advised to aim at *tayyib* as an optimal category of food, as well as its products in other sectors, such as medicine, cosmetics, pharmaceuticals, and tourism, that can eventually even be certified and labeled as such.

## Tayyib *in Halal Standards Malaysia*

Halal industry regulations in Malaysia have already adopted the *halalan/tayyiban* concept into a regulatory requirement that must be fulfilled, thereby elevating this to a rank more than optional advice or *mandub*. There are no less than three Malaysian standards devoted to the various aspects of *halalan-tayyiban* and its regulatory requirements. The first is on the transportation of halal goods, the second on warehousing and related activities, and the third on retailing. The first of these standards is clearly compulsory, as it provides at the outset that "this Malaysian Standard consists of requirements which are industry specific and intended to be applicable to [all relevant] organisations . . . to establish a management system based on *halalan-toyyiban* [*sic*] requirements."[11] Here we provide an outline of the first of these three standards (i.e., MS 2400-1, 2010) with regard to transportation of halal food and *halalan-tayyiban* management and regulatory requirements; the other two (MS 2400-2 and MS 2400-3)[12] follow parallel and similar approaches with regard to warehousing and retailing, respectively.

Spelling out the basic concepts, MS 2400-1 provides that halal/*halalan* signify "things or actions which are permitted or lawful in Islam. It conveys basic meaning and defines the standard of acceptability in accordance to shariah requirements."[13] *Halalan/toyyiban* as a combined phrase occurs regularly in all three documents, and it is described as that which "complements and perfects the essence (spirit) of the basic standard or minimum threshold (halal), i.e. on hygiene, safety, sanitation, cleanliness, nutrition, risk exposure, environmental, social and other related aspects in accordance to situational or application needs and wholesomeness."[14] *Halalan-tayyiban* (henceforth HT) is thus a value-added concept that ensures the purity of halal foods and services during transportation, warehousing, and retailing. The relevant standards set in place a management system to ensure that the movements of halal products and cargo at all points retain their purity and cleanliness. Organizations and transport and handling agencies are accordingly expected to "inculcate shariah requirements into their quality management practices," so that products produced, handled, and delivered are "halal, clean, safe and hygienic."[15] To this effect the standard envisages a chain management system, or a supply chain that conforms to

---

11. *Halalan-Toyyiban Assurance Pipeline- Part 1: Management System Requirements for transportation of Good and/or Cargo Chain Services:* MS 2400-1:2010 (Clause 1.2.1).

12. MS 2400-2:2010 is titled *Halalan-Toyyiban Assurance Pipeline—Part 2: Management System Requirements for Warehousing and Related Activities,* p. 34; whereas MS 2400-3:2010 bears the title *Halalan-Toyyiban Assurance Pipeline—Part 3: Management System Requirements for Retailing,* 40.

13. MS 2400-1, Clause 2.19.

14. Ibid., Clause 2.3.7.

15. Ibid., Clause 0.3.

the HT principles and guarantees that both "*halalan* and *toyyiban* are integrated into holistic and balanced requirements."[16] A series of requirements
are then spelled out, which include appointment by the organization of a
HT leader, committee, and shariah advisor for execution of the HT management system in the organization. The HT leader must have appropriate
qualifications, education, and experience on halal and non-halal aspects of
processes, products, and services, and be well-qualified in halal management techniques. The HT committee must also have equivalent knowledge
and training as HT leaders. These too may refer to a HT Shariah Advisor
as a reference point on the implementation of an HT management system,
especially when decisions need to be made with regard to the handling of
contaminated and affected products.[17]

The MS 2400-1 also establishes a risk-management process that requires
detailed documentation on all inbound and outbound transportation services, on risk analysis, and on checking containers and equipment, mode of
transportation, and stacking and storage conditions, which are to be checked
prior to dispatch and receiving, handling and distribution. The organization must keep this information available and updated. The standard also
specifies depot and warehouse layout, such as receiving areas, quarantine
areas, sorting areas, sanitary facilities, pest control points, waste disposal
areas, and lighting, temperature, humidity, cold-rooms, etc., so as to prevent
contamination with non-halal, harmful, and unhygienic substances.[18]

We now advance a brief analysis of *tayyib* from a slightly different angle.

## Tayyib, *Spirituality, and* Fitrah

*Tayyib* is often used in juxtaposition with halal and often as synonymous with
it. But a less well-known aspect of *tayyib* is its role as a conduit between the
physical and the spiritual dimensions of halal—that of the body and the soul.
"Intelligent people know that seeking salvation in the hereafter," wrote the
twelfth-century polymath Abu Hamid al-Ghazali, "depends on learning and
practice." For only a healthy body can provide consistency for salvation of
the soul. Al-Ghazali added that serenity of the body is not possible without

---

16. Ibid., Clause 2.20.

17. For further details, see MS 2400-1:2010 (Clauses 3.1 through to 3.2.2.4).

18. See MS 2400-1:2010, Clause 4, 15–18.

food and nourishment. In light of this wisdom, some pious ancestors held that eating is part of the teachings related to salvation in religion.[19]

Qur'anic dispensations on *tayyib* also imply that lawful things and foods that are appealing to the senses should be enjoyed and celebrated. Philologists helpfully and interestingly point out that the elements of pleasure and delight are included within the ideas of purity and lawfulness. Thus, the crucial responsibility of caring for the body involves both an element of observing ethics and an element of pleasuring the body. Since body and soul are not essentially separated, caring for the body is like caring for the soul. In other words, the integrity of the soul becomes manifest and takes form in the integrity of the body. Hence, there is an elaborate practice of caring for the body, starting with the nourishment of the body in Muslim practice.

The reasoning goes like this: If the body is the vehicle for the soul, then it attains the same inviolability as the soul. However, Muslim teachings differ as to whether the body attains sanctity on its own, irrespective of the soul, or whether the body is instrumental to the needs of the soul. Since the purpose of human existence in Muslim thought is related to an after-worldly salvation, the body and its needs have also become an important aspect of the same, according to some Muslim thinkers at least. In order to attain salvation, the body has to be disciplined through learning and practice. Since the body is the locus of such discipline, the etiquette of consuming food also acquires a certain importance in the overall scheme of salvation.[20]

The spiritual dimension of food is further expressed by Islam's outlook on food, which views food as a manifestation of divine mercy and beneficence. The devout in Islam express their gratitude to God by upholding the dignity of food and showing respect for the sources and means of sustenance. Whether it is to safeguard food sources or for aesthetic purposes, or perhaps for both reasons, Muslim teachings also strongly advocate the protection and preservation of the natural environment. The protection of trees, agricultural land, and sources of food and water (and their purity) are all vital components of a balanced Muslim environmental ethics through which the human body and self can obtain felicity and fulfilment.

This ties in with Islamic teachings on the preservation of naturalness (*fitrah*). To preserve uncontaminated nature coupled with the celebration

---

19. al-Ghazali, *Ihya' 'Ulum Al-Din*, as quoted in Moosa, "Genetically Modified Foods and Muslim Ethics," 138.

20. Cf., Moosa, "Genetically Modified Foods," 137.

of a healthy and sound human nature is viewed as one of the Islamic ideals. The human *fitrah* has many dimensions, one of which is the inborn, intuitive ability to discern between right and wrong, and is therefore of central importance to Muslim physical and ethical integrity. "So direct your face steadfastly to faith," enjoins the Qur'an, "as God-given nature (*fitrah*), according to which God created humanity: there is no altering the creation of God" (al-Rum, 30:30). God in the Qur'an is also described as the Original Creator (*Fatir*—which is also the name of sura 35 in the Qur'an), Who created the heavens and the earth without any model. *Fitrah* is essentially supra-religious and permanently inclined to the *Fatir*, the Creator of *fitrah*, as in the Qur'an (al-An'am, 6:79). Preservation of *fitrah* thus becomes an indispensable part of Islamic spirituality and ethics. Further endorsement of this is seen in Islam's identification of itself as *din al-fitrah*, a religion inherently inclined to *fitrah*; that is, to protecting the natural *fitrah* in all things. *Fitrah* in bodily terms is best preserved through consumption of food that preserves its natural goodness to qualify as *tayyib*. One of the principal attributes of *fitrah*, or sound human nature, that the Tunisian scholar Muhammad Tahir Ibn 'Ashur (d. 1974) has underlined in conjunction with his pioneering work on the higher purposes, or *maqasid*, of shariah, is that it shuns severity and extremism and favors moderation in all things.

To understand *fitrah*, for the most part, also implies understanding the limits of human intervention in God-ordained nature and inherent qualities of food and beverage. Human intervention through scientific methods, as in the case of genetically modified food, is thus acceptable within the inherent limitations of *fitrah* and clear understanding thereof. Some of these limitations are also imbedded in the shariah conceptions of halal and *haram* and of *fitrah*-based naturalness. As for the rest, intervention in the natural endowment of victuals must pass the tests of rationality, human need and benefit, and avoidance of harm to the natural purity of food and that of the natural environment which is necessary for nurturing it. For without these limits, the *fitrah* is also known to be susceptible to distortion and corruption through bodily indulgence in transgression and disobedience.

# 5

# *The Principle of Original Cleanliness (*Taharah*)*

THE PRINCIPLE OF cleanliness (*taharah*)[1] in shariah is in many ways supplementary and parallel to that of original permissibility (*ibahah*, or *mubah*), yet there are differences between them. Juridically, *taharah* means cleanliness from impurity and filth in both the physical and nonphysical senses (i.e., *hadath* and *khabath*). Both of these can be temporary or permanent, although *hadath* is more inclined to temporality. *Taharah* is inclusive of both the religious and temporal dimensions of cleanliness. In the religious context proper, for instance, the requirement in shariah of ritual prayer (*salah*) is that anyone who prays must be clean from both *khabath* and *hadath*, which means cleanliness of the body through ablution, of attire, and of place where *salah* is offered—and also that the attire is both physically and spiritually clean. *Salah* is not valid, for instance, in stolen clothes. With regard to victuals (food and drink), and the utensils used, the shariah requirement is also inclusive of both the physical and nonphysical aspects of cleanliness in that the food and drink that are consumed must be clean, both physically and from the religious purity perspectives. *Taharah* is thus a juridical attribute specified and determined by the Lawgiver with reference to devotional and nondevotional aspects of human conduct, as well as regarding animals and objects. Hence not all aspects of purity are required in the same way for all activities— whereas some aspects of cleanliness may be obligatory (*wajib*), others may be only recommended (*mandub*) or permissible (*mubah*).[2]

---

1. Other Arabic synonyms: *nizafah, nazahah*.

2. Cf. al-Jaziri, *al-Fiqh 'ala'l-Madhahib*, 9–10.

*Shariah and The Halal Industry.* Mohammad Hashim Kamali, Oxford University Press. © Oxford University Press 2021. DOI: 10.1093/oso/9780197538616.003.0006

A general position of note here is that whatever the shariah has made halal is also pure and clean, and all that which is made *haram* is also most likely to be impure (*najis*).[3] Original cleanliness also means that the normative position of shariah with regard to all things is that of cleanliness.[4] It tells us that God Most High has created all things clean for the use and benefit of human beings, unless there be evidence to suggest otherwise. All things, be they solid or liquid, are therefore clean, and this is a general presumption of shariah that is rebutted only by clear proof. The solid category includes all the components of the earth and that which is hidden underneath, such as minerals, gold, silver, copper, iron, and the like. Also included are all plants, even if they be narcotic, such as opium and hashish, or poisonous. All of these are clean, even though consuming them may be prohibited on various grounds. Liquids naturally include waters, oils, juices and liquid tapped from plants, and syrup of flowers, perfume, vinegar, and the like, all of which are clean. This also includes tears, sweat, saliva, mucous, and arguably semen of all living animals, notwithstanding differences of opinion over details that exist among the schools of law. Solid matter is all clean unless tainted by filth, which is also evident to the senses. This also extends to eggs and milk obtained of halal animals, including humans: they are clean, as are the hair, wool, fur, and feathers obtained from living or dead animals, halal or non-halal, provided that the bodies from which they are obtained have not become putrid or decomposed.[5]

Filth is also divided into two types: sensible (*hissiyyah*), such as the filthy objects detectable by the senses, and putative (*hukmiyyah*), which are not. Thus, it is reported that when the Prophet visited the sick, he would say "never mind; it is a cleanser God willing—*la ba's, tahurun in sha' Allah*," which means that illness cleanses its victim of the impurity of sins he or she might have committed. Idols that are worshipped (*athnaam*) are held to be unclean, and that only means putatively unclean.[6]

---

3. Muslim jurists draw a subtle distinction between *najis* and *najas*. *Najis* is the wider expression of the two in that it includes both temporary and permanent impurity, whereas *najas* applies to that which is inherently and permanently unclean. Pig meat and blood shed forth are thus both *najis* and *najas*, whereas dirt that can be cleaned easily is *najis*. Cf. al-Jaziri, *al-Fiqh 'ala'l-Madhahib*, 11–12.

4. Wizarat, *al-Mawsu'ah al-Fiqhiyyah*, vol. 40, 75.

5. al-Jaziri, *al-Fiqh 'ala'l-Madhahib*, 10–11; See also Abu Zayd, *al-Intifa' bi'l A'yan al-Muharramah*, 26–28.

6. al-Jaziri, *al-Fiqh 'ala'l-Madhahib*, 7.

Whereas the Maliki school, has, on the whole, upheld an unqualified and general understanding of the principle of original cleanliness, the Shafiʿi and Hanbali schools specify the basic premise that all things are presumed to be clean, by saying that cleanliness is the norm with regard to all tangible objects (*al-aʿyan*), including solid matter and animals, except for two: pigs and dogs. Dead carcasses are all unclean except for three: the human body (Muslim and non-Muslim alike), the fish, and the locust. What is emitted from living animals, such as bodily fluids and sweat, also falls under the principle of original cleanliness, but, according to an alternative view, only of the clean and "slaughterable" (i.e., "permitted") animals.[7] The Hanafis are in agreement with the majority on this, with one exception, which they make concerning dogs, by holding the view that dogs are not intrinsically unclean.

The Malikis widen the scope further by holding that the shariah presumption of cleanliness subsumes all things, including land and sea animals, dog and swine included. For life itself is the effective cause (*ʿillah*) and criterion of cleanliness. What is prohibited is the flesh of these animals for consumption, but they are not intrinsically unclean when alive. The body fluids of dogs and pigs, whether emitted in the state of wakefulness or sleep, except for the contents of their bellies, excrements, and vomit, are also clean.[8]

Cleanliness thus becomes an attribute of the created world and life forms therein. This is a corollary also of the basic Qurʾanic position, which is one of specification concerning things that are unclean. Filth and impurities of things thus need to be specified and determined by a clear text, failing which they are presumed to be clean. The leading Shafiʿi jurist Imam al-Haramayn al-Juwayni (d. 478/1085), the teacher of the renowned al-Ghazali, thus held that the norm of shariah is cleanliness generally, and that which is unclean is limited in scope and has also been specified. He further wrote that this norm becomes the basis for the application of the shariah presumption of continuity, or *istishab*, that establishes everything remains in its original cleanliness unless there is decisive evidence that it has become unclean.[9] The limitation expressed in the shariah sources on the scope of *najis* and *haram* is confirmed by the fact that the Qurʾan specifies only ten items as *najas* for

---

7. al-Jaziri, *al-Fiqh ʿala'l-Madhahib*, 7.

8. al-Jaziri, *al-Fiqh ʿala'l-Madhahib*, 40:79 and 85.

9. As quoted by Hammad, *al-Mawad al-Muharramah*, 18, from al-Juwayni, *Ghiyath al-Umam fi Iltiyath al-Zulam*, 439.

human consumption (cf. al-Ma'idah, 5:3–4)[10] and then declares in an open address to the Prophet Muhammad: "They ask you what is made lawful for them. Say (all) that is good and wholesome is made lawful" (5:4). Thus, it is not for us to expand the range of prohibitions, *haram* and *najis*, beyond the textual specifications.

Affirmative shariah evidence on the original permissibility and cleanliness of all things is found in the Qur'anic verse, wherein God Most High ingratiates his human servants that "He it is who created for you (your benefit) all that is (there) in the earth. (al-Baqarah, 2:29). Muhammad Rashid Rida (d.1935), the author of *Tafsir al-Manar,* comments that ingratiation (*al-imtinan*) is highly unlikely to proceed over things that are illegal or unclean. Hence all things are made permissible for human benefit, including eating, drinking, medication, wearing, riding, and beautification. Original permissibility also goes hand-in-hand with original cleanliness.[11] This combination of permissibility and cleanliness is also found in several Qur'anic verses where halal and *tayyib* (permissible and pure/clean) are juxtaposed and mentioned together, the one establishing permissibility and the other cleanliness. Ibn Taymiyyah has gone on record to observe that "the norm in all things found in the existential world is that notwithstanding their diversities and differences in attributes and substance, they are absolutely permissible for human use; they are all clean and nothing of it is precluded from the all-encompassing scope of this principle."[12] Yet it is noted that cleanliness and permissibility do not necessarily go together. So it is possible that something is clean yet not halal due to its inherent harm and its adverse consequences if consumed.[13]

Only a clear text, and, failing that, factual evidence that makes dirt and impurity detectable by the senses determines that something is impure/*najis*. Water is generally clean, for instance, for purposes of ablution, drinking, and other uses unless one detects dirt and impurity therein, either physically or through a change of color, smell, etc. Water is clean and also cleansing (*tahir wa mutahhir*) if it has remained in its natural purity and nothing has been mixed or added that would compromise its original purity, and as such it is

---

10. The ten items include pork, blood, dead carcasses, animals that had been strangled, beaten, fallen, gored, or partly eaten by wild beasts, and animals slaughtered in the name of deities other than Allah.

11. Rida, *Tafsir al-Manar,* vol. 1, 247.

12. Ibn Taymiyyah, *Majmu'at Fatawa Shaykh al-Islam Ibn Taymiyyah,* vol. 21, 535—as also appear as part of longer quotation in Hammad, *al-Mawad al-Muharramah,* 17–18.

13. Wizarat, *al-Mawsu'ah al-Fiqhiyyah,* vol. 5, 153.

good for ablution and removal of putative impurity (*hadath*) and physical impurity (*khabath*). The original purity of water is diminished, and cleaning with it becomes reprehensible when animals drink from it. Thus, when a cat, dog, free-ranging chicken, rat, snake, donkey, or predatory bird drinks from a small quantity of pure water, it is still classified as clean but not recommended for cleansing or for ablution unless there be no other clean water available, in which case it may be used for cleaning purposes and ablution. However, if the water is of a large quantity, its purity is not affected in the first place.[14]

The natural purity of water also remains intact when the smallest quantity, say a single drop of unclean liquid, falls into it and does not change its color or other natural attributes. It is also reprehensible to use the water from a well in the midst of a cemetery, or one located in usurped land, or one suspected to be unclean. The original purity of water is diminished also when a clean substance, solid or liquid, is mixed with it and changes its characteristics such that it can no longer be called water, but something else, such as juices, or medicine of some kind. The majority of jurists maintain that such a mix may not be used for ablution, except for the Hanafis, who allow it.[15] The *fiqh* scholars have recognized other manners of cleansing, such as long exposure to the sun that dries up and purifies land surfaces that may have been polluted by urination or other pollutants. Rain water that falls on such surfaces and washes away its impurity is also accepted as a natural cleanser.[16] In addition to text and palpable evidence, Muslim jurists have held that general consensus (*ijma'*) and inherited wisdom across the generations can also determine what is unclean for human consumption and use. Thus, only a clear text, factual evidence, and general consensus can rebut and set aside the presumption of original cleanliness.[17]

Arab linguistic usage and Islamic texts use a variety of expressions to signify defilement and dirt, whether inherent or putative, including *najis, qadhir, khubth, rijs,* and *rikz*. *Fiqh* scholars have divided the *najis* into two types, as earlier mentioned, physical (*'ayniyyah, hissiyyah*) and fictitious (*hukmiyyah*). Physical impurity is real and palpable to the senses and often inherent in the object itself. The shariah also corresponds, for the most part, with sense perception, and has in most cases identified inherently unclean substances.

---

14. Wizarat, *al-Mawsu'ah al-Fiqhiyyah*, vol. 29, 96.

15. Wizarat, *al-Mawsu'ah al-Fiqhiyyah*, 97–98.

16. Wizarat, *al-Mawsu'ah al-Fiqhiyyah*, 106.

17. Cf. al-Ashqar and Shabir, *Dirasat Fiqhiyyah*, 317.

Physical dirt has been subdivided into three categories of intense, light, and average. If there is total consensus among juristic schools and scholars on the impurity of something, it is intense (*mughallaz*). Differences of opinion among them reduce that level to either average or light (*mutawassit* and *mukhaffaf*, respectively). Without entering into details, these categories are often relevant in determining the legality or otherwise of the sale and other uses of the items concerned. The basic position concerning *haram* and *najis* is that, barring dire necessity, they may neither be consumed nor sold nor used for food, medicinal, cosmetic, or other purposes, and that any contact with them is also likely to interfere with the integrity of one's ritual prayer (*salah*).[18]

Fictitious impurity is essentially a juridical attribute that may or may not be visible to the naked eye, but which the shariah has identified as such, and it nullifies ablution for ritual prayer—for example, defecation, urination, or sexual intercourse. The state of cleanliness is restored either through taking a minor ablution (*wudu'*) or full bath (*ghusl*) and washing generally with clean water. Other methods of purification of *najis* that the *fiqh* texts have recorded include drying and tanning, as in the case of animal hides, heating by fire and burning, pouring away certain quantities of water from a polluted water well, and ritual cleanliness through dry ablution (*al-tayammum*).[19]

The shariah has also identified other varieties of impurity, such as the denial of faith (*kufr*), crime, and sin, which are deemed to pollute and compromise the purity of one's personality and character. This pollution may be removed by embracing the faith, or, in the case of crime and sin, through prosecution and punishment, or through expiation (*kaffarah*) involving charity, fasting, and sincere repentance (*tawbah*).[20] The consequence of declaring something as *najis* may be that this substance becomes wholly unlawful, even when mixed with other substances, for human consumption, or that it vitiates the ritual prayer when present on one's person, clothes, or place of worship.[21]

The question as to precisely what items are *najis*, apart from the ones mentioned in the clear text, is a subject of juristic disagreement. The first point of disagreement arises over the authority of determining the purity or impurity

18. Muslim jurists are thus unanimous on the filth of human excrement and excrement of carnivorous animals, and also on their urine, although on the latter with some differences of opinion. They have differed more widely on the excrements and urine of "slaughterable" animals, noncarnivorous animals, and birds.

19. Cf. al-Kurdi, *Buhuth wa Fatawa Fiqhiyyah Mu'asirah*, 29–31.

20. Ibid., 313.

21. Wizarat, *al-Mawsu'ah al-Fiqhiyyah*, 40:74 and 77; see also 40:101–103.

of objects, acts, and conduct. Is it only the shariah, or also popular custom and the natural predilections of people, that can detect and determine legality and cleanliness? The *fiqh* scholars generally maintain that *najasah* (filth) from the viewpoint of shariah is a particular category, which does not always correspond with what people may normally think. For example, the shariah declares alcohol as unclean (*rijs*; cf. Qur'an al-Ma'idah, 5:90), a declaration that does not coincide with popular perceptions among the Arabs. In addition, the Arabs consider certain things to be unclean that are not necessarily so in the shariah. Included among these are certain human bodily emissions, such as semen, spit, and mucus, which are not textually declared to be unclean. People's perceptions thus vary according to their respective culture, climate, and customary habits and do not always correspond with shariah positions.[22]

Many *fiqh* scholars have drawn the conclusion that everything the shariah has made *haram* is also *najis*. Yet a closer analysis would show that even this is likely to be less than accurate. For example, shariah prohibits marriage to one's mother or sister, which is *haram* without question, yet the objects of that prohibition, namely the women involved, cannot be said to be *najis* in themselves. In response, it has been stated that these prohibitions are not concerned with objects or persons, as it were, but with relations, which are undoubtedly abhorrent, but that there is no issue over inherent dirt and uncleanliness of objects or persons in this case. Yet the argument is further extended to other items such as poison, which may not be dirty as such, but which the shariah prohibits for consumption. Many scholars of the leading *fiqh* schools have also gone on record to say that even the birds and animals that the shariah has prohibited for consumption, such as predatory animals and birds with claws and other characteristics, are not necessarily dirty in themselves, but that they have been declared prohibited for reasons most likely other than impurity (*najasah*). This level of divergence is acknowledged in the *fiqh* maxim that "everything *najis* is *haram*, but not all *haram* is *najis*."[23]

The question still remains as to what exactly is the effective cause (*'illah*) of determining something as unclean/*najis*. If one could identify that the presence of a certain factor, substance, or attribute means the presence of impurity/*najasah*, and its absence also means that *najasah* is absent, then one would have a formula and guideline to operate on. It is admitted, however,

---

22. al-Ashqar and Shabir, *Dirāsāt Fiqhiyyah*, 318.

23. al-Ashqar and Shabir, *Dirāsāt Fiqhiyyah*, 314.

that we are unable to identify an effective cause or meaning of that kind. "Since this is a grey area and points of doubt still remain in the whole debate over *najasah*, the *ulama* have held that we can only look at the textual injunctions of shariah and other rational evidence to tell us what is *najis*. This is the only way and the best guideline to be applied."[24]

---

24. al-Ashqar and Shabir, *Dirāsāt Fiqhiyyah*, 317.

# 6

# *The Prohibited (*Haram*)*

HARAM, ALSO KNOWN as *mahzur, mamnuʿ* and sometimes as *muharram* (*muharramat* in the plural form is more common among the ulema of *usul al-fiqh*), may be defined as "all that which the Lawgiver (*al-shariʿ*) has prohibited in definitive terms, and its perpetrator is liable to a punishment in this world or the Hereafter." *Haram* is thus a binding demand from the Lawgiver in respect of abandoning something, and it is conveyed in a variety of linguistic expressions, as will presently be elaborated. A perusal of the Qur'an and hadith would indicate that a *haram*, or a prohibition amounting to *haram*, is conveyed in numerous linguistic expressions, particles, and phrases, which convey *haram* but may also add nuances as to their intensity, conditionality, and other characteristics. The text may clearly use the word *haram* or its derivatives, as in the Qur'anic phrase "*hurrimat ʿalaykum* (forbidden to you) is the carrion, blood shed forth and pork, etc." (al-Ma'idah, 5:4), or in its reference to usury (*riba*): "*wa harrama al-riba*" (al-Baqarah, 2:275). When the text declares, for instance, that a certain conduct is impermissible (*la yahillu*), this also conveys *haram*, as in the Qur'anic verse (al-Baqarah, 228, with reference to a prospective divorce wherein it is not permissible for the wife to conceal her possible pregnancy), but also many hadith reports that record the expression (*la yahillu li'l-Muslimin*). The Arabic expression *al-nahy* ("prohibition," as opposed to *al-amr*, "command") also conveys the meaning of *haram*, as in the Qur'an when it is declared "*wa yanha ʿan al-fahsha' wa'l-munkar*"—on the prohibition of lewdness, lawlessness, and evil (al-Nahl, 16:90). In the hadith literature, the Companions are often quoted as saying that "the Messenger of God prohibited such and such (*naha Rusul Allahi ʿan kadha*)". This can also be said of Arabic expressions such as *la tafʿal* (do not do) such and such, which signifies a *haram*. An example is the phrase *la ta'kulu* (eat not your properties wrongfully among yourselves) (al-Baqarah, 2:188). Another variation of the use of the Arabic particle "*la*" that signifies prohibition is when it is said

*Shariah and The Halal Industry.* Mohammad Hashim Kamali, Oxford University Press. © Oxford University Press 2021.
DOI: 10.1093/oso/9780197538616.003.0007

by way of denial or negation of a certain conduct, as in the Qur'anic phrase "*la yarith al-qatil*—the murderer does not inherit" the relative he has slayed. A similar expression in the Qur'an is *ijtanibu* (avoid), as with regard to the prohibition of wine drinking and gambling (al-Ma'idah, 5:90). One of the clearest expressions of *haram* in the Qur'an, however, is when the text stipulates a severe punishment for a certain conduct, as in the case of the prescribed crimes of murder, theft, adultery, and slander, known as the *hudud*.[1] Broadly, the shariah emphasis on *haram* can be gauged from the following hadith, which juxtaposes the *haram* with a command and then speaks of the manner of their observance. The Prophet thus addressed the believers, saying, "When I forbid you from something, avoid it completely, and when I command you to do something, do it to the extent you can." There is thus no flexibility in the observance of a *haram*, but some flexibility would seem to exist in the fulfilment of a command. A command usually conveys an obligatory order (*wajib*), which would appear to take a lower degree of emphasis to that of the *haram*.[2]

*Haram* may be an act, object, or conduct that is forbidden by clear evidence in the Qur'an or hadith. The conduct may consist of acts or words as they are commonly understood by the general usage and custom of people—should there be a question, for instance, as to what exactly amounts to *action* or *word*, it will be referred to customary usage. Acts may also involve the avoidance of doing something, just as words may be understood in their secondary or metaphorical sense—although the literal meaning is normally preferred.[3] Committing *haram* is punishable and omitting it is rewarded. This is the position of the majority of the Islamic legal schools (*madhahib*). The Hanafi school has added the proviso that if the source evidence in question is anything less than definitive in respect of both authenticity and meaning, the *haram* is downgraded to the category of *makruh tahrimi* (*makruh* close to *haram*) and no longer *haram* in the full sense. These last two resemble one another in that committing either of them is punishable and omitting is rewarded, but they differ insofar as a willful denial of the *haram* incurs infidelity (*kufr*), which is not the case with regard to *makruh tahrimi*.[4]

---

1. For details, see Kamali, *Principles of Islamic Jurisprudence*, 421–425, 187–202. See also al-Raysuni, *al-Haram fi'l-Shariah*, 49761.

2. Cf. al-Raysuni, *al-Haram fi'l-Shariah*, 34.

3. Cf. Abu Zayd, *al-Intifa' bi'l-A'yan al-Muharramah*, 22.

4. Cf. al-Qaradawi, *al-Halal wa'l-Haram*, 15; Shabbir, *al-Qawa'id al-Kulliyyah*, 324; Kamali, *Principles*, 421.

In the order of shariah values, *haram* is the strongest expression determined by the clear text independently of inference and *ijtihad*. *Haram* cannot, as such, be established by means of interpretation or *ijtihad* in the absence of a definitive text. The Qur'an provides the primary proof in respect of *haram*, as the text itself declares: "He (God) has explained to you in detail what is forbidden (*harrama*) to you" (al-An'am, 6:119), which means that a vague and inconclusive text is not enough to establish a *haram*. With regard to prohibited foods, for instance, the Qur'an has specified ten items:

> Carrion (*al-maytatu*), blood, the flesh of swine, the animal slaughtered in any name other than Allah's, the animal which has either been strangled, killed by a violent blow, has died of a fall, or by being gored to death; that which has been partly eaten by a wild animal, unless you are able to slaughter it (in due form- *illa ma zakkaytum*),[5] and that which is sacrificed on stone (altars). . . . But if any is forced by hunger, with no inclination to be a rebel or a transgressor, God is indeed Oft-Forgiving, Most Merciful. (al-Ma'idah, 5:3)[6]

The subject also occurs in two other verses that actually summarize the ten items into four (cf. al-An'am, 6:145 and 2:172) as the last six items in the list of ten are actually included in the category of carrion. Wine drinking has also been declared forbidden (5:90). This is the sum total of clear prohibitions found in the Qur'an. As for the rest, it is ordained: "And do not utter falsehoods by letting your tongues declare: this is halal and that is *haram*, thus fabricating lies against God" (al-Nahl, 16:116). All other foodstuffs, animals of land and sea, harmful or unclean substances, and so on that are

---

5. Disagreement has arisen among Qur'an interpreters and jurists as to whether this exception is a connected exception (*istithna' muttasil*) or disconnected exception (*istithna' munqati'*). If the former, it would mean that slaughter also subsumes the five preceding types and animals in these categories, hence they should also be slaughtered if still alive, for prohibition is attached to *al-maytatu*, that is death prior to slaughtering, not to animals that may still be alive. But those who maintain that it is a disconnected exception hold that strangled and gored animals, etc., are forbidden regardless of slaughter. Al-Qurtubi, who discusses both these views, is inclined to the first view, saying that slaughter can apply before the animal dies or to one that is not too close to the point of dying. For details, see al-Qurtubi, *Bidayat al-Mujtahid*, vol. 1, 322–323.

6. Abdullah Yusuf Ali's translation. The Qur'anic prohibition of pig meat represents a continuation of the Judaic tradition. Similarly, the negative view of the Islamic tradition toward dogs is attributed to the fact that canines were often seen as carriers of rabies and best kept at a safe distance.

discussed in the *fiqh* manuals are subject to disagreement due mainly to the different perceptions of jurists concerning "the grounds of *haram*" as elaborated below.

Carrion or carcass (*al-maytatu*), being the first word in the verse (5:4) subsumes, as already noted, most of the other categories, such as animals that are strangled, killed by a blow, gored, or died of a fall. The animal may have died by itself or through a human act other than a valid slaughter. Beyond the confines of this text, carrion also includes the slaughter of an idol worshipper, an apostate, or follower of a non-monotheistic religion—since their slaughter fails to be a valid slaughter in Islam and therefore falls under carrion in the verse under review. *Al-maytatu*, moreover, includes forbidden game, such as hunting a bird or animal by one who is in the sanctified state of *ihram* for the haj pilgrimage. Since *al-maytatu* actually subsumes death by strangulation, fall, death by a violent blow, or when gored to death, it may be asked why the text goes on to mention them separately. The reason is not clear, although it is suggested that it is probably because the pre-Islamic Arabs held them all as permissible meat.[7] In an earlier sura (al-Baqarah, 2:172-173) the Qur'an only mentions *al-maytatu* without these additions, but sura 5:4 itemizes these other varieties for emphasis and the removal of doubt. Another Qur'anic verse on the subject of prohibited meat refers to hunting during the time of haj (al-Ma'idah, 5:95). This same prohibition is then extended to hunting in the actual precinct of the mosque of Ka'bah, or the *Haram* (sacred precinct), at all times, not confined to the duration of state of sanctity, or Ihram, for the haj. Added to these are also animals, birds, sea creatures, and insects that are prohibited by clear hadith reports for various reasons: they may be predatory, poisonous, or inherently objectionable and the like. In addition to their rationally understood benefits and harms, these prohibitions are also manifestations of the Qur'anic vision of human dignity, as well as aspects of the purity and cleanliness (*tayyibat*) that is a recurrent theme of the Qur'an and hadith.[8] That said, while most of the instances of *haram* in victuals are due to identifiable rational causes, this is not always the case. *Haram* is an obligatory law (*hukm taklifi*) that carries legal and religious consequences, and the faithful are expected to follow it whether or not they are able to understand the reason behind it. The prohibitions for Muslims to avoid consuming pig meat, carrion, and blood shed forth are strict and absolute; they are *haram*

---

7. Cf. 'Assaf, *al-Halal wa'l-Haram fi'l-Islam*, 285.

8. 'Assaf, *al-Halal wa'l-Haram fi'l-Islam*, 279.

in the full sense, regardless of whether one understands the reason for it or not—one must still comply.[9]

Slaughter is only valid of an animal that is still alive. In the event that an animal has fallen from a height, or been strangled or gored, it may only be slaughtered if it shows signs of life. In a report from 'Ali ibn Abi Talib, it is recorded that if the slaughtered animal does not move its eye or foot, or tail or ear, even if there is ample flow of blood but no movement, it is non-halal.[10] In response to a question regarding *mutaraddiyah*—that is, if an animal that falls from a height—suppose that the animal has been slaughtered and then falls into water and drowns, or falls in fire, is it still halal? The majority of Sunni schools and the sixth Shia Imam Ja'far al-Sadiq maintain that only if the slaughter has been duly completed and the vital passages were cut, would it then be halal.[11] The Qur'anic concept of dead carcass (*maytatun*), which is *haram*, also includes severed limbs or parts of an animal while still alive. This is unlawful and not fit for consumption. But if the same animal is then duly slaughtered, whatever is left of it becomes halal.[12]

Some members of a focus study group of Muslims in Vancouver, Canada, offered medical and scientific rationales as to why Islam forbade the consumption of carrion, blood, and pork. Blood contained harmful pathogens, they claimed, which could in turn be harmful to the body. For this reason, Islamic slaughtering methods of allowing the blood to drain from the meat were viewed to have health benefits. Participant (only referred to as) V8 succinctly conveyed the prevailing attitude toward food: "The philosophy of Islam is to save the human body from any dangers. So Islam prohibited ... different food[s] [since] they are injurious to human health."[13] Regarding pork, participant V3 claimed to have learned from his son, who was also a neurologist, that it contributed to the parasitic infection of the brain, neurocysticercosis, with symptoms similar to epilepsy.[14] The same participant explained

---

9. Cf. Abu Zayd, *al-Intifa' bi'A'yan al-Muharramah*, 36–38.

10. al-Tabarsi, *Mustadrak al-Wasa'il*, vol.16, 137, sec. 19394. Muslim scholars and jurists are hesitant to use the word haram when there is an element of doubt—hence may prefer to use an alternative expression, such as non-halal.

11. al-Tabarsi, *Mustadrak al-Wasa'il*, vol.16, sec. 19396.

12. al-Tabarsi, *Mustadrak al-Wasa'il*, vol.16, 152, sec. 19439.

13. "Epilepsy," *Encyclopaedia Britannica*.

14. *Muslim Focus Group*, May 30, 2005, Vancouver, BC. Viewpoints from both the managed risk approach and the precautionary approach percolated the opinions canvassed at the focus group on the question of the relationship of religiously informed dietary practices with food.

that to observe a religious diet was to seek God's love, friendship, proximity, and wisdom. Another participant, referred to as V2, provided a more dogmatic response, arguing that the dietary prescriptions of Islam dating back to antiquity contained wisdom that even science could not fathom very well.[15]

On the interpretation of that which has been "slaughtered in any name other than Allah," the Shia scholars quote Imam 'Ali ibn Abi Talib to have said concerning the verse under review that "the Prophet, pbuh, prohibited the slaughter of jinn (*dhaba'ih al-jinn*), but when he was asked 'O Messenger of God, and what is the slaughter of jinn,' to which he replied: 'when it is done by the occupant of a house who fears the ghosts, and slaughter an animal for them.'"[16] Added to this are also cases when slaughter is done to gain closeness to an idol, the object of one's devotion, a tree or the like (*sanam, wathan, aw shajar*)."[17] One may add to this animal slaughter for the sea in order to keep the sea calm. In pre-Islamic times, the Quraysh tribe used to worship certain trees and rocks and also slaughtered animals to extinguish fire at burning premises on fire. A "rebel" (*baagh*) in the verse under review is one who exits obedience to the imam (or lawful government), and "transgressor" (*'aad*) here is understood to mean an oppressor (*zalim*), thief, and usurper. These acts of transgression also include, according to the Shia, one who claims prophethood for someone who is not a prophet, or imamate for one who is not an imam. All of these also disentitle their perpetrators from taking advantage of the concessions, of consuming prohibited meats under stressful situations granted in the verse under review.[18]

As for the full Qur'anic phrase, "if any is forced by hunger, with no inclination to be a rebel or a transgressor," although the hadith plays an important role in determining what is *haram*, or explaining the Qur'an on this subject, the scope of *haram* is generally quite limited. This is also indicated in the following hadith: Salman al-Farisi narrated that the Prophet was asked a question about the wild ass (zebra), quails, and curdled milk, and he gave this response: "Halal is that which God has permitted in His Book, and *haram* is that which God has prohibited in His Book. As for what He has chosen to

---

The focus group elicited a series of very productive and interesting responses as to how communities relate to food. See also Moosa, "Genetically Modified Food," 150.

15. Cf. Muslim Focus Group, May 30, 2005, Vancouver, BC.

16. al-Tabarsi, *Mustadrak al-Wasa'il*, vol. 16, 200, sec. 19582.

17. al-Tabarsi, *Mustadrak al-Wasa'il*, vol. 16, 200, sec, 19581.

18. al-Tabarsi, *Mustadrak al-Wasa'il*, vol. 16, 200, secs. 19583–19588.

remain silent about, it is exonerated."[19] Since there was no particular text in the Qur'an on the three items in question, they were consequently declared to be halal. In this hadith the Prophet himself referred the determination of *haram* to the Qur'an, so there is little scope for anyone else, including the jurist, the *mujtahid* (one who exercises *ijtihad*), the *mufti*, and government authorities to play a significant role in the determination of *haram*. Yet there is some flexibility for the head of state to prohibit what has already been determined as reprehensible (*makruh*), or to elevate the recommendable (*mandub*) to the level of an obligatory command in order to realize a manifest *maslahah* (public interest), or prevent a manifest *mafsadah* (corruption, harm). This kind of discretionary power and its proper exercise is often subsumed under the Islamic public law principle of shariah-oriented policy (*siyasah shar'iyah*).[20]

Identifying something as *haram* is not confined, as already noted, to the prohibition of eating, drinking, and wearing, but also includes other aspects of conduct and transactions, such as sale and purchase, or even giving something as gift and charity. Yet being haram does not mean that the object has no market value. The market value of that object is not, in other words, nullified by its prohibition. For it may still be a valuable item for a non-Muslim, even if it is not a valuable object (*maal*) from the Islamic point of view. Yet there is some disagreement to the effect that a slightly less emphatic *haram*, or when there is some doubt in the component elements of the *haram* at issue, may be given in charity. An example of this may be non-halal money gained on certain *riba*-oriented accounts or investments by an Islamic bank or institution, which is usually given to charity. This has, in fact, become a common practice among shariah advisors and committees in Malaysia and elsewhere. Al-Qaradawi has also given a *fatwa* in support of this. Yet the same cannot be extended to giving *haram* meat in charity or gift.

## Classifications of Haram

*Haram* has been classified into several types, depending on the purpose, subject matter, and the researcher's viewpoint. Some of the juristic discussion on the typology of *haram* runs into technicality that may not be of immediate interest to our context here. Yet understanding the halal and its manifestations

---

19. Ibn Majah, *Sunan Ibn Majah*, vol. 3, 367; al-Qaradawi, *al-Halal wa'l-Haram*, 23.

20. For details on *siyasah shar'iyah*, see Kamali, *Shari'iah Law*, 225–245.

in the halal industry is, in many ways, also a study about the *haram* even more than that of the halal itself. It is important therefore to expound the classifications of *haram*, which is followed, in turn, by an exposition of the grounds or causes of *haram* from the shariah perspective. Three main classifications of *haram* are discussed in the following pages.

## *Haram* in Itself and *Haram* Due to an Extraneous Factor

This classification looks into the intrinsic characteristics of *haram* as opposed to any extraneous factors and influences that turn something that is essentially permissible into *haram*. Muslim schools and scholars have thus divided the *haram* into two types: (a) *haram* for its own sake (*haram li-dhatih*), such as theft and murder, carrion, blood shed forth, and so forth, which the Lawgiver has forbidden explicitly for their inherent enormity, and for reasons that may also be known to us, such as filth, intoxication, and harm (as elaborated below), or which may not be so known; and (b) *haram* due to the presence of an extraneous factor (*haram li-ghayrih*), such as sale that is used as a disguise for securing usury (*riba*), and the sale of stolen goods. Sale in itself is permissible in shariah, but it is unlawful in these two instances because of usury and theft. A consequence of this distinction is that *haram* for its own sake is null and void (*batil*) *ab initio* in all of its applications, whereas violation of a *haram li-ghayrih* renders its subject matter into a *fasid* (voidable, irregular) but not null and void, and a transaction over it may fulfill some of its legal consequences. For instance, if the subject matter of a contract of sale is carrion or wine, the contract will be null and void (*batil*) and would produce no legal effect. But a contract of sale of permissible meat or animal when concluded immediately after the call to Friday prayer and while the prayer is still in progress is not null and void, but irregular (*fasid*), and it does produce some of its legal effects. Yet this is basically a Hanafi distinction. The Shafiʿi, Hanbali, and also Zahiri, schools maintain that all of these are null and void, as they do not recognize the validity of the distinction between *batil* and *fasid*. Similarly, a contract with an unlawful condition, or a usurious contract that involves unequal countervalues, is not null and void, according to the Hanafis, but irregular (*fasid*), because it can be rectified by removing the unlawful elements even after its conclusion. A typical example of this is a marriage contract concluded without the presence of witnesses, which can, however, be supplied after the contract, or publicizing the marriage in other ways—for the purpose of witnesses is to publicize the marriage. Food consumed by a hungry person that belongs to another without the owner's permission is unlawful, but it can be legalized by a belated permission. Most other schools do not recognize *fasid* as a separate category and would subsume the violations in question all as null and void. *Haram* for its own sake does not become permissible save in cases of dire necessity (*darurah*), such as imminent death from starvation that allows the person to consume *haram* substances. *Haram* due to extraneous factors becomes permissible, however, in cases of manifest need (*hajah*) that is a rank below necessity, and when it prevents hardship (*haraj*). Should there be a choice between one or the other of these two types of *haram* in situations of necessity—as to which one may be consummated for instance—then the *haram* for an extraneous reason is to be preferred over *haram* for itself, as the former is a lighter variety of *haram*. For instance, eating pig meat is *haram* in itself and may not be violated except in situations of dire necessity to save one's life, whereas consuming halal meat that belongs to another person is *haram* for that very reason, but it can be made halal by obtaining the owner's permission.

According to a legal maxim of *fiqh*, "the means to *haram* also partakes in *haram*—*al-wasilah ila'l-haram haram*."[21] What the maxim means is that when the end result is *haram*, the same also applies to its means, regardless of whether the means in question was originally permissible, recommendable, or reprehensible. This is the basic rule and it applies, in some cases at least, even if the end result is not secured. For instance, illicit retirement (*khalwah*) with a stranger who is a member of the opposite sex is forbidden, even if it does not lead to *zina*. This is because the shariah seeks to obstruct the ways and means that beget *haram*. For if the shariah permitted the means to *haram*, it will run into contradiction and controversy. When the shariah forbids usury (*riba*), the means to *riba* is also forbidden. In a similar vein, the sale of arms to the enemy of Muslims in wartime is forbidden, and so is the sale of grapes to a winemaker or factory owner. If theft and murder are *haram*, the means toward procuring them are also *haram*, and if pig meat is *haram*, then trading, processing, exporting, and promoting it are as well.

As for the question of reward and punishment, Muslim scholars have recorded the view that abandonment of the *haram* earns a spiritual reward only when it is accompanied by the intention (*niyyah*) to seek closeness to God, but that without such a state of mind, the Muslim merely fulfills his duty and is consequently absolved of it as a result and there is no further reward nor

21. Cf. al-Qaradawi, *al-Halal wa'l-Haram*, 34; al-Qurtubi, *Bidayat al-Mujtahid*, vol. 1, 242; Shabir, *al-Qawa'id al-Kulliyyah*, 324. See also Hasan, *Principles of Islamic Jurisprudence*, vol. c 1, 121; Abu Zayd, *Al-Intifa' bil A'yan al-Muharramah*, 62–63.

punishment. This is because avoidance consists of mere abnegation (*al-kuff*), which is not an act in itself.[22] Yet according to a minority, and probably preferable, opinion, avoidance is an act and merits spiritual reward. The advocates of this view illustrate this by citing the example of fasting (*al-sawm*), which consists mainly of avoidance, yet it is rewarded. Further in support of this is cited the hadith, recorded by al-Bayhaqi,[23] wherein the Prophet, pbuh, responded to a question put to him: "Which act is most liked by God Most High?" The Prophet paused a little and then responded, "It is to guard one's tongue—*qala huwa hifz al-lisan.*" It is then stated that "guarding one's tongue is an act and it earns a reward." The end result of this discussion still does not change the basic position that, in both cases, be it an act, or avoidance from acting, it must be accompanied by correct intention. Avoiding the *haram* itself, and also the means which begets it, thus consist of a duty fulfilled, and it earns a spiritual reward if it is done with the intention of earning God's pleasure, or helping another living soul, a harmless animal, or insect, for instance, out of compassion and with a good intention.[24]

Some of the more consequential applications of the foregoing in a contemporary context may be as follows: if the use of narcotics is forbidden, then one should also block the means that lead to their production, processing, transportation, and marketing. If adultery, gambling, and narcotics are forbidden, then one should also disallow rental of houses and premises to brothels and drug-making factories. In a similar vein, sorcery and pornography are forbidden, so one should also disallow the publication of magazines, electronic media, and books that promote them.[25]

## Major and Minor Haram (*al-kaba'ir wa'l-sagha'ir*)

From the viewpoint of its ranking on the renowned binary scale of transgressions in shariah, namely of major sins and minor sins (*al-kaba'ir wa'l-sagha'ir*), *haram* is also divided into the two corresponding categories of major *haram* and minor *haram*, although there are differences of opinion on the attributes of each. *Haram* that falls under the *kaba'ir* is greater in enormity to that which may fall under the *sagha'ir*. The basis of this classification is given

---

22. Cf. al-Raysuni, *al-Haram fi'l-Shariah*, 99.

23. al-Bayhaqi, *Sunan al-Bayhaqi: Bab fi Hifz al-Lisan: Fasl fi Fadl al-Sukut*, hadith no. 4950.

24. For details, see al-Raysuni, *al-Haram fi'l-Shariah*, 213–215.

25. Cf. al-Raysuni, *al-Haram fi'l-Shariah*, 190–191.

in the scripture. In several places the Qur'an, and also the Sunnah, refer to major sins, which has prompted Muslim scholars and jurists to distinguish these from the minor ones. Thus, one reads in the Qur'an in an address to the believers:

> If you eschew the most heinous of the things which are forbidden to you (*kaba'ira ma tunhawna 'anhu*), We shall conceal your evil deeds (*sayyi'atikum*) and admit you to a Gate of great honour. (al-Nisa', 4:31)

> Those who avoid great sins (*kaba'ir al-ithm*) and shameful deeds, only (falling into) minor faults, verily your Lord is ample in forgiveness. He knows you well. (al-Najm, 53:32)

Commenting on the first of these, the Qur'an commentator Ibn Kathir explained that avoiding the major sins acts as a concealer of the minor ones; God forgives, out of His grace and mercy, the minor failings of those who are assiduous in refraining from the major sins.[26]

Hadith reports provide more details on the identification of major sins. Thus, according to a hadith on the authority of Abu Bakr, the Prophet has said: "Should I inform you what the greatest of all major sins (*akbar al-kaba'ir*) are? These are three: Associating another deity with God, offending one's parents; the Prophet was leaning [on a pillow, took a pause] and sat upright, and [added], beware, it is perjury or telling a lie."[27] In another hadith, narrated by the Companion Abu Hurayrah, the Prophet is also reported to have said: "Refrain from seven devastating sins (*al-sab' al-mowbiqat*), that doom a person to Hell. We asked then: What are they, O Messenger of God? He said: Associating others with God (*shirk*); witchcraft (*sihr*); killing a soul whom God has forbidden to kill, except in the cause of justice; devouring usury (*riba*); consuming orphans' wealth; fleeing from the battlefield; and slandering chaste and innocent women."[28] The fact that the Prophet has spoken of major sins in terms of a specific number has prompted Ibn Kathir to say that these are the major *harams* based on clear text, but the Prophet has

---

26. Ibn Kathir, *Tafsir al-Qur'an al-'Azim*, vol. 2, 255 as quoted in al-Raysuni, *al-Haram fi'l-Shariah*, 75. The hadith is also recorded in al-Bukhari and Muslim.

27. Wizarat, *al-Mawsu'ah al-Fiqhiyyah*, vol. 34, 153. Al-Bukhari has recorded this hadith under "*ala 'unaibbi'ukum bi-akbar al-kaba'ir.*"

28. Wizarat, *al-Mawsu'ah al-Fiqhiyyah*, vol. 34, 151–152. The hadith is also recorded in al-Bukhari under "*ijtanibu al-sab' al-mowbiqat,*" and in Muslim under "*al-zawajir.*"

not ruled out that there may also be others.[29] 'Ali ibn Abi Talib, 'Ata ibn Abi Rabah, and 'Ubayd b. 'Umayr from among the Companions are also quoted to have confirmed the number of *kaba'ir* at seven. Others have said that they are eight in number, adding "offending one's parents" to the seven. Other scholars have looked at the wider evidence in the sources, especially in hadith, and record different numbers of the *kaba'ir*, at nine, ten, fourteen, seventeen, twenty-five, and even higher numbers, all of which are *haram* of the major type. Al-Shatibi, along with some other scholars, has observed that neither the major sins nor the *haram* can be specified by number, adding that it is perhaps better to classify them in a different way: The *kaba'ir* are mainly concerned with destruction and attack on the five essential objectives (or *maqasid*) of Islam, which are also similarly recorded in almost all major traditions/ religions: these are protection and preservation of religion, and of life, intellect, lineage, and property. All the textual references to *kaba'ir* are concerned with serious attacks on and violation of these higher objectives (*maqasid*) and those which stand in parallel with them.[30] The Tunisian scholar Ibn 'Ashur (d. 1974), who is author of an important book on the higher purposes, or *maqasid*, of shariah has also concurred and observed that the *kaba'ir* are primarily concerned with attacks on the sanctity of the *maqasid*.[31] Abu'l-Hasan al-Mawardi (d. 450/1058) of the Shafi'i school, and Abu Ya'la al-Farra' (d. 458/1066) of the Hanbali school have held that *haram* in the *kaba'ir* category include all acts which carry a punishment in the sources and are the subject also of warning and threats to its perpetrators of the wrath of God and painful punishment in the hereafter.[32]

Then the question has also arisen as to which are the minor sins. Many responses are given, but none seems any more definitive than the ones already examined concerning the major sins.

The renowned Shafi'i scholar 'Izzuddin Abd al-Salam al-Sulami (d. 660/ 1262) has held that any sin that is lesser than the lowest of the major sins is a minor sin.[33] While confirming this, al-Raysuni has added, provided also that the minor *haram* in question has not been the subject of a prohibition, punishment or threat of punishment, cursing, or wrath and anger in the scriptural

---

29. Ibn Kathir, *Tafsir*, vol. 2, 256 as quoted by al-Raysuni, *al-Haram fi'l-Shariah*, 80.

30. al-Shatibi, *al-I'tisam*, vol. 2, 57; al-Shatibi, *al-Muwafaqat*, vol. 2, 299.

31. 'Ashur, *Maqasid al-Shari'ah al-Islamiyyah*, 1998, 290.

32. As quoted in Wizarat, *al-Mawsu'ah al-Fiqhiyyah*, vol. 34, 150.

33. al-Salam, *al-Qawa'id al-Ahkam*, vol. 1, 22.

sources. Some of the examples of the minor sins or *sagha'ir* include looking at a stranger who is a member of the opposite sex, exiting a mosque after the call to prayer, looking around during the prayer, cursing and insulting the wind or (God-ordained) natural phenomena, consuming raw garlic prior to congregational prayers, and the like.[34] The key Hanbali scholar Ibn Qayyim al-Jawziyyah (d. 751/1350) has gone on record to say that that which is prohibited in the Qur'an is a major sin, and that which the Prophet has prohibited is a minor one.[35]

According to another opinion, attributed to Ibn Abi'l-'Izz al-Hanafi (d. 1390/1970), a major sin is one on which all the major traditions are in agreement, but those on which differences of opinion are recorded are minor ones.[36] Some scholars of *usul al-fiqh*, including Abu Bakr ibn Tayyib al-Baqillani (d. 1013/1604), Imam al-Haramayn al-Juwayni, and others, have recorded the view that the minor *harams* are all attached to the major *harams*, such as kissing and playing that precede adultery (*zina*), preparations that lead to the crime of theft, plotting to kill and other acts that actually lead to murder, all acts that lead to perjury, deliberate mixing of *haram* meat with halal meat, or of stolen food with halal food without announcing it, and so forth. The act of mixing is not *haram*, as it can be to feed animals, but when it is done to feed the unsuspecting public, or when intended to sabotage the halal market, then the act of mixing becomes a minor *haram*, and the accomplished act is *haram* major.[37]

There are also situations wherein a minor sin/*haram* can change into a major one, such as in the following: (1) Persistence in minor sins while belittling the enormity of doing such. This is the purport of a hadith on the authority of Sahl ibn Sa'd, which warns that repetitions in "belittling the enormity of sins can lead their perpetrators into perdition."[38] Although the hadith is about all sins, major and minor, but with regard to minors sins, if the perpetrator persists and does so with boastfulness and disdain, it will amount to a major sin. A statement of the renowned Companions Ibn 'Abbas is also quoted in this connection, wherein he said "there is no minor sin without

---

34. al-Raysuni, *al-Haram fi'l-Shariah*, 85–86.

35. al-Jawziyyah, *al-Jawab al-Kafi*, 136.

36. In Abi'l-'Izz al-Hanafi, as cited in al-Raysuni, *al-Haram fi'l-Shariah*, 85.

37. Wizarat, *al-Mawsu'ah al-Fiqhiyyah*, vol. 34, 149.

38. Hadith recorded in Ibn Hanbal, *Musnad*, vol. 2, 313, and included in al-Albani's *Silsilah al-Ahadith al-Sahihah*, no. 389. Al-Albani, Muhammad Nasir al-Din. *Silsilah al-Ahadith al-Sahihah*. Riyadh: Maktabah al-Ma'arif, 1995.

persistence and no major one with [asking for] forgiveness."[39] (2) Belittling and denigrating the minor sins and habitual commitment that emanate from a certain blackness of the heart turns them into major ones. Abu Hamid al-Ghazali has similarly written that "when the sweetness of minor sins overwhelms a servant [of God] it becomes bigger and bigger until it blackens his heart."[40] The difference between a faithful Muslim and a sinner is that the former feels remorseful and fears God even when committing a minor sin, whereas the latter denigrates it until he feels no guilt about it.[41] (3) Openly declaring the minor sin (al-mujaharah) and taking pride in committing it also raises it to the level of a major sin. (4) Perpetration of minor sins by one who is learned and respected by others is tantamount to setting bad examples for others. To this effect, 'Abd al-Salam al-Sulami authored a legal maxim, stating that "a minor sin from the notables are counted as a major one—al-saghirah min al-amathil ta'uddu kabiratan."[42] Quoted in authority for this is the Qur'anic verse which, in an address to the wives of the Prophet, says that their punishment for any act of lewdness shall be double that of the other believing women (al-Ahzab, 33:20), which is evidently on account of the exemplary status they held in the eyes of others.

## Haram That Admits Concession and Haram That Does Not

From the viewpoint of its openness to concession (rukhsah) and omission (suqut), haram is again divided into three types. The first is haram that is not open to concession or omission whatsoever, even in situations of necessity or compulsion. An example of this is slaying another person, Muslim or non-Muslim, or severing his or her limbs. This is also said of the perpetrator of adultery (zina) under duress that even if he is exonerated from punishment, he remains a sinner, as the consequences of the shame he inflicts and illegitimate offspring he may beget cannot be easily wiped out. Hence, no amount of compromising conditions, necessity, or compulsion exonerates the perpetrator of murder and zina. As for the minority view that permits committing these in situations under absolute duress, they still say that the sin committed

---

39. As quoted in al-Raysuni, al-Haram fi'l-Shariah, 86. See also Wizarat, al-Mawsu'ah al-Fiqhiyyah, vol. 34, 156.

40. al-Ghazali, Ihya' 'Ulum al-Din, vol. 4, 32.

41. al-Raysuni, al-Haram fi'l-Shariah, 87.

42. 'Abd al-Salam, al-Qawa'id al-Ahkam, vol. 1, 98.

is not forgivable in the eyes of God, even if the person is not punished by the prescribed (*hadd*) punishment. Muslim jurists have also differed as to whether the person who kills another under duress is liable to retaliation (*qisas*), or is it the agent of duress who is so liable, or both. This will not be explored here any further, as it falls outside our scope.[43]

Second is the type of *haram* that is not open to omission and not permissible for a competent Muslim to commit, but which is open to concession under necessity and compulsion, although it still remains *haram* in principle. An example of this is utterance of the word of disbelief (*kalimat al-kufr*) while the person doing so is still a believer at heart. This is only allowed when the person is subjected to life-threatening duress, or mutilation of limbs and the like, and he utters the word of *kufr* in that situation. Provided that the threat is immediate and there is no other way out of that situation, the person may pronounce it. The concession here is granted in the Qur'an (al-Nahl, 16:106), but it is understood that the concession so granted is an exception, which means that the *haram* does not cease to be *haram* and continues to be *haram* in principle. The concession here, moreover, manifests a combination of two rights: one of which is the Right of God,[44] in respect of the integrity of a Muslim's faith, and the other is the Right of Human regarding the preservation of life, and the latter takes priority over the former. The *haram* remains *haram* in that God Most High never in principle permits disbelief and *kufr*, but only grants a concession in situations of absolute duress. If the person under duress does not give way and persists in his faith, he will earn a great reward. Another example of this is consuming the food that belongs to another person without that person's permission in situations of imminent starvation or death. This is permissible as an exceptional concession, without, however, compromising the sanctity of the private property, which remains intact in principle.[45]

The third variety of *haram* is that which is open to omission (*al-suqut*) altogether, and it is no longer *haram* for the person that qualifies for it in

43. For details, see al-Raysuni, *al-Haram fi'l-Shariah*, 89–90.

44. Muslim jurists envisage a division of rights into two types: Right of God and Right of Man/Human (haq al-Allah, Haq al-'Abd). This is not an all-inclusive division, but, broadly, Haq Allah is tantamount to community right/public right, worship matters (*'ibadat*), dogmatics, halal and *haram*, and certain penalties that are meant to protect the public or have a religious dimension. The Right of Man/Human broadly includes civil transactions (*mu'amalat*) and personal rights. Sometimes the two may coexist in an act or a claim, however, in different proportions that the court of shariah may ascertain.

45. Cf. al-Haaj, *al-Taqrir wa'l-Tahbir*, vol. 2, 146; al-Raysuni, *al-Haram fi'l-Shariah*, 91.

situations of necessity. Examples of this are the concession for the starving person to consume pork or carrion in order to save his or her life, or for one to drink wine to quench a life-threatening thirst when no other alternatives are available. The concession here is based on the clear text of the Qur'an reviewed earlier (al-Anʿam, 6:119). What the distressed person is doing is a permissible or *mubah* act, one that is regulated, however, by certain rules and a number of legal maxims on the subject. If the starving person refuses to eat anything to save his or her life, that person is committing a sin and the advice is for one to take advantage of the available concession. One is exonerated for not eating to save one's life if it is done out of ignorance, but not otherwise.[46]

Thus, it seems certain that not all varieties of *haram* are of the same degree of enormity, and that some are more heinous than others. If one takes one of the higher objectives, or *maqasid*, of shariah as a criterion, than one can apply the order of priority that exists among the *maqasid* also to *haram*. *Haram* that attaches to the sanctity of life is thus of greater severity than that which attacks the sanctity of religion, reason, property, and family lineage. Protection of religion is a higher purpose or *maqsad* of the first order, and will have to be placed first in certain situations. But one also knows from one's general knowledge of the shariah that in the event of conflict between the Right of God and Right of Man (*haq Allah, haq al-adami*), the latter takes priority. Hence *haram* that pertains to survival or destruction of a person's life is of greater severity than that which violates a religious duty. *Haram* that attaches to the destruction of property may be said to be of lesser gravity than *haram* that threatens the destruction of one's life and religion, and so forth.

The rules of *haram* are applied equally to all persons and places. It would thus be unacceptable, barring situations of dire necessity, to make concessions in favor of particular individuals and groups, localities, climatic conditions, and the like. Muslims may not relax the rules of *haram* in their dealings with non-Muslims either, nor would it be valid to make concessions on the ground merely of common practice among people over something that is *haram*.[47] Recourse to legal stratagems and ruses (*hiyal*) that seek to procure *haram*

---

46. Cf. al-Raysuni, *al-Haram fi'l-Shariah*, 92–93.

47. Cf. al-Qaradawi, *al-Halal wa'l-Haram*, 37–38. Minor exceptions exist here in the case, for instance, of *riba* (usury) that a Muslim may practice, in relationship to a non-Muslim. But this too, is a disputed opinion. While the Shia Imamiyyah permit this, other schools and jurists consider it invalid. Yet another opinion adds the proviso that only if the non-Muslim is a *harbi*, enemy at war and resident of a hostile country, may a Muslim may charge the person interest.

under a different guise or name is also forbidden.[48] Good intentions do not justify the *haram* either: In response to the question whether a *haram* act can be combined with one that is intended to seek closeness (*qurbah*) to God Most High—such as giving stolen food, or the proceeds of *riba*, in charity—it is stated that the *haram* overrides and suppresses the *qurbah*. As noted earlier, halal and *haram* are not always self-evident or clearly identified in the sources, and gray areas do persist between them that may fall under the rubric of doubtful matters (*mashbuhat,* also *al-shubhat*), which are addressed separately below. But before that, we explore the grounds of *haram* (*asbab al-tahrim*), especially with reference to foodstuffs.

## *The Grounds of* Haram

Muslim jurists have identified four grounds of *haram* in foodstuffs: manifest harm, intoxication, filth/natural repulsiveness, and encroachment on the rights of others. It may be noted at the outset that this four-fold identification of the grounds of *haram* is based on juristic research and the understanding of Muslim jurists of the guidelines of the Qur'an and hadith on the subject—there being no categorical identification of such grounds in the said sources. It is not necessary that all the grounds of prohibition should simultaneously exist to prove something *haram*, although one often finds more than one ground to be present in most of the haram substances. The four grounds are now examined.

### Manifest Harm (*Darar*)

Poisonous plants and flowers, snakes, scorpions, poisonous fish, and arsenics are included in this category. Poison is forbidden for human consumption absolutely, according to the majority of the leading schools of Islamic law. However, the Maliki and Hanbali schools have held that some quantities of it may be used in medicine and the treatment of disease.[49] This addition is generally agreeable, as exceptional uses of poison are also covered under the subject of necessity (*darurah*). Harmful substances also include objects that may be harmful, even if not poisonous, such as the eating of mud, charcoal,

---

48. al-Qaradawi, *al-Halal wa'l-Haram*, 34. Al-Qaradawi illustrates this by say calling casino dance as a form of art, or *riba* as permissible profit.

49. Cf. Wizarat, *al-Mawsu'ah al-Fiqhiyyah*, vol. 5, 125.

harmful plants, insects, and animals, etc. The Shafi'is hold that these may not be *haram* for someone who is not harmed by them, whereas the Hanbalis classify these objects under the category of reprehensible (*makruh*). Added to this is the proviso that identifying the harm in an object is not always self-evident and may need an expert opinion.[50] The preferred view, according to Wahbah al-Zuhaili, is that consumption is forbidden of dirt, mud, bones, and charred bread that is burnt by fire so as to prevent harming oneself.[51] The Ja'fari Shia are in agreement on the prohibition of eating mud generally, but they record the following report from their sixth Imam, Ja'far al-Sadiq: "All mud is *haram* for the children of Adam (to eat), except for clay taken from the grave of al-Hussein, pubh. One who eats that finds relief from pain."[52]

In principle, the shariah forbids all that which is purely harmful and permits all that which is purely beneficial. The *haram* category may also include substances whose harm outweighs their benefit, as in the case of wine, which is described in the Qur'an as being sinful even if it has some benefit, but that its harm is greater by far (al-Baqarah, 2:219). That said, al-Qaradawi makes the point that it is not necessary for a Muslim to know all the harms and benefits of things. Muslims are to take God Almighty's commands and prohibitions at face value and accept them as a matter of faith, and not necessarily based on their benefits and harms. For the shariah may impose prohibitions, as in the case of pig meat, whose harm may not be obvious to the naked eye, but which must still be taken at face value and obeyed.[53]

Inflicting harm and perdition on oneself is forbidden by the clear text of the Qur'an, which states, "Throw not yourselves in perdition by your own hands" (al-Baqarah, 2:195), and in another simply declares, "And kill not yourselves" (al-Nisa', 4:29). Inflicting harm is generally forbidden, not only on oneself but also on others. This is the clear message of the renowned hadith: "Harm may neither be inflicted nor reciprocated in (the name of) Islam."[54]

Combining harm with a lawful act suppresses the latter and the whole act becomes unlawful. An instance of this would be to slaughter a healthy animal

---

50. Cf. Wizarat, *al-Mawsu'ah al-Fiqhiyyah,* vol. 5, 125.

51. al-Zuhayli, *al-Fiqh al-Islami,* vol. 3, 511.

52. al-Tabarsi, *Mustdrak al-Wasa'il,* vol. 16, 203. A variation of the same report also appears on 205.

53. al-Qaradawi, *al-Halal wa'l-Haram,* 29–30.

54. al-Hakim, *al-Mustadrak,* vol. 2, 66, hadith no. 2345; also quoted in Abu Zayd Jumanah, *al-Intifa' bi'l-A'yan al-Muharramah,* 27.

with a poisonous tool, which would raise the possibility of poison spreading through the flesh of the animal so that it becomes non-halal, especially if one is inclined to think that the animal died due to poison. It is noted further in this connection that poison infiltrates with the completion of slaughter with the poisonous tool, not just with a light touch.[55]

Permissible for human consumption are, on the other hand, all that which are harmless, beneficial, and clean, as is conveyed in the clear text of the Qur'an in several places.

The Ja'fari Shia take similar positions on *darar* to those of the Sunni schools. It is reported from Imam Ja'far al-Sadiq, who said it on the authority of hadith from the Prophet, that plant yields, grains, and pulses that are harmful are forbidden for consumption, unless it be for medicinal purposes.[56]

Prevention of harmful and hazardous food has become a major theme of the applied laws of Malaysia, and also of most other countries, due partly to the continuous addition of new food varieties in the marketplace. The Food Act of Malaysia 1983 (Section 13) is in line with the shariah principles and even takes them a step further to impose a penalty on anyone who prepares or sells food that is injurious to health. This is the principal legislation that regulates the safety of food sold in Malaysia. This act, along with the Malaysia Food Regulations 1985, which supplements the Food Act 1983, prescribe a series of safety standards that ensure wholesomeness in food supplies. They ensure that food supplies are clear of pesticide residue, drug residue, and other contaminants. All in all, the applied laws of Malaysia go a long way to uphold the shariah principle of wholesomeness (*tayyib*) in food production and supplies. The 1985 regulations further require that foods which contains beef, pork, and alcohol are to be clearly labeled as such.[57] The Malaysian standards add the provision that plants and microorganisms on land, air, and water, as well as all sources from soil and water and their byproducts, including minerals, are halal for use, except for those that are harmful or mixed with *najis*.[58] Mushroom and microorganisms of all types (i.e., bacteria, algae, and fungi)

---

55. Wizarat, *al-Mawsu'ah al-Fiqhiyyah*, vol. 21, 182–183.

56. al-Tabarsi, *Mustadrak*, vol. 16, 207, sec. 19610.

57. For details, see Ramli, "Legal and Administrative Regulation," 93–94. The Ministry of Health Malaysia and the Ministry of Agriculture have introduced a series of other regulations that ensure food safety in agriculture and hygiene control at various levels of food production and marketing.

58. Malaysian Standard. *MS 2200: PART 1: 2008 Islamic Consumer Goods – Part 1: Cosmetic and Personal Care – General Guidelines*. Cyberjaya: Department of Standards Malaysia, 2008 (Clause 4.1.2 and 4.1.3).

and their byproducts and/or derivatives are halal except for those that are poisonous, intoxicating, or hazardous to health. The same provision is extended to natural minerals and chemicals, which are all halal except for those that are poisonous, intoxicating, or hazardous to health.[59]

Foods and drinks containing products and/or byproducts of genetically modified organisms or ingredients made with the genetic material of animals that are non-halal under shariah law are not halal. Notwithstanding the foregoing, products from hazardous aquatic animals or plants are halal when their toxin or poison content has been eliminated during processing.[60]

## Intoxication

Intoxicants of all kind, including alcohol and all varieties of narcotics, whether liquid or solid, are forbidden on the basis of the clear textual mandate of the Qur'an, which enjoins the believers to refrain (*fa-jtanibu*) from wine and gambling (al-Ma'idah, 5:90), and the hadith which declares that "every intoxicant is like *khamr* [wine obtained from grapes] and all *khamr* is *haram*."[61] The prohibition conveyed in the Qur'an (i.e., avoidance or *ijtinab*) is held to be comprehensive in that "avoidance" not only relates to wine drinking but also all aspects of dealing, transaction, gift-giving, etc., of alcohol and other intoxicants.[62] According to a hadith Abu Dawud has recorded on the authority of Umm Salmah, the Prophet's widow, "the Messenger of God prohibited all that intoxicate and cause inertia" (*naha Rasul Allah 'an kull musakkir wa mufattir*). *Mufattir* is seen as a preliminary to intoxication and includes substances that blur clarity of the mind and its faculty of judgment.[63] This extends to the prohibition to such substances as opium, hashish, and their derivatives in the hard drugs category.

Since alcohol is a *haram* for its own sake (*haram li-dhatih*), it is prohibited regardless of the quantity used, whether by itself or mixed with other substances and diluted, unless the mixture is such that it alters the nature of the

---

59. MS 2200: 2008, Part 1 (Clause 4.1.5).

60. MS 2200: 2008 (Clause 5.5.1.2–3.5.1.7).

61. al-Qushairi, *Mukhtasar Sahih Muslim*, hadith no. 1262, 342.

62. al-Qurtubi, *Tafsir al-Qurtubi*, vol.6, 288—as quoted in Abu Zayd, *Al-Intifa' bil A'yan al-Muharramah*, 28.

63. Abu Dawud, *Sunan Abu Dawud*, also quoted in Abu Zayd, *Al-Intifa' bil A'yan al-Muharramah*, 28.

substance and it no longer intoxicates—such as when wine that has turned into vinegar. Alcohol may not be used in medicine at first recourse, as per general agreement of the leading schools, although they all allow for situations of absolute necessity when, for example, it is known for certain that alcohol or its derivatives provide the cure for a disease and no other alternative can be found.[64] All other intoxicants, such as opium, heroin, cocaine, barbiturates, etc., that are known to be even more dangerous and severe are prohibited, not only through analogy to alcohol, but also by direct shariah evidence that prohibits infliction of harm on oneself and on others, including one's own safety and sanity. The hadith of Umm Salmah, reviewed above, that "The Prophet prohibited every intoxicant and debilitator," is cited as textual authority for the prohibition of all the above-mentioned narcotics.[65] Commenting on this hadith, the contemporary scholar Shaykh 'Assaf has quoted Ibn Taymiyyah (d. 728/1328) in support of his own conclusion to say concerning some of the more severe intoxicant varieties that "they inflict harm and corruption greater than *khamr*, and are therefore prohibited all the more so." Umm Salmah's hadith clearly widens the scope of shariah prohibitions and is inclusive of all varieties of narcotics and intoxicants.[66] Moreover, consumption of *khamr* and its derivatives is *haram*, regardless of the quantity—large or small, all are included. Hence the alcohol percentage in its derivatives has no bearing on the basic prohibition in shariah—which clearly subsumes the position on beer that may have only 1 or 2 percent alcohol content.[67] But see further details on this below.

The majority of Muslim jurists have held, nevertheless, that narcotics derived from plant sources, such as hashish, opium, and their derivatives, such as morphine, heroin, henbane (*banj*), and cocaine, are clean in themselves. The Maliki jurist Shihab al-Din al-Qarafi (d. 684/1283) and the Shafi'i Ibn Daqiq al-'Id (d. 625/1228) have mentioned a consensus to that effect. This is because all plants are clean from the shariah perspective, and nothing in them is found to be filthy. Added to this is the proviso that prohibition does not necessarily imply filth, hence they remain in their original condition of

---

64. al-Kasani, *Bada'i' al-Sana'i' fi Tartib al-Shara'i'*, vol. 5, 114; al-Zuhayli, *al-Fiqh al-Islami*, vol. 3, 5.

65. Dawud, *Sunan Abu Dawud*, vol. 3, 329, hadith no. 3686. *Mufattir* is that which debilitates one physically and intellectually; all that which makes one languid and listless. For details, see Abu Zayd, *Al-Intifa' bil A'yan al-Muharramah*, 28.

66. 'Assaf, *al-Halal wa'l-Haram fi'l-Islam*, 264.

67. Cf. 'Assaf, *al-Halal wa'l-Haram fi'l-Islam*, 257.

cleanliness. This may also be said with regard to lethal poisons and intoxicants in that consuming them is prohibited but they are not filthy/*najis*.[68] A dissenting opinion in the Hanbali school attributed to Ibn Taymiyyah is also quoted on this to the effect that these are all *najis* like "wine, and wine is like urine, and hashish is like dirt." Yet having quoted this view, Nazih Hammad has observed that no credible support can be found for the validity of it.[69] Prohibition does not necessarily imply filth. This is also extended to stolen goods; if it is food, it will be prohibited for consumption without the permission of its owner, or of the Lawgiver, but that does not necessarily mean that it is filthy/*najis*. In a similar view, blood shed forth is forbidden for a Muslim to consume, but that too does not mean that blood is *najis*, as blood, being of human beings or animals, is not *najis* in itself. It is reported in this connection from the learned Companion 'Abd Allah ibn Mas'ud, who said that on a certain occasion he was in close vicinity to slaughtering of some animals and their blood spattered and soiled his clothes. Then he stood up and performed his prayer without washing it off.[70]

As for the use of narcotics, including consumption, drinking, sniffing, enema, and injection, be it for pleasure-seeking, fun, or intoxication, all of them are equated, by the majority of Muslim jurists, to *khamr*/wine by way of analogy. It is often added that the harmful effects of these substances on the human body and mind are in many ways greater and more severe than alcohol, and they are all prohibited. Ibn Taymiyyah has similarly said, concerning hashish, that "hashish and cannabis is also *haram*, and anyone who uses it is liable to the punishment of whipping in the same way as the wine drinker; it is even more objectionable (*akhbath*) than wine-*khamr*."[71]

The Malaysian authorities, have, however, determined a certain quantitative exemption limit of 1 percent alcohol content in food items. Speaking during the state-level *fatwa* seminar in Kuching, Russly Abdul Rahman of Universiti Putra Malaysia's Halal Products Research Institute said that many Malaysian Muslims were unaware of this and tend to think that anything with alcohol content is *haram* or illicit according to Islamic law. He said that the

---

68. Hammad, *al-Mawad al-Muharramah*, 49, also quoting al-Qarafi, *Kitab al-Furuq*, vol. 1, 218, and others.

69. Hammad, *al-Mawad al-Muharramah*, 49.

70. Cf. al-Raysuni, *al-Haram fi'l-Shariah*, 169.

71. Ibn Taymiyyah, *al-Siyasah al-Shar'iyyah*, 144; as also quoted in Hammad, *al-Mawad al-Muharramah*, 50. See also Wizarat, *al-Mawsu'ah al-Fiqhiyyah*, vol. 5, 126.

Malaysian Fatwa Committee of the National Council for Islamic Affairs had earlier declared that any food items which were not of alcoholic beverage or type (i.e., *arak*) would be considered halal if the alcohol content therein did not exceed 0.01 percent. Thus, food items such as some bicarbonate drinks, cooking sauces, ketchups, and *tapai* (fermented rice)" were halal. "Essentially, not all food items with alcohol are alcoholic beverages like liquor or beer. Alcohol sometimes exists naturally in many natural and organic food items such as fruits due to natural fermentation." Russly Rahman then added that due to a common misunderstanding among consumers, the Malaysian Fatwa Committee made a revision and raised the limit to 1 percent. Any food item containing not more than 1 percent alcohol content and not meant to be alcoholic is thus halal. Examples would include sauces, ketchups, and any permitted food additives. Medication and perfume products with small amounts of alcohol not intended to be alcoholic beverages were also deemed halal.[72] In Islamic juristic terms, this will arguably be also subsumed by the principle of extreme dilution (*istihlak*), which is the subject of a separate chapter below.

## Filth, Impurity, and Natural Revulsion (*Najis, Rijs, Khaba'ith, Mustaqdharat*)

*Najis* (filthy) is the opposite of clean (*tahir*), and it is of two types, *najis* in itself (*najis dhatiyyah*), that is, items that are inherently filthy, which are either identified in the clear text, such as carrion, spilt blood, pig meat (Qur'an, al-An'am, 6:145), or when people of sound mind and nature consider them as such. The object concerned may be solid or liquid, animate or inanimate—all are included. Filth may also be temporary due to an extraneous factor, which is the second of the two types under review. This would include a clean garment that is made unclean but can be washed and made clean again, or when a rat falls into fat—if the fat happens to be solid, it is made clean by removing the rat and all the surrounding surface that has come into contact with it, and the rest is clean. But if the fat is liquid then it must be poured away and disposed of.

Another somewhat overlapping classification of filthy/*najis* is that of the two varieties of literal/original (*najis haqiqi*), which is palpable to the senses, such as spilt blood or a carcass that falls into clean water, and putatively unclean (*najis hukmi*), such as disbelief (*kufr*) or adultery—as in the Qur'anic

---

72. Halal Focus, "Many Still Confused."

verse stating that "truly the pagans are unclean" (al-Tawbah, 9:28), which means in a nonphysical sense, as otherwise all human beings, alive or dead, are deemed to be clean on account of the inherent dignity God has endowed in all equally, which is recognized for all human beings absolutely in the clear text (al-Isra', 17:70). Carcass is *najis* of land animals, with the exception again of human beings, and in particular animals that have fluid blood in their bodies and blood runs out when there is an injury, contrary to sea creatures, which are declared clean, whether alive or dead. For, according to a hadith text, "the sea water is clean and so is the dead of the sea."[73]

The Hanafi school has subdivided najas (unclean) into the two types of intensely unclean (*najasah mughallazah*) and lightly unclean (*najasah mukhaffafah*). The intensely unclean is that which is established in a clear text and no other text/evidence exists to dispute or derogate from it. The light variety of *najis* is that over which two different texts or lines of evidence may exist and each conveys a different message. This is the case, for instance, of the urine of halal animals. On this there is a hadith enjoining the Muslims to "cleanse yourselves from urine—*instanzahu min al-bawl*," which is understood to mean that all urine is unclean, and the hadith of 'Urainah that, although it declares only the camel urine as clean, is understood more generally to mean that the urine of halal animals may either be regarded clean or a lighter variety of *najis*. Hence the *najasah* here belongs to the second type (i.e., *mukhafafah*). The bile of animals generally follow the ruling that applies to their urine.[74]

Beyond these basic essentials, the schools of law have differed over many details. Pig and dog are *najis* in themselves and there is no disagreement on this, but disagreement is recorded over some related details. Whereas the majority consider the body emissions of non-halal animals, such as tears, sweat, saliva, and mucous, also to be *najis*, the Maliki school maintains that all of them are clean, based on the principle that all living animals and whatever that emits from them (except for vomit and feces) are clean.[75]

Carcass (*al-maytah*) linguistically describes any animal that dies without the ritual purification/slaughter. The animal may have died through natural causes and without any human intervention, or it may have died due to the act of a human when this act is other than by way of ritual purification/slaughter.

---

73. Cf. al-Jaziri, *al-Fiqh 'ala al-Madhahib al-Arba'ah*, 11–12; hadith on the dead of the sea is quoted on p. 12. See also Abu Zayd, *al-Intifa' bi'l- A'yan al-Muharramah*, 27.

74. For details, see al-Jaziri, *al-Fiqh 'ala'l-Madhahib*, 10, 14.

75. Ibid., 12–13.

The death may be the result of strangulation, a heavy blow, or a lethal fall, or the animal may have been gored by other animals, or killed and partially eaten by predatory animals. All of these fall under *maytah*, as is also seen in the Qur'anic verse (5:3) that specifies ten items of prohibited meat. All of these are declared forbidden. The meaning of carcass is also extended to include the slaughter of a halal animal slaughtered by someone who deliberately precludes recitation of *tasmiyah* (short for Bismillah al-Rahman al-Rahim), or one who cites the name of an idol or of a deity other than God Most High.[76]

*Khabith* (pl. *khaba'ith*, revolting, impure), being the antonym of *tayyib* (pure, wholesome, clean) is a degree lower than both the *najis* and *rijs*. *Khaba'ith* accordingly subsume predatory animals and birds as well as certain insects, such as lice and worms. They may or may not be *najis* in themselves, but they are subsumed, nevertheless, under the Qur'anic prohibition of *al-khaba'ith* (al-A'raf, 7:157). Some substances are declared unclean because of the repulsion they may invoke, even if they are not filthy in themselves, such as human saliva, mucous, sweat, and semen, all of which are clean, notwithstanding some differences of detail regarding them among the various schools of Islamic law, but are declared non-halal for consumption on grounds of their natural repulsion.

Muslim jurists have held different views regarding insects. Except for the locust (and desert lizard, a reptile) which are declared permissible on the authority of hadith, all other insects and reptiles are forbidden for human consumption, as they are among the *khaba'ith*, deemed to be dirty and naturally repulsive. This is the Hanafi position on the subject. The second view is that of the Maliki school, which is that they are all permissible except for those that are harmful, on condition, however, that they are duly slaughtered, especially those among them that have fluid blood in their bodies. The Shafi'is have held that they are generally non-halal except for some among them that are not unclean, such as jerboa, rock hyrax, hedgehog, and weasel. The Hanbalis disagree with regard to the hedgehog and weasel, which they consider forbidden, but agree otherwise with the Shafi'is.[77]

It is generally correct to say that all filth and impurity, and all that which is *najis* and *khabith*, are most likely also to be harmful, yet it is possible that something that is unclean and objectionable may be harmless, which is why

---

76. Abu Zayd, *Al-Intifa' bil A'yan al-Muharramah*, 35–36.

77. For details on all the scholastic positions in Wizarat, see *al-Mawsu'ah al-Fiqhiyyah*, vol. 5, 143–144.

harm and filth are recognized as two separate grounds of prohibition under shariah, notwithstanding the fact that they often overlap.[78]

Muslim jurists have differed on the status of agricultural crops and fruits that are watered with filthy waters and fertilizers (such as human feces), whether they are *najis* and therefore *haram*, or merely reprehensible. Ibn Qudamah looks into this and comments that the evidence on their reprehensibility tends to be stronger. The reason given is that the filth is transformed through internal changes within the plants and crops, and that the process amounts to substance transformation (*istihalah*) and the produce becomes clean. This is somewhat similar, it is added, to internal organisms of animals, such as sheep and cows, which transform blood that circulates in their bodies and is then converted into milk, which is then lawful for human consumption.[79]

From the juxtaposition of halal and *tayyib* in the Qur'an and the foregoing analysis, it is also understood that *haram* in shariah is not meant to be a punishment from God; rather, it partakes in guidance that involves avoidance of filth and corruption infiltrating the Muslim person and upbringing, and a manifestation as such of divine grace and mercy on people. From our understanding of the evidence discussed, we can also conclude that consumption of good and wholesome animal food and agricultural produce is also an aspect of human dignity in Islam. The shariah encourages that food taken by Muslims is lawful, pure, and wholesome. This too is another side of the same coin of guidance for Muslims to lead a clean life, while enjoying the bounties of God Most High to lead a life of purity and excellence (*hayat tayyibah*) in this world that earns God's pleasure and compassion for the hereafter.[80]

*Najis* under the Halal Standard Malaysia, MS 1500-2009, includes all that is *najis* under shariah law, which includes dogs and pigs and their derivatives and halal food that is contaminated or comes into direct contact with non-halal objects, as well as alcoholic beverages and intoxicants and carrion of halal animals not slaughtered under shariah rules. Also included under *najis* is any "liquids and objects discharged from orifices of human beings or animals, such urine, blood, vomit, pus, placenta and excrement, sperm and ova of pigs and dogs, excepting sperm and ova of other animals" (clause 2.4).

---

78. Cf. Abu Zayd Jumanah, *al-Intifa' bi-A'yan al-Muharramah*, 27–28.

79. Ibn Qudamah, *al-Mughni*, vol. 13, 92.

80. Cf. Fadlullah, *Fiqh al-At'imah*, 34.

There are three types of *najis*: (a) *mughallazah*, which is considered intense *najis*, such as dogs and pigs, including any liquids and objects discharged from their orifices, descendants, and derivatives; (b) *mukhaffafah*, which is considered light *najis* (the only *najis* in this category is urine from a baby boy [or girl] at the age of two years and below who has not consumed any other food except his mother's milk); and (c) *mutawassitah*, which is considered medium *najis* that does not fall under either intense or light *najis*, such as vomit, pus, blood, *khamr*, carrion, and liquid and objects discharged from the orifices.[81] Any level of contact with *najis* in the manufacture, packaging, and transportation of halal food must also be avoided.

These precautions are articulated as follows: Halal food shall be suitably packed. Packaging materials shall be halal in nature and shall fulfill the following requirements: (a) the packaging materials shall not be made from any raw materials that are decreed as *najis* by shariah law; (b) it is not prepared, processed, or manufactured using equipment that is contaminated with things that are *najis*; (c) during its preparation, processing, storage, or transportation, it shall be physically separated from any other food that does not meet the requirements stated in items a or b, or any other things that have been decreed as *najis* by shariah law. Any food item that does not meet the requirements specified in items a, b, and c, or any other things that are decreed as *najis* by shariah law are also considered *najis*.[82]

## Unlawful Acquisition

Forbidden foodstuffs and beverages also include unlawfully acquired property, such as stolen or usurped food and objects obtained through gambling, bribery, fraud, and other unlawful means that are *haram* under shariah. This is the purport of the Qur'anic address to the believers to "devour not one another's properties wrongfully, unless it be through trading by your mutual consent" (al-Nisa', 4:29).[83] An exception is granted in this connection to certain individuals, such as one's parent and guardian, a charitable endowment or *waqf* administrator,

---

81. Malaysian Standard. *MS 1500:2009 Halal Food – Production, Preparation, Handling and Storage – General Guidelines.* Cyberjaya: Department of Standards Malaysia, 2009 (Clause 2.4.2).

82. MS 1500-2009 (Clause 3.7.1).

83. The substance of this is also conveyed in a hadith: "It is forbidden to take the property of a Muslim without his consent." See al-Bayhaqi, *Sunan al-Bayhaqi*, vol. 6:100, hadith no. 11, 325. We also read in another hadith: "You and your property both belong to your father." See al-Tabrizi, *Mishkat al-Masabih*, hadith no. 3, 354.

and one compelled by dire necessity and threat of starvation. These are made exceptional based on available evidence in the scriptural sources. As for an un-lawfully acquired animal that has then been slaughtered by its usurper, Muslim jurists have disagreed as to whether the slaughter can amount to a valid purifica-tion (*tadhkiyah*). For instance, when a Muslim usurps a goat, or steals it from its lawful owner and then slaughters it, in accordance with the shariah guidelines, the slaughter is deemed to be valid and the meat is also lawful for consumption, except that the slaughterer remains responsible for his act of usurpation or theft, as the case may be, and bears responsibility to compensate the owner. It is like-wise not permissible for that person to consume the meat or other parts of the animal unless a valid permission is granted by its owner.[84]

If necessity renders the prohibited substance lawful, does this justify encroaching on another person's rights? In other words, if a person consumes food that belongs to someone else due to circumstances beyond his or her con-trol, would the consumer be liable to compensate the owner? The majority of Muslim scholars, including the Malikis and Hanbalis, are reported to have rejected any claims of compensation if the consumer was driven by necessity under the legal maxim that "necessity renders the prohibited permissible." The Hanafi school of thought has held, on the other hand, that the person con-suming the food must compensate for the loss. Necessity, in other words, does not overrule the right of another person. The majority view maintains, how-ever, that the Lawgiver has permitted consumption of what is unlawful under necessity, and that this nullifies any demand for compensation, provided that necessity is not exploited in order to transgress the limits.[85] However, if gen-uine necessity does not exist, there must be compensation according to the general consensus of all schools.[86] If the owner of foodstuffs also happens to be in dire need of that food for sustenance—that the person is, in other words, also faced with necessity, then no one else may take it under any condition. This may happen, for instance, when a group of people are traveling together in a remote place and are all running into starvation, although differences of opinion exist to the effect that one who is in a critical condition may still take what may save his or her life.[87] Unlawful acquisition does not, it seems, vitiate

84. For details, see Wizarat, *al-Mawsu'ah al-Fiqhiyyah*, vol. 5, 127.

85. Al-Makdisi, 'Abd al-Rahman bin Ibrahim. *Al-'Uddah Sharh al-'Umdah*. Cairo: Dar al-Hadith, 2003, 307–308.

86. al-Maqdisi, *al-'Uddah*, 319. See also Kamali, "Principles of Halal and Haram," 51.

87. For details, see Ibn Qudamah, *al-Mughni*, vol. 13, 103.

a slaughter, although it does render it reprehensible. This is because valid ownership is not a prerequisite of purification (*tadhkiyah*). This is based on the authority of a hadith that the Prophet, pbuh, was informed that a certain roasted meat was of a goat that was slaughtered without the permission of its owner, and the Prophet said to "feed the prisoners [of war] with it."[88]

The Shia Imamiyyah take a strictly prohibitive position on taking other people's food without their invitation and consent. Quoted in authority for this is a hadith from the Prophet on the authority of 'Ali ibn Abi Talib that "one who attends someone's place uninvited and helps himself to eat food that belongs to others, he has entered as a transgressor, and what he eats is haram to him, and he exits that place as a transgressor."[89] In a similar hadith report attributed directly to the Prophet, without mentioning any narrator, it is provided: "The Prophet, pbuh, said: one who eats the food of another without being invited to it, he would have devoured a burning piece of fire into his belly."[90] It is further added that Hasan b. Fadl al-Tabarsi reported in *Makarim al-Akhlaq* that the Prophet, pbuh, was invited by some residents of Medina to a meal they had prepared for him and five of his Companions; he accepted the invitation and when he was on his way, a sixth person joined them and started walking with them. When they reached the house, the Prophet turned to the sixth person and told him, "The host has not invited you, so stay here until I mention where you are and ask for his permission on your behalf."[91]

That said, there are numerous hadith reports in recorded Shia sources on the virtue of feeding the hungry. According to a saying of 'Ali ibn al-Hussein, "One who feeds a believer suffering from hunger, God will feed him of the fruits of Paradise."[92] In a hadith reported from the Prophet, pbuh, he said, on a broader note, "There is no virtue greater than satisfying the hunger of a hungry stomach,"[93] which is inclusive, it seems, of all living humans, even animals. In a chapter on "the obligation of feeding the hungry when in need," five hadith reports are recorded through different channels, all conveying more or

---

88. As quoted by al-Zuhayli, *al-Fiqh al-Islami*, vol. 3, 649. Hadith is also recorded in al-Shawkani, Nayl al-Awtar, vol. 5, 321.

89. al-Tabarsi, *Mustadrak al-Wasa'il*, vol. 16, 206, sec. 19603.

90. al-Tabarsi, *Mustadrak al-Wasa'il*, vol. 16, 206, sec. 19606.

91. al-Tabarsi, *Mustadrak al-Wasa'il*, vol. 16, 207, sec. 19607.

92. al-Tabarsi, *Mustadrak al-Wasa'il*, vol. 16, 253, sec. 19777.

93. al-Tabarsi, *Mustadrak al-Wasa'il*, vol. 16, 253, sec. 19778. See also http://library.islamweb.net/hadith/display_hbook.php?bk_no=4182&pid=927175&hid=688, 69, 70.

less the same message with various degrees of emphasis; one of which states, "He is not a believer in me who sleeps the night well-fed while his neighbor is hungry, nor does he believe in me who sleeps the night clothed while his neighbor is naked."[94]

Since there is the basis of an obligation, it may be difficult under Shii law to justify penalizing a hungry person in need for helping himself to food that belongs to someone else without even a prior permission. If permission is granted by the owner, after the event, that would resolve the issue. Should there be a claim, however, by the owner, and the claim is for a larger amount than needed for a single feeding, the judge may deem it fit to order compensation.

## Mixing of Halal and *Haram*

According to a legal maxim of Islamic law, "when the halal and *haram* are mixed up, the *haram* prevails."[95] The maxim means that when the halal and the harm are mixed in the same place, at the same time, and with the same subject matter, such as when water and wine are mixed and there is no possibility of separating the one from the other, then the whole of it must be abandoned simply because the haram dominates the whole. Put simply, when the available evidence can imply both permissibility and prohibition, the latter prevails. While quoting this in his *al-Ashbah wa'l-Naza'ir*, al-Suyuti (d. 911/1505) mentions that this maxim is based on a hadith to the same effect. The hadith thus provided that "[w]hen there is a mixing of halal and *haram*, the latter prevails—*ma ijtama'a al-halal wa'l-haram illa ghuliba al-haram.*" However, Abu'l Fadl Zayn al-'Iraqi (d. 1403/806) wrote in his *Takhrij Minhaj al-Usul* that there is no basis for this hadith (*la-asla lahu*), and Nasir al-Din al-Albani (d. 1999) included this in his Weak and Fabricated Hadith Series (*Silsilah Ahadith al-Da'ifah wa'l-Mawdu'ah*). Taj al-Din al-Subki (d. 1369/771) and Abu Bakr al-Bayhaqi (d. 1064/456) considered this to be a weak hadith too, due to a disruption in its chain

---

94. al-Tabarsi, *Mustadrak al-Wasa'il*, vol. 16, 265, sec. 19820.

95. The Arabic version reads *"idhā ijtama' al-ḥalāl wa'l-ḥarām, ghuliba al-ḥarām."* Jalal al-Din al-Suyuti, *al-Ashbah wa'l-Naza'ir*, Beirut: Dar al-Kitab al-'Ilmiyah, 1994, 151. Shabbir, *al-Qawa'id al-Kulliyyah*, 325. Interestingly enough, al-Qaraḍāwī does not refer to this maxim in his brief discussion of "avoidance of the doubtful—*ittiqā al-shubhāt*," which is perhaps not accidental, due to some weakness in its evidential basis and also another line of evidence that advises taking that which is the easier course and brings facility and relief. This may also explain why al-Qaraḍāwī subsumes the issue under the rubric of *sadd al-dharā'i'*.

of transmission.[96] 'Abd al-Razzaq al-San'ani (d. 211/826) in his *Musannaf*, concludes that it is a statement of the Companion, 'Abd Allah ibn Mas'ud, and not a hadith of the Prophet. Al-Raysuni examines the evidence and concludes that the hadith is definitely unreliable, yet the legal maxim under review is still valid and that a vast majority of leading scholars have upheld it. Al-Raysuni adds, however, that the maxim in question should not be applied literally but rationally and with due regard to its surrounding circumstances. Hence, in circumstances where the amount of mixing and scope of confusion is slight to negligible, the legal maxim under review may also be of doubtful application. Some scholars have gone on record, moreover, to exonerate altogether situations that involve minimal and sometimes unavoidable amounts of mixture with forbidden stuffs. This is because the normative state in shariah is that of permissibility, and it is only abandoned when there is clear evidence to the contrary. But those who have preferred abandoning the mixture have done so on the basis of caution and piety and a preferable course of action.[97]

It is further stated that the basic norm with regard to preference of the halal and *haram* to one another when they are inseparably mixed is that of preponderance: if the *haram* is the larger part, the whole becomes *haram*, but when the *haram* is of a small quantity and the much larger part is halal, the whole is regarded as halal. According to 'Izzuddin al-Sulami, in situations of this kind, it is not just the halal and the *haram* that one must consider, but also what may come between them. The intervening categories he mentions between the halal and *haram* are the reprehensible (*makruh*) and permissible (*mubah*, or halal). The *makruh* side tends to become stronger when the *haram* amount is the larger part, and it becomes weaker when the halal quantity is larger. He then illustrates this as follows: if doubt arises over two dinars, one of which is lawful and the other unlawfully earned, one must clearly prefer the *haram* side, but not if only one or two non-halal dinars are mixed with a thousand lawfully earned dinars. The issue of mixture is thus not as black and white as many have made it out to be, but one that poses questions regarding which is the larger and predominant part until there is parity, in which case the doubt becomes of equal proportions on both sides.[98] It would similarly

---

96. See for a discussion, al-Raysuni, *al-Haram fi'l-Shariah*, 109 ; Securities Commission, *Resolutions of the Securities Commission*, 158.

97. Cf. al-Raysuni, *al-Haram fi'l-Shariah*, 107–108.

98. 'Abd al-Salam, *al-Qawa'id al-Ahkam*, vol. 1, 84, also quoted in al-Raysuni, *al-Haram fi'l-Shariah*, 108.

seem inadvisable to reject 99 out of 100 duly slaughtered sheep for a doubt over one of them, and thus take a literal approach to the maxim under review. Muslim jurists have applied the maxim in many situations, including the following:

- When a game hunter sends a trained dog to catch a game bird and then finds an untrained dog next to the trained one, and doubt occurs as to which actually did the catch or kill, the game is non-halal.
- In the event where a Magian puts his hand on top of the hand of the Muslim slaughterer, the slaughtered meat becomes non-halal due to the mix.
- In the event that the slaughterer doubts whether the slaughtered animal was already dead, the slaughter is non-halal—none of it may be consumed, not even due to *ijtihad.*
- In hybrid animals, if one of the parents is halal but the other non-halal, the offspring is non-halal—such as the mule.[99]

Muslim jurists have allowed, on the other hand, the following by way of exceptions to the maxim under review:

- In the event that a head of cattle grazes and consumes non-halal grass that belongs to someone else without the owner's permission, its meat and milk are still halal, but may be abandoned on grounds of piety.
- When a game bird is shot and falls to the ground and found to be dead, it is still halal, as it would be difficult to avoid such fractions of delays in permissible hunting.
- When the ruler/government sends a donation/gift to a person, and most of the assets involved are *haram,* it may be taken and utilized, although many have also held it to be reprehensible (*makruh*).[100]

The more modern applications of the maxim under review include implantation, be it through traditional or modern genetic engineering techniques. When, for example, a scientist produces an organ or skin tissue by implanting a pig or rat tissue or gene for use in human body, the product is non-halal. This can also be said of one who produces a hybrid plant by implanting an

---

99. al-Raysuni, *al-Haram fi'l-Shariah*, 112—quoting them from al-Hajji, Iydah al-Qawa'id al-Fiqhiyyah.

100. al-Raysuni, *al-Haram fi'l-Shariah*, 112.

intoxicating or poisonous plant gene in another plant, the hybrid is held to be non-halal. Exceptions in both cases may be made in situations of absolute necessity, such as when it may be necessary to save human life.[101]

According to another legal maxim of *fiqh*, "prevention of harm takes priority over the realization of benefit."[102] Should there be confusion due to the existence of two divergent hadith reports, for instance, or two conflicting analogies for that matter, one prohibitive, and the other permissive, the former prevails over the latter, which means that prohibition is given priority over permissibility. The doubt that arises over the understanding of a text may be genuine (*haqiqi*), such as ambiguity in the actual wording of a hadith, or it may be relative and metaphorical (*idafi, majazi*), and doubt arises in their application to a particular case. In all of these, an opportunity may arise for fresh interpretation and *ijtihad*, which should be attempted, and an effort should be made to secure that which is closer to the higher purposes (*maqasid*) of shariah and the public interest, or *maslahah*. Thus, in cases of confusion between lawfully slaughtered meat and carrion, the prohibitive position prevails and consumption is consequently not recommended. Similarly, in the case of confusion arising between revenues from *riba* and from a lawful sale, one should exercise caution on the side of avoidance. In the case of the hybrid breeding of animals, such as between a horse and a mule, the offspring is considered to be non-halal. Most jurists would, however, take the mother's side as the stronger indicator of permissibility: If the mother is the horse, which is halal, the offspring is also considered halal in this view. In the event that a goat sucks the milk of the swine to the extent that its flesh becomes firm, then the goat and its offspring become non-halal. However, if the suckling is only temporary and stops prior to muscle growth and firming, then it should suck the milk of another goat for a minimum of seven days. But if it is out of the suckling stage, it should be brought up on grass in the open field, and it is halal afterward.[103]

Should there be a mixture of two varieties of food, one halal and the other *haram*, two situations may initially arise: Either the separation of the two parts is unfeasible, such as when wine, blood, or urine are mixed with water—then the *haram* prevails over the halal; but if the two parts can be separated, the object is removed and the rest becomes halal. However, if the mixture is

101. Cf. al-Ghazali, *Ihya' 'Ulum al-Din*, vol. 2, 89; al-Raysuni, *al-Haram fi'l-Shariah*, 114–115.

102. The legal maxim in Arabic reads: "*Dar' al-mafasid awlā min jalb al-manafia.*"

103. Fadlullah, *Fiqh al-At'imah*, 124.

of a very small quantity that is hardly detectable, and establishment of complete purity is not devoid of hardship, such as the remains of small amounts of alcohol in cooking utensils in big hotels, the doubt in them is overlooked but avoidance is preferable.[104]

In large slaughterhouses and situations where halal meat is mixed with non-halal meat, or meat slaughtered by Muslims is mixed with meat slaughtered by Magians and idol-worshippers such that they cannot be distinguished from one another, the following may apply: Should there be any signs by which they can be distinguished, they should be separated and the halal meat is good for consumption. However, if no such signs can be found to exist, then two situations may be considered, one of which is the situation of necessity, in which case the meat may be consumed after due diligence and reasonable guessing (*al-taharri*) at separation. In normal situations, however, when a choice may exist and there is no necessity, three possibilities are again envisaged as follows: (1) the halal is predominant, in which case it is permissible to consume; (2) the *haram* is predominant, in which case the whole is presumed to be non-halal; and (3) the two are about equal, in which case the *haram* prevails again based on the maxim that when halal and *haram* are mixed, the latter prevails.[105] Differences of opinion have, however, been recorded over these positions. Apart from the situation of necessity on which there is consensus, when duly slaughtered meat is mixed with carrion or non-halal meat, many jurists among the Shafi'i and Hanbali schools and the Shia Imamiyyah hold that all of it is presumed non-halal and none may be consumed. The preferred opinion seems to be permissibility when the halal is the larger and predominant part, but caution and *taharri* are advised generally.[106]

According to yet another legal maxim, which is often thought to be contradictory to the one just reviewed, but which is actually supplementary to it, "*haram* does not turn the halal into *haram—al-haram la yuharrimu al-halal*."[107] What this means is that a slight quantity of *haram* does not change a much larger quantity of halal into *haram*. Otherwise, people would be placed into hardship, whereas the shariah generally advises removal of hardship (*raf'*

---

104. Cf. Shabir, *al-Qawa'id al-Kulliyyah*, 326–328

105. For details, see al-Ramlawi, *al-Halal wa'l-Haram*, 384–385.

106. al-Ramlawi, *al-Halal wa'l-Haram*, 386.

107. al-Suyuti, *al-Ashbah wa'l-Naza'ir*, 115. See also al-Raysuni, *al-Haram fi'l-Shariah*, 116.

*al-haraj*) from the people.[108] The maxim just reviewed, which gives preference to *haram* when it is mixed with halal, would evidently apply to situations
when the quantities on both sides are about equal, or when *haram* constitutes
the larger part. But when the *haram* portion is minute or negligibly small, the
halal prevails. We shall not, however, enter into further details, as much of
this discussion relates to the principle of "extreme dilution," or *istihlak*, which
is the subject of a separate chapter.

With reference to Malaysia, mixing of halal and non-halal meat is normally
not expected to be a frequent occurrence: the Animals Importation Order
1962 requires that all imported meat and livestock imported into Malaysia
must be halal, safe and disease-free. Section (3.2) of the order also provides
that all imports for human consumption are subject to certain restrictions as
are set out in its Second Schedule.[109]

Furthermore, The Control of Slaughter Act 1975 that regulates livestock slaughter within Malaysia provides that livestock slaughter is allowed
at approved abattoirs but outside slaughter is permitted only under certain
conditions. Section 8.2 of the act thus provides that livestock slaughtered for
human consumption outside the approved abattoir is prohibited unless it is
accompanied with a warranty that such an animal is free from disease and safe
for consumption.[110]

---

108. Cf. al-Raysuni, *al-Haram fi'l-Shariah*, 116–119.

109. Cf. Ramli, "Legal and Administrative Regulations," 102.

110. Cf. Ramli, "Legal and Administrative Regulations," 102.

# 7

# Haram, *Permanence*, and Change

## THE PRINCIPLE OF SUBSTANCE TRANSFORMATION (*ISTIHALAH*)

HALAL AND *HARAM* are basically permanent and unchangeable. What the shariah has made *haram* thus remains so for all time, regardless of personal preferences, custom, and culture. Shariah rules on halal and *haram* are also all-inclusive in that Muslims do not have the privilege of making something *haram* for others and halal for themselves, or vice versa. These shariah designations are meant to be for everyone, although certain exceptions have been made for non-Muslims and even for Muslims themselves under stressful circumstances that endanger life. Shariah also provides for situations whereby the *haram* can change into halal, and vice versa, under certain circumstances that are expounded under the principle of *istihalah*. *Istihalah* may be characterized as a nonreversible change of a substance to a different substance with differences in taste, color, and odor. The changes that so occur include a change of salient properties and the transformation of impure materials into pure ones. It is further added that *istihalah* is a change of *najis* or *haram* into something else with a different physical appearance and properties, such as name, odor, taste, color, and characteristics.[1] *Istihalah* can thus be understood as a complete physical and chemical transformation of one substance into another substance.

The principle of necessity (*darurah*) plays a similar role, although necessity can change the *haram* into halal without, however, changing the nature of the substance concerned. The renowned legal maxim of *fiqh* that "necessity

---

1. Hammad, *al-Mawad al-Muharramah*, 30. See also Malaysian Standard. *MS 2393: 2013 Islamic and halal principles - Definitions and interpretations on terminology*. Cyberjaya: Department of Standards Malaysia, 2010 (Clause 2.17).

*Shariah and The Halal Industry.* Mohammad Hashim Kamali, Oxford University Press. © Oxford University Press 2021. DOI: 10.1093/oso/9780197538616.003.0008

makes the unlawful lawful"[2] has wide-ranging applications to conditions of illness, advanced age, pregnancy, emergencies, and even traveling as a hardship category in its own right. Another basic position of shariah concerning halal and *haram* to be noted is that small and large amounts all fall under the same rules. This is based on the authority of a hadith to the effect that when something is made *haram*, even the smallest quantity of it partakes in the same. Muslims are thus prohibited from consuming even small quantities of pork or alcohol. A legal maxim conveying the shariah position thus provides that "prohibition of something absolutely demands that all parts of it is prohibited, unless there be an exception."[3] The only exception taken by the Hanafi school that may be mentioned here involves the consumption of a very small quantity of wine that does not reach the digestive system or intoxicate. In this instance, the perpetrator is deemed to be guilty, yet not punishable with the prescribed punishment, or *hadd*, of wine drinking.[4]

That said, however, any amount of consuming *haram* becomes sinful even if it does not pollute or intoxicate, on grounds of caution and the shariah principle of blocking the means to *haram*, known as *sadd al-dharaʾiʿ*.[5] The leading schools of law have taken a similar position over the taking of opium, other herbal intoxicants, and the smoking of hashish, which are deemed harmful and thus fall under the ruling of the renowned hadith "*la darar wa la dirar fiʾl-Islam*—harm must neither be inflicted nor reciprocated in [the name of] Islam."[6] Harm must, in other words, be avoided, whether it is inflicted on oneself or someone else. All intoxicants are deemed to be harmful for human consumption. Yet the perpetrator, or one who consumes these substances, is not held liable to the application of the prescribed *hadd* punishment of wine drinking. This is because of an element of uncertainty that is obtained in the ruling of analogy (*qiyas*), which in this case has been drawn between wine

---

2. Shabir, *al-Qawaʿid al-Kulliyyah*, 213.

3. The Arabic version of the maxim reads "*tahrim al-shayʾi mutlaqan yaqtadi tahrim kull juzʾin minhu illa ma-istathna.*" The actual wording of this maxim is attributed to Ibn Taymiyyah and appears in his *Majmuʿat al-Fatawa*, vol. 21, 85. Two exceptions mentioned in this connection concern the wearing of silk and gold for men, which is prohibited on the authority of hadith, yet very small amounts have been exonerated in both cases. for a discussion, see also al-Raysuni, *al-Haram fiʾl-Shariah*, 124.

4. Cf. al-Zuhayli, *al-Fiqh al-Islami*, vol. 6, 161f.

5. al-Kasani, *Badaʾiʿ al-Sanaʾiʿ*, vol. 5, 113, claims a conclusive consensus (*ijmaʿ*) on the prohibition of even a smallest quantity of alcohol. For a discussion of *sadd al-dharaʾiʿ*, see Kamali, *Principles*, 397–410.

6. Al-Nawawi. *The 40 Hadith*. Norwich: Diwan Press, 1981.

and these other intoxicants. For the Qur'an only refers to wine but not to the other items mentioned—hence the uncertainty of extending the punishment of one to the other.[7] One may add, however, that if fresh research and customary practice arrive at different positions based on stronger evidence, the *fiqh* rules may be adjusted accordingly.

Literally, *istihalah* has two meanings, one of which is *impossibility*, when something is said to be impossible, or *mustahil*, but this meaning is of little concern to our discussion here. The second meaning of *istihalah* is transformation of something from one state to another. Internal changes that alter the essence and basic properties of objects, such as chemical permutations occurring with or without human intervention, may alter the *haram* and convert it to halal—such as the transformation of wood into ash, of semen into an animal, of impure liquid into vapor, or when pig meat falls into salt and over time becomes an indistinguishable part of it. This transformation can occur naturally, as in the case of alcohol when it is left in an open place or exposed to the sun and it changes into vinegar, or when other substances, such as onion, bread, or yeast, are immersed into it.[8] While giving these examples, Sayyid Hossain Fadlullah adds that if transformation or change of features does not reach the extent of changing the nature of the substance—such as when milk becomes cheese, wheat becomes dough or bread, and so on, it is not *istihalah* and does not make the thing pure.[9]

The *fiqh* principle of *istihalah*, or transformation, is nowadays more frequently practiced in the context of food augmentation or alteration due to chemical treatment and industrial intervention for trading, nutrition, medicinal, and other purposes. According to the Islamic Organization for Medical Sciences (IOMS), *istihalah* is transformation of the natural characteristics of a forbidden substance to produce another substance with a different name, properties, and characteristics. Substance transformation here refers to a chemical permutation, such as the process that changes oil and fat into soap or the decomposition of fats into fatty acids and glycerol through scientific intervention.[10]

---

7. Cf. al-Zuhayli, *al-Fiqh al-Islami*, vol. 6, 166.

8. Cf. *al-Sharq al-Awsat* (London), no. 9173, July 9, 2004, 11; Awang, "Istihalah and the Sunnah of the Prophet," 58; Fadlullah, *Islamic Rulings*, 58–59.

9. Fadlullah, *Islamic Rulings*, 59.

10. al-Kurdi, *Buhuth wa Fatawa*, 29. See also Fadlullah, *Islamic Rulings*, 59.

Juristic opinion tends to differ over the legality and effects of *istihalah*. Can a Muslim consume or use an unclean substance if its chemical properties have changed? The majority opinion of the Hanafi, Maliki, Hanbali, Shafi'i, and Shia Imamiyyah schools hold this to be permissible based on the reasoning that *haram* exists due to unclean properties, and when they cease to exist, the normative shariah state of permissibility is restored—as in the case of alcohol changing into vinegar. For the rulings (*ahkam*) of shariah are founded in their proper and effective causes (*'ilal*). When the effective cause of a ruling collapses and is no longer found, its relevant ruling (*hukm*) also collapses and may be replaced with another suitable one. The main exception to this is devotional practices (*'ibadat*), whose effective causes cannot be accurately identified by the human intellect.

Two opinions of note have been recorded on the application of *istihalah*. According to the first opinion, *istihalah* can be applied in different circumstances involving both natural and synthetic changes. Many prominent scholars, past and present, have subscribed to this view, including Ibn al-Qayyim al-Jawziyyah, whose views on this may be summarized as follows:

> If the cause behind a substance being viewed as impure is not present, then it is considered pure. This is the basic premise of shariah and the premise of punishment and reward. Therefore, this ruling may be pertinent to every other impurity if it has undergone *istihalah*. God Most High says of milk that it comes "from between discharges and blood" (al-Nahl, 16:66). Muslim jurists have also held unanimously that if a creature eats unclean things, then it is confined and nourished with clean things, its milk and meat become halal as a result. The same applies to fruits and crops: if they are watered with impure water, but are then watered with pure water, they become halal as a result of the *istihalah* in the impure thing, which then becomes pure. The opposite also applies: if a pure thing changes into something impure, then it becomes *najis*; for instance, when water and food change into urine and feces. So, God Most High brings forth *tayyib* things from *khabith* and *khabith* things from *tayyib*. It is not the origin of a thing that matters, but rather its current state. It is not possible for the ruling of *khabith* to remain when its name and properties have completely changed. Those who recognized the *istihalah* of wine and other things said that it becomes *najis* due to the process of change [from grapes into wine], and then it may become pure if it undergoes another *istihalah*. It was said to them that blood, urine and feces became *khabith*

due to the *istihalah* of water and food and may become pure as a result of a further *istihalah*.[11]

The second opinion of note on *istihalah* is held by some scholars of the Shafi'i school who restricted the use of *istihalah* to natural transformation with no synthetic intervention, like the natural change of wine to vinegar. The first opinion, which has a much wider base of support, including from the Hanafi and Hanbali schools, would appear to be more suitable for contemporary research, as it extends the scope of food processing that undergo chemical and physical transformation.

There is yet a third opinion, though a minority one, on *istihalah;* it has been held by a number of jurists within the leading schools to the effect that inherent impurity remains even after *istihalah*—as transformation is often partial and not absolute and often unclear in some respects. The majority view has, however, the support of most contemporary scholars and scholarly organizations, including the Eighth Fiqh-Medical Seminar of the IOMS held in Kuwait (May 1995), which held that additive compounds extracted from prohibited animals or prohibited substances that have undergone *istihalah* are clean and permissible for consumption or medication. According to a statement issued by the seminar, "*Istihalah* is a process that causes an object to change into another, totally different in properties and characteristics, it turns the unclean, or what is deemed to be unclean, into a clean object, and therefore turns prohibited things into things permissible by the shariah."[12]

The next topic that merits attention is that of extreme dilution and perishment (*istihlak*), which is in many ways a natural follow up on *istihalah*.

---

11. al-Jawziyyah, *I'lam al Muwaqqi'in*, vol. 2, 14–15.

12. For the IOMS resolution, see Hammad, *al-Mawad al-Muharramah*, 61.

# 8

# *Perishment, Extreme Dilution (Istihlak)*

SOME TEXTBOOK WRITERS have considered *istihlak* as a variety of *istihalah,* yet there is a difference between them. Whereas *istihalah* is concerned with internal chemical changes in haram substances such that no trace of the latter remains, *istihlak* is primarily concerned with the mixing of quantities such that it reduces the smaller quantity into total insignificance. An example of *istihalah* is when wine is converted into vinegar through chemical changes, while an example of *istihlak* would be when a drop of wine falls into a large quantity of clean water. Both seem to be coterminous as far as the ruling of shariah is concerned, in that the *haram* element is considered virtually non-existent and ignored.

*Istihlak* has two meanings. One is the linguistic meaning of *istihlak,* which refers to everything that undergoes destruction, perishes, or is consumed. For example, so and so consumed *(istahlaka)* his wealth, which means that he spent or squandered his wealth and finished it. Second, from the *fiqh* point of view, *istihlak* refers to the "mixing of one substance with another such that its properties and features in the larger mix becomes non-existing or negligible despite its nominal presence." The relevant Malaysian Halal Standard[1] defines *istihlak* as "decomposition of a substance in a dominant medium which transforms the substance into the nature of the latter." An example would be the mixing a drop of alcohol or milk with a large quantity of fluid.[2] When a very small quantity of a forbidden or impure substance is mixed with a large

---

1. MS 2393-2013 (Clause 2.18).

2. Hammad, *al-Mawad al-Muharramah,* 30.

*Shariah and The Halal Industry.* Mohammad Hashim Kamali, Oxford University Press. © Oxford University Press 2021.
DOI: 10.1093/oso/9780197538616.003.0009

quantity of a pure and permissible substance such that the properties of the
pure substance overwhelm the properties of the impure substance in terms of
taste, color, and smell, then the *fiqh* process of *istihlak* has occurred, and none
of the properties of the larger mix can consequently be characterized as *haram*
or *najis*. The key Hanbali scholar Ibn Taymiyyah went on record to say that
"God Most High has forbidden unclean things (*khaba'ith*), such as blood,
carcass, pork, and so forth; if any of these substances fall into water or something else and completely disappears, so that there is no blood, dead meat, or
pork left at all, the position becomes similar to the case where wine disappears
in a liquid, then the one who drinks it is not drinking wine."[3]

It is also held that the prescribed punishment for wine does not apply to
the individual who drinks it when it has already perished in the water and
nothing of its taste, color, and smell remains, or if one eats bread that was
kneaded with wine and is then baked, there is no prescribed punishment due
to *istihlak* of the wine.[4]

Of the two main sources from which the principle of *istihlak* is derived,
the first is a renowned hadith of the Prophet. When he was asked a question
regarding water found in a remote place that was frequented by predatory and
other animals, the Prophet said, "When the volume of water reaches two *qullahs (qullatayn)*, it does not carry dirt."[5] In another hadith, the prophet said
that "water is clean, it is not made dirty by anything unless there is a change in
its smell, taste, and color."[6] Ibn Taymiyyah commented on this hadith, saying
that when the water is of a large quantity, that is, two *qullahs* (roughly one
meter in depth), then it is not affected by impurities, provided that no obvious impurity is detectable in its color, taste, and smell, in which case it is
presumed to be pure. The whole idea of *istihlak* is that pure water, drinks, and
liquid food are not polluted by a minute quantity of an impure substance if
there is no visible evidence of any change in the color, taste, and smell. Ibn
Taymiyyah states categorically that there is no evidence from the Qur'an, the

---

3. Ibn Taymiyyah, *Majmu'at Fatawa*, vol. 21, 501–502.

4. Abu Zayd, *al-Intifa' bil A'yan al-Muharramah*, 239.

5. Wahbah al-Zuhayli, who quotes this hadith narrated by 'Abd Allah ibn 'Umar, also adds that
it is recorded in *Sunan Abu Dawud: Kitab al-Taharah: Bab Ma Yunajjasu min al-Maa'*, and *al-
Mustadrak* of al-Hakim, and that the latter also said that the hadith is sound/*sahih* and fulfills
the conditions of al-Bukhari and Muslim. Al-Zuhayli has also ascertained the precise meas-
urement of a *qullah*, which tends to vary slightly in Egypt, Syria, and Iraq, but concludes that
water contained in a pond of about one meter in length, width, and depth would qualify: *al-
fiqh al-Islami*, vol. 1, 122 (the text of the hadith appears in vol. 1, 128).

6. al-Faqi, Muhammad Hamid. "Hadith: Inna al-Ma' Tahur la Yunajjisu Shai'." al-Alukah.net.
February 21, 2014. https://www.alukah.net/sharia/0/80067/.

Sunnah, consensus (*ijma'*), or even analogical reasoning (*qiyas*) to suggest otherwise. This is also Wahbah al-Zuhayli's conclusion, who then remarked that even if the quantity of water is two *qullahs* or more, if there is a change in the color, taste, and smell due to any impurity that may have fallen in it, then it is dirty by virtue of general consensus and remains so for as long as the impurity and its consequent changes remain.[7]

The second position on the subject under review is that *istihlak* may be considered a form of *istihalah*: If a small quantity of *haram* and impure substance is mixed in a large quantity of pure and halal substance such that nothing of the impure matter—its color, taste, and smell—is present, then its name too disappears due to a lack of its obvious properties, and therefore the *haram* status also collapses, as the rulings of shariah are normally attached to the names and characteristics of things.[8] This is the view also of Ibn Hazm al-Zahiri, who made the observation that if the properties of a substance whose name is classified as *haram* by the text change, then the name also changes; when the name changes the *haram* ruling associated with it is not applicable to it anymore because it no longer carries the name under which it was originally forbidden. An example is when wine transforms into vinegar.[9] Ibn Hazm also stated, "If a drop of wine falls into water or a drop of water falls into wine, it will be of no effect, and the water remains pure despite the drop of wine therein, and so is the wine which remains *haram* despite the drop of water therein—and this equally applies to all other substances. For the legal rulings append to the names and the names are also attached to the [presence of certain] characteristics."[10]

According to 'Abdul Razzak Abu Zayd, there is a similarity between *istihlak* and *istihalah*, both of which imply removal and disappearance of the properties of the impure substances such that no effect of any kind with regard to color, taste, or smell in the larger mix of the two substances is detectable.[11] Yet there are dissimilarities between them. First, the characteristics of the impure substance in *istihalah* undergo internal change or transformation, unlike *istihlak*, in which it only remains hidden from the naked eye; second, the *haram* substance undergoing *istihalah* acquires new properties and a new

---

7. al-Zuhayli, *al-Fiqh al-Islami*, vol. 1, 128.

8. Hammad, *al-Mawad al-Muharramah*, 33.

9. al-Zahiri, *al-Muhalla*, vol .7, 422.

10. al-Zahiri, *al-Muhalla*, vol. 1, 138.

11. Abu Zayd, *Al-Intifa' bil A'yan al-Muharramah*, 239.

name, whereas in *istihlak* no new substance is formed but the impure substance merges with the substance of the larger quantity.[12]

There is no doubt among the people of knowledge that *istihlak* is indeed one of the well-founded principles of Islamic law. Muslim scholars have only differed in respect of either restricting or broadening its application. Among the leading schools of law, the Hanafi, Shafi'i, and Hanbali schools restricted the application of *istihlak* to certain matters, whereas its wider application is recognized by Ibn Hazm, Ibn Taymiyyah, and Imam Malik.

Ibn Taymiyyah has stated that if a drop of alcohol falls into water and dissolves, and then someone drinks it, the person is not drinking alcohol and is not liable to punishment for drinking alcohol. If a woman's milk is poured into water and it perishes such that no trace of it is left, and a child drinks that water, he does not become the foster son or daughter of that woman through breastfeeding.[13]

Regarding this, Ibn Hazm wrote, "Every liquid such as water, olive oil, butter, milk, rose water, honey, stew, perfume, etc., in which an impurity or a *haram* substance falls, it is compulsory to abstain from it if it changes the color, taste, or odor of the liquid. The entire liquid is affected and consuming it is *haram*. It is neither permissible to use it nor to sell."[14]

In sum, any *haram* substance added to a halal substance will not make it *haram* if either the haram substance undergoes a complete change (*istihalah*) or is completely diffused and mixed in the halal substance, such that its presence becomes totally insignificant (*istihlak*).

The foregoing analysis on *istihlak* may be extended to the water purification processes attempted in countries facing water shortages. The present writer read a news item a few years back with a picture of the then incumbent prime minister of Singapore, who appeared in a Kuala Lumpur newspaper drinking a glass of purified sewer water. The newspaper caption added that the refuse water had undergone reliable purification processes such that it was good for drinking and completely safe. It was clearly stated that any elements of impurity and filth that had existed and polluted the water were subsequently taken out through scientifically proven methods, and the water was consequently purified and made clean for human consumption. The process of purification in this case is not, strictly, that of *istihalah*, as water remains

---

12. Abu Zayd, *Al-Intifa' bil A'yan al-Muharramah*, 240.

13. Ibn Taymiyyah, *Majmu'at Fatawa*, vol. 21, 33.

14. Al-Zahiri, *al-Muhalla*, vol .1, 135.

water and has not changed into something else, which is why, in the present writer's view, the impurity therein has completely perished through a process that more likely amounted to *istihlak*.

The issue over the permissibility of using such water had actually arisen much earlier, in 1989, before the Islamic Fiqh Academy of the Muslim League at its eleventh session in Mecca. The issue put before the Academy was over the permissibility of using refuse water for ablution after it had undergone chemical processes of purification. Specialist opinion was solicited and it was ascertained that the chemical purification process of polluted water occurs in four different stages: sedimentation (*al-tarsib*), ventilation (*al-tahwiyah*), elimination of microbes (*qatl al-jarathim*), and sterilization (*ta'qim*), and the whole process is such that it leaves no traces of impurity in the water. Its taste, color, and smell become that of pure clean water. The Fiqh Academy thus reached the conclusion that water purified in this way became pure for all purposes.[15]

It is then added that this matter was also considered by the Leading Ulama Council (*Hay'at Kibar al-'Ulama*, or LUC) of Saudi Arabia eleven years earlier, in 1398/1978. The LUC had determined that polluted water is purified in various ways, both naturally (e.g., exposure to sun rays and winds for a long period), or through chemical processes that involve total cleansing and purification according to modern scientific methods. Polluted water so purified by scientific methods becomes pure and its purity is known from its taste, color, and smell, in which case it may lawfully be used for all cleaning purposes, including ritual ablution and drinking. The LUC added, however, that the use of such water is permitted when there is a need for it or when there is shortage of natural clean water.[16]

At its ninth session, held in Casablanca in July 1997, the Medical Fiqh Association of the Islamic Medical Organization (al-Munazzamah al-Islamiyyah li'l-'Ulum al-Tibiyyah) held that "additives to food or medicine which originate in unclean or unlawful substances convert and become permissible in two ways, either through substance transformation (*istihalah*), or through extreme dilution (*istihlak*). The latter takes place when a small amount of unclean or unlawful substance is mixed with a very large amount of a clean substance such that all the original properties, including taste, color,

---

15. Islamic Fiqh Academy resolution at its 11th session in Mecca 13–20 of Rajab corresponding to February 19–26, 1989—also quoted in Hammad, *al-Mawad al-Muharramah*, 90.

16. The text of the LUC resolution appears in Hammad, *al-Mawad al-Muharramah*, 90.

and smell of the smaller substance perish and are completely overwhelmed by the larger mix, then credibility, from the shariah point of view, is given to the larger substance. Instances of this include composite food products that involve minute amounts of alcohol. This very small amount may even be an inseparable part of coloring, preservative, emulsifier, or anti-rancid (these are further discussed in another section below).[17]

17. Al-Nadwah al-Fiqhiyyah al-Tibiyyah al-Tasi'ah li'l-Munazzamat al-Islami li'l-'Ulum al-Tibiyyah, al-Dar al-Bayda, July 1997 as quoted in al-Harithi, *al-Nawazil fi'l-At'imah*, vol. 2, 926.

# 9

# *Necessity (*Darurah*) and Forgetfulness (*Nisyan*)*

*DARURAH* IS A broad concept and has been extensively treated in the *fiqh* literature. What is said here briefly specifies its applications to food and medicine.

To begin with, juridical necessity is not very different from the common man's perception of necessity. *Darurah* is defined as a situation that entails fear for loss of one's life, affliction with grave bodily injury, or loss of property and honor with a degree of certainty that arises from one's knowledge of the situation such that it leaves the victim with no choice for an alternative. Yet it is still a fear of death or injury. It is not necessary, in other words, that one waits until meeting one's death or injury, but one is permitted to act in self-defense, or, if necessary, commit what is normally unlawful.[1] Two conditions must be fulfilled, one of which is that there is no permissible alternative to fulfil one's pressing need. Should there be any permissible alternative accessible to the distressed person, there will be no case for *darurah*. The other condition is that the forbidden substance is taken to the extent only necessary for survival but no more. This is the purport of a legal maxim that states, "What is permitted in necessity must be measured according to its true proportions."[2]

A leading legal maxim on necessity that is commonly cited, as mentioned earlier, also provides that "necessity makes the unlawful lawful,"[3] provided

---

1. Ibn Qudamah, *al-Mughni*, vol. 8, 596; al-Zuhayli, *al-Fiqh al-Islami*, vol. 3, 515.

2. Wizarat, *al-Mawsuʿah al-Fiqhiyyah*, vol. 5, 160; *Majallah al-Ahkam al-Adliyyah* (Art. 22); Hammad, *al-Mawad al-Muharramah*, 40. The maxim in its Arabic wording: *"al-daruratu tuqaddaru bi-qadriha."*

3. *Majallah al-Ahkam al-Adliyyah* (Art. 21); Hammad, *al-Mawad al-Muharramah*, 39.

*Shariah and The Halal Industry.* Mohammad Hashim Kamali, Oxford University Press. © Oxford University Press 2021.
DOI: 10.1093/oso/9780197538616.003.0010

that the aforementioned conditions are also fulfilled. Another maxim states that, "Harm must be eliminated—*al-dararu yuzal.*" The victim of a distressful situation is often faced with intolerable harm, which need not be tolerated.

Basic Qur'anic authority on *darurah* is found in the following verses:

But if one is forced by necessity without willful disobedience or transgressing due limits, then he is guiltless. For God is forgiving, most merciful. (al-Baqarah, 2:173)

But if anyone is forced by hunger, with no inclination to transgress, then God is indeed forgiving and merciful. (al-Ma'idah, 5:4)

He (God) has explained to you in detail what is forbidden to you, except under compulsion of necessity. (al-An'am, 6:119)

The message thus conveyed is that the Lawgiver makes concessions in situations that involve grave danger or infliction of intolerable suffering on the individual. This is also the purport of a parallel and supplementary shariah principle of facilitation and ease (*al-takhfif wa'l-taysir*), to the effect that people who are afflicted with illness or life-threatening danger and loss should be afforded the opportunity to find a way out of their intolerable predicament.

All the foregoing evidence is clear on the permissibility of consuming forbidden substances due to necessity and duress. The two provisos attached, namely the absence of willful transgression and disobedience, as well as observance of a carefully measured approach and certain other details specified in the legal maxims have been interpreted and presented by jurists and commentators in different ways. Some differences of opinion have thus arisen on the details of fear for one's life and safety, and how the afflicted person may actually feel: should this reach certain knowledge (*'ilm*), or would a strong probability (*zann*) also be sufficient? The Maliki and Hanbali schools, and some Shafi'i jurists, have held that the fear for one's loss of life must reach certain knowledge or strong probability, whereas the Hanafis maintain that a genuine fear, even if not amounting to positive knowledge of the expected consequences for one's life or loss of limb, would qualify. A minority view in the Shafi'i and Hanbali schools also hold that the fear of death or affliction with a grave illness, or severe hardship that disables a person to walk or to move, also qualifies.[4] The whole of this discussion seems to be premised on

---

4. al-Qurtubi, *Bidayat al-Mujtahid*, vol. 1, 476; Hammad, *al-Mawad al-Muharramah*, 40–41.

an acknowledgment that fear is a somewhat subjective variable that tends to differ from person to person, notwithstanding the recognition that fear can also be objectively assessed.

The leading schools of Islamic law have also differed regarding the question of whether it is a juridical obligation for one to eat forbidden substances to save one's life, or a mere permissibility for one to so. The majority view inclines toward obligation, as this is how they understand the Qur'an, especially the verses "Throw not yourselves into destruction by your own hands," and "Kill yourselves not, for God is truly merciful unto you" (al-Baqarah, 2:195 and al-Nisa', 4:29, respectively).[5] Hence anyone who refuses to eat and drink until he dies is guilty of a violation. To this effect, the renowned Shafi'i scholar 'Izz al-Din 'Abd al-Salam wrote that "if someone has to eat prohibited substances, it is an obligation for him to do so in order to keep alive, for causing the loss of one's own life and limb is a greater evil than eating a forbidden substance."[6] The Hanbali school as well as Abu Yusuf (d.182/798) of the Hanafi, and Abu Ishaq al-Shirazi (d.476/1083) of the Shafi'i school, have held, however, that eating forbidden substances under such conditions is permissible only. It is quite possible that the person is extremely repulsed by the idea of eating a carcass, for instance. Then it is added that eating forbidden substances at times of necessity is a concession (*rukhsah*), and, like all other concessions, taking advantage of it is permissible (*mubah*) only. Thus, it is reported that when one of the Prophet's Companions, 'Abd Allah b. Hudhafah al-Shami, was captured by the tyrants of Rome, he was incarcerated in a house and made only wine mixed with water and roasted pig meat available to him. He was held for three days, during which he did not eat or drink until his head drooped from hunger and thirst and they let him go when they feared his death. He said later that God Most High had permitted him to eat as he was starving, yet he did not wish to go against his faith, but also that this permissibility to eat was a concession and in the nature of *mubah*.[7] It is a totally different issue if one denies oneself food and goes on in a state of hunger for some reason that does not amount to necessity until one dies. This is held to be sinful. Hence

---

5. Hammad, *al-Mawad al-Muharramah*, 39. See for an analysis of these verses Kamali, *The Right to Life*, 30f.

6. 'Abd al-Salam, *al-Qawa'id al-Ahkam*, vol. 1, 141. See also Hammad, *al-Mawad al-Muharramah*, 41.

7. Ibn Qudamah, *al-Mughni*, vol. 13, 95.

it is impermissible for prisoners and others in similar circumstances to go on a hunger strike until they die.[8]

All that which is made *haram* under shariah is addressed to competent persons who are in possession of their faculties. The shariah expounds the *haram* in detail but makes exceptions in cases of necessity and irresistible duress. Hence, for someone who is exposed to conditions of necessity and duress while not intending to violate the law or to be sinful, flexibility is granted to do what is necessary.[9] Eating food is a necessity of life, and *darurah* in this case aims at curbing starvation, which sets in, according to some Muslim jurists, after a day and a night when nothing can be found to eat or drink other than forbidden substances. The Maliki school and a minority opinion in the Shafiʿi and Hanbali schools have held that one may then take of what is available to the extent of satisfying one's hunger until one finds permissible food. The majority position is, as already mentioned, that one may take only an amount that is necessary for survival.[10]

Schools and scholars of Islamic law have recorded the following conditions for necessity (*darurah*):

1. That it is irresistible (*mulji'ah*). This is when the distressed person is certain or thinks with strong probability that he will lose his life or limb or will be afflicted with fatal illness.
2. That it obtains in the present and it is subsistent.
3. There is no permissible means available to satisfy the necessity.
4. The distressed person does not indulge in the forbidden substance/act more than repelling the anticipated danger/harm.
5. The person in distress is not guilty of transgression.
6. That one who is compelled duly observes the order of intensity in the prohibited substances that may be available: thus, one should avoid taking a deceased human's flesh if there is animal carcass available, and take the flesh of another animal in preference to the swine carcass, and so forth.
7. That the forbidden substance is taken with the intention of removing the stressful condition.
8. What is being taken does indeed remove the stressful condition.[11]

---

8. Cf. al-Zuhayli, *al-Fiqh al-Islami*, vol. 3, 516. See also Abu Zayd, *al-Intifaʿ bil A ʿyan al-Muharramah*, 283

9. Cf. Q. al-Anʿam, 6:119; al-Baqarah, 2:172; al-Maʾidah, 5:3.

10. Cf. Abu Zayd, *al-Intifa 'Biʾl Aʿyan al-Muharramah*, 269.

11. al-Sharbini, *al-Iqnaʿ*, vol. 2, 584; Abidin, *Hashiyah Radd al-Mukhtar*; Abu Zayd, *al-Intifaʿ bil Aʿyan al-Muharramah*, 266ff.

Similar questions have arisen with regard to medicine that is derived from forbidden substances. Whereas some jurists do not see medicine as being of the same rank of necessity as food for survival, the correct view is that both are requirements of human survival, and may thus be taken when no halal alternative is available. However, the concession that shariah has granted regarding medicine is contingent on the fulfilment of the following conditions: (1) that there is a real health risk if the medicine in question is not taken—such as the taking of insulin for a diabetic; (2) that the danger is in the present and not in the future; (3) that it is certain knowledge that taking the forbidden substance will cure the illness at issue; (4) that no halal alternative is found; (5) that one stops at the minimum necessary to prevent self-destruction—according to the majority view; and (6) that a trustworthy Muslim physician prescribes it.[12] In the event that a Muslim physician is not available, a trustworthy non-Muslim physician is an acceptable substitute.

Necessity may occur when one is at one's normal residence or when traveling. This is because the concession granted in the Qur'an (al-Ma'idah, 5:4) is unqualified and does not stipulate one or the other, and the effective cause of the concession is protection of life, which can materialize even when one is at home, such as in the year of drought (*'aam al-maja'ah*) during the time of 'Umar b. al-Khattab, during which the protection of life took priority over the enforcement of the prescribed punishment for theft.[13] A question does arise, however, regarding travel for unlawful purposes, as in the case of bandits and those who commit crimes: Are they equally entitled to the shariah concessions? The answer to this is indicated in the Qur'anic verse that allows one who is compelled, provided one is not a rebel or bent on committing transgression (al-Ma'idah, 5:4). This is the majority position, but the Hanafi school would treat transgressors and nontransgressors on the same footing. The Hanafis refer in this connection to other Qur'anic verses (i.e., 2:195 and 4:29—that one should neither court danger nor kill oneself), saying that these directives do not make any distinction and are addressed equally to all.[14] The Hanbali school takes the opposite view and

---

12. Cf. al-Qaradawi, *al-Halal wa'l-Haram*, 52–53; al-Zuhayli, *al-Fiqh al-Islami*, vol. 3, 17.

13. Ibn Qudamah, *al-Mughni*, vol. 13, 95.

14. Cf. Abu Zayd, *al-Intifa' bil A'yan al-Muharramah*, 275 also referring to al-Baji, *al-Muntaqa Sharh al-Muwatta'*, vol. 3, 141. The Hanafis also add that the reference to transgression and lawlessness in the main verses on *darurah* is to the eating itself of forbidden substances such that one does not eat the latter when permissible food is available nor does so to excess.

denies the starving bandit, for instance, the ability to take advantage of the concession.[15]

As for the actual substances taken under necessity, the Malikis and some other jurists have excepted the human flesh. The majority have also prohibited killing and dismembering a human being, whether Muslim or non-Muslim, in order to be consumed under any conditions. The Hanbalis have excepted the taking of poison on medicinal grounds.[16] Muslim jurists have also disagreed on taking alcohol, its derivatives, and other intoxicants, although somewhat less emphatically in the case of taking other intoxicants for medication, due mainly to a hadith stating that "God does not make the *haram* a means of healing for you."[17] Another supplementary hadith also provides that "God has created ailments and cures, and has created cure for every ailment. So seek cure [for your ailment] but not with what is *haram*."[18]

Whereas the majority proscribes it, the Hanafis have held alcohol-based medication to be permissible if it is known for sure to offer a cure and no halal alternative can be found, but not if it is doubtful. The majority of Maliki and Hanbali jurists have held that medication with *haram* is proscribed absolutely and without exception. However the Maliki scholars Ibn al-'Arabi (d.583/1140) and Abu'l-Walid ibn Rushd al-Qurtubi (d.520/1126) have also concurred with the Hanafis, provided that all the aforementioned conditions are satisfied. Some have added the proviso that medication with prohibited substances is allowed under necessity if it is mixed with lawful substances, but not otherwise.[19]

The scope of this discussion becomes considerably wider in view of the new knowledge expansion, especially in respect of food and medicine varieties derived from chemical and synthetic sources that are also mass produced in Western factories and elsewhere. Questions have arisen, in this connection, over the use of juridically impure and doubtful substances,

---

15. Cf. Ibn Qudamah, *al-Mughni*, vol. 13, 96.

16. al-Zuhayli, *al-Fiqh al-Islami*, vol. 3, 520.

17. The Arabic version of the hadith reads: *"inna Allaha lam yaj'al shifa'ukum fima hurrima 'alaykum"*; al-Bukhari has recorded this hadith on the authority of 'Abd Allah ibn Mas'ud. See al-Zuhayli, *al-Fiqh al-Islami*, vol. 3, 522.

18. al-Sijistani, *Sunan Abu Dawud*, vol. 4, 312, hadith 3875. The *isnad* of this hadith is noted to be weak (*da'if*).

19. al-Zuhayli, *al-Fiqh al-Islami*, vol. 3, 523. See also al-Hajji al-Kurdi, *Buhuth wa Fatawa*, 25.

such as lard, alcohol derivatives, and heparin obtained from the swine's intestines. A variety of medicines that contain these are in use for heart and kidney diseases, blood ailments, congestion of the arteries, and so forth. It is all the more advisable therefore to observe the prerequisite conditions of *darurah* carefully and under supervision or recommendation of qualified physicians. A suggestion is also made that in doubtful situations it is preferable to have an opinion from two qualified physicians, based on the idea that one person's opinion may fall below the juridically credible evidence of two witnesses.[20]

Muslim jurists have recorded several exceptions to the originally prohibited positions in shariah based on necessity in the following cases:

- Burning of trees and slaying of animals of the warring disbelievers by the Muslim army, when this is deemed necessary or when conducive to breaking enemy superiority.
- Opening the grave of a deceased person after burial for reasons of necessity and crime investigation.
- Viewing the private parts of a woman due to medical reasons or ascertaining her condition only to the extent necessary.
- A Muslim who stays in a place where *haram* prevails and no halal food can be found, a small amount of non-halal food is allowed in order to survive without excessive indulgence.
- A person in a state of major impurity (*al-junub*) or a menstruating woman may enter a mosque to take refuge from an enemy or someone forcing him or her into wrongdoing.
- Issuance of a *fatwa* based on opinion in the absence of any shariah evidence in exceptional cases.
- Notwithstanding disagreement by some and claims of its outlandishness, the Malikis have allowed a woman to commit *zina* in order to save herself from starvation and imminent death. This may, according to the proponents of this view, also be extended to providing the essentials of life for her child. This position is held apparently notwithstanding the Qur'anic verse earlier reviewed concerning rebels and transgressors.[21]

---

20. *Al-Sharq al-Awsat*, 16 Dhu'l-Qa'dah 1424/9 January 2004, serial no. 9173 reporting proceedings of Islamic Fiqh Academy of the Muslim League session.

21. al-Raysuni, *al-Haram fi'l-Shariah*, 177–178.

Some of the more modern applications of the shariah principle of necessity include the following:

- Opening a deceased person's body for autopsy due to a valid *maslahah* such as criminality research or similar other situations.
- Permissibility of medication by filthy (*najis*) substances in the event that no clean alternative can be found to replace it. This is because fighting illness takes priority over the benefit of avoiding consuming filth.
- It is permissible to open a pregnant woman's belly when childbirth becomes intolerably difficult. For saving the life of the infant takes priority over observing the bodily integrity of its mother, provided that the surgical operation does not endanger the mother's own life.
- Permissibility of price control ( *al-tas'ir*) when food suppliers engage in aggressive profiteering and price distortion, notwithstanding the impermissibility of price control under normal conditions.[22]

## Forgetfulness (Nisyan)

The shariah recognizes forgetfulness as a ground of exoneration for committing something unlawful or omitting a required element in the completion of halal ritual slaughter. In cases of genuine and innocent forgetfulness, the perpetrator is not taken to task and is not held to be a transgressor. For forgetfulness is tantamount to absence and renders the perpetrated act or omission as if it did not occur in the first place. Yet there are some limitations to this, one of which is that the exemption due to oblivion applies mainly to the Right of God aspects of conduct in matters, for instance, of worship and religious performances that do not concern the rights of other human beings. Thus, if one eats out of forgetfulness during daytime in Ramadan, the fast remains intact, and if one performs the obligatory prayer (*salah*) without *wudu* due to forgetfulness, the prayer is not vitiated. This is the purport of a legal maxim: "One who commits a prohibited act due to oblivion is not a transgressor."[23] Quoted in authority for this maxim is the Qur'anic verse "God does not burden a soul beyond its capability" (al-Baqarah, 2:286; al-Talaq, 65:7) And also the elevated hadith of Ibn 'Abbas

---

22. al-Raysuni, *al-Haram fi'l-Shariah*, 178–179.

23. al-Suyuti, *al-Ashbah wa'l-Naza'ir*, 207; al-Raysuni, *al-Haram fi'l-Shari'ah*, 151. The Arabic version of the maxim is: "*man fa'ala al-mahzura nasiyyan la ya'uddu 'aasiyan.*"

from the Prophet: "God Most High has exonerated my community for mistake, forgetfulness and duress."[24]

Rights of God are singled out in this connection, as it is said that God Most High is in no need of such performances and His mercy and compassion is beyond bounds. That said, the Right of God and Right of Man/Human division is not always clear-cut and not mutually exclusive. It would appear, nevertheless, that the halal slaughter rituals, *tasmiyah*, and certain other requirements fall in the category of the Right of God, and as such would attract the above-mentioned exemptions over forgetfulness. In the event, however, where the Right of God subsumes the right of humans, then the latter is likely again to dominate the former. For instance, if a person takes food belonging to another person due to forgetfulness, the person is arguably liable to compensate the owner. Taking someone else's food because of to extreme hunger is exonerated based on necessity and God's grant of forgiveness not to penalize it, but then it has subsumed the right of a human, which in this case takes priority and generates liability for compensation.

But in regard to the rights of humans, forgetfulness is of little effect and does not provide a valid excuse either. Thus, if someone destroys another person's property due to forgetfulness, he is still liable for compensation, unless the owner exonerates him. For the shariah more diligently protects the rights of individuals and only the right bearer has the privilege to grant exemption or release.[25]

24. Ibn Majah, *Sunan Ibn Majah, Kitab al-Talaq, Bab Talaq al-Mukrah wa'l-Naasi*, hadith 2054.

25. al-Raysuni, *al-Haram fi'l-Shariah*, 152–153.

# 10

# *The Reprehensible (Makruh)*

MAKRUH (LIT. DISLIKED, from the root word *kariha*) is the opposite in Arabic of *mahbub* (liked or loved). Juridically, according to the
majority of the leading schools of law, *makruh* refers to an act, object, or
conduct that should be avoided, but whose perpetrator is not liable to
punishment and does not incur moral blame. The Hanafis are in agreement with the majority position in respect of only one of the two varieties
of *makruh*, namely that of *makruh tanzihi* (*makruh* for the sake of purity), but not with regard to what the Hanafis classify as *makruh tahrimi*
(*makruh* closer to *haram*), which does entail moral blame but not punishment. The leading schools are in agreement that one who avoids *makruh*
merits praise and gains closeness to God.[1] *Makruh* is often described as
the lowest degree of prohibition, and in this sense it is used as a convenient category the jurists have employed for matters that fall between the
halal and *haram*, matters that are definitely discouraged but where the
evidence to establish them as *haram* is less than certain. Matters of this
kind are conveniently placed under *makruh* mainly for lack of a better
alternative. The Hanafi category of *makruh tanzihi* is subsumed under
*mubah* by the majority.

According to the Hanafi position, an act is *haram* when it is prohibited in definitive terms, but when there is an element of weakness in the
prohibitive language of the Qur'an or hadith, the matter falls under *makruh tahrimi*, or *makruh* close to *haram*. For example, it is *makruh tahrimi* to make an offer of betrothal to a woman who is already betrothed
to another man. The reason for this is that the hadith proscribing this is a

---

1. For details, see Zahrah, *Usul al-fiqh*, 424.

*Shariah and The Halal Industry*. Mohammad Hashim Kamali, Oxford University Press. © Oxford University Press 2021.
DOI: 10.1093/oso/9780197538616.003.0011

solitary (*ahad*) hadith, which is not altogether devoid of doubt in respect of authenticity.[2]

On a historical note, the leading imams of jurisprudence have often used *makruh* to actually convey what they had meant to be forbidden, or *haram*, but they often labeled it *makruh* out of piety and the emphatic Qur'anic reminder to the believers to exercise extreme caution in declaring that "this is *haram* and that is halal." For if this is less than accurate it would be tantamount to attributing lies to God Most High (al-Nahl, 16:116). It was in due regard for this very restrictive Qur'anic approach to *haram* that the leading Imams and pioneers pronounced hardly anything as *haram* without clear textual evidence. Ibn Qayyim al-Jawziyyah has confirmed this and added that the juridical meaning of *makruh* that is now commonly accepted was actually an invention of the *Muta'akhkhirun* (later-day jurists) among the *fiqh* scholars; that is, the later-day jurists who applied *makruh* to that which was below the level of *haram*. This was actually a departure, in Ibn Qayyim's view, and also that of his teacher, Ibn Taymiyyah, from the position of the pioneers, al-Mutaqaddimun. It is then added that the pioneers' usage of *makruh* was in greater harmony with the language of the Qur'an and hadith, but the later jurists then changed that and used *makruh* for that which fell below the *haram*.[3]

Imam Abu Hanifah's disciple al-Shaybani reported that the Imam saw the *makruh* closer to *haram*. For instance, Abu Hanifah and his disciples wrote that "profiteering (*al-ihtikar*) in foodstuffs of humans and animals is *makruh*, especially when it causes them hardship and harm."[4] By this they evidently meant that it was *haram*. They also wrote that "sale of arms [to the warring parties] during conflict is *makruh*."[5] This too meant that it was *haram*. This is also the case with Imam Shafi'i, who was most careful not to employ *haram* in his expressions. He would use *makruh* that carried the meaning of *haram*.[6] The same is true of Imam Malik, who would use the phrase "I dislike this—*akrihu hadha*" in places that actually conveyed *haram*. Many examples are also found in Imam Ibn Hanbal's writings and *fatwa* where *makruh* is used to convey *haram*. His son 'Abd Allah thus reported what his father said: "I

---

2. Cf. Kamali, *Principles*, 426.

3. Ibn Qayyim, *I'lam al-Muwaqqi'in*, vol. 1, 39–40.

4. al-Kasani, *Bada'i' al-Sana'i'*, vol. 5, 129.

5. al-Kasani, *Bada'i' al-Sana'i'*, vol. 7, 147.

6. Ibn Qayyim, *I'lam al-Muwaqqi'in*, vol. 1, 39.

dislike (*akrihu*) the flesh of snake and scorpion, for the former has canine teeth and the latter has poison." He is also reported to have said "I dislike the flesh and milk of *jallalah* (animal that feeds on filth)," by which he meant all of them were forbidden (*haram*).[7] All of this, it is added, was due to the afore-mentioned Qur'anic verse (al-Nahl, 16:116) and the caution it conveyed over the facile use of *haram* and halal.[8]

There is much disagreement among jurists about the *makruh* in foodstuffs and other substances for human consumption, but most would include rotten meat that develops an offensive smell, water from a well in the midst of a graveyard, and unsupervised cattle and poultry that feed on impurities and filth such that changes of taste and smell in them may be detectable. The relevant hadith also includes the milk of such animals.[9] This impurity is, however, removed when such animals are kept away from their dirty habitats for a number of days (three for poultry, four for sheep and goats, and ten for camels and cows). The preferred position of the majority of schools on this issue, however, departs from these specifications and merely advises isolation until the offensive signs and smells are no longer present.[10] The Shia Imamiyyah position on *jallalah* animals resembles that of the majority of Sunni schools, excepting the Malikis, in regards to the methods of purification it proposes for *jallalah* animals and birds. Thus it is stated, on the authority of Imam 'Ali ibn Abi Talib, who is quoted to have said that the flesh of *jallalah* chicken is not to be eaten until the expiry of three days, of *jallalah* duck until five days, and of sheep and goats until ten days. Cows and bulls must be kept away in clean conditions for twenty days, and camels for forty days. These rules also apply to the milk of bovine animals and camels. Some Shia sources add that they should not be used for riding as well, for the same length of time.[11] The Shia scholars have differed on whether consuming the flesh of *jallalah* animals is *makruh* or *haram*, but the preferred position is that it is *makruh*.[12] It

---

7. Ibn Qayyim, *I'lam al-Muwaqqi'in*, vol. 1, 39.

8. Cf. al-Raysuni, *al-Haram fi'l-Shariah*, 43–45.

9. Thus, according to one hadith, "The Prophet proscribed eating the flesh of a *jallalah* camel," and according to another "The Prophet proscribed drinking the milk of a *jallalah*." These hadiths are quoted in *Sunan Daraqutni* and *Sunan Abu Dawud*, respectively, and in Wizarat, *al-Mawsu'ah al-Fiqhiyyah*, vol. 5, 149.

10. al-Kasani, *Bada'i' al-Sana'i'*, vol. 5, 39–40; Muhammad Amin, *Hashiyah Radd al-Mukhtar*, vol. 5, 194.

11. Fadlullah, *Fiqh al-At'imah*, 120–121.

12. Fadlullah, *Fiqh al-At'imah*, 120.

is *makruh* to consume the meat of donkeys and drink their milk; drinking the urine of camel and consumption of horse meat is likewise disapproved—especially in wartime, when horses may be needed in *jihad*.

Some food varieties that are basically good for consumption are held to be reprehensible if taken under certain circumstances. The Prophet (pbuh) thus said, "Whenever you consume raw onion or garlic, you should not go to the mosque for congregation prayers."[13] These items should not be consumed when their odor becomes offensive to others in the mosque setting, as is stated in the hadith, but also elsewhere, when close contact with others is likely to have a similar effect.

While it is reprehensible to use the tusk of an elephant as a tool for slaughter, there are conflicting views on the matter. The Shia position on this is more specific and relies on a hadith they quote from the Prophet, who has "prohibited slaughter with any tool that is not iron—*annahu naha 'an al-dhabh bi-ghayr al-hadid*." Imam Ja'far al-Sadiq has also said in confirmation that "slaughter is not valid by other than an iron tool."[14] It is also reprehensible to slaughter an animal without the intention of having it as food for consumption, for it would mean killing an animal without a valid purpose. Furthermore, the hunting of birds for pleasure is reprehensible, for all living beings have their own worth in the order of creation, and humans are responsible for the protection of animals at their disposal and control, including their health and adequate feeding. It is a part of human responsibility as God's vicegerents on the earth to care for the natural environment and the well-being of all of earth's inhabitants.

It is reprehensible, moreover, to swallow fish while still alive, and to grill or roast it in that condition, for it involves the infliction of torture unnecessarily. This is also the position with regard to the locust and other halal insects, although a variant view recorded by the Hanbali school and some Shafi'i jurists draws a distinction between fish and insects. For fish have no certainty of remaining alive outside water, whereas the insects may have, or may take a long time if one had to wait for its natural death to occur—hence it is permissible to be taken alive.[15] There is disagreement on the basic permissibility or otherwise of human consumption of the desert lizard. Those who say it is permissible refer to a report that it was eaten by one of the Companions, Khalid

---

13. al-Mawsili, *al-Jam'u Bain al-Sahihayn*, vol. 2, 38.

14. al-Tabarsi, *Mustadrak*, vol. 16, 131, sec. 19367 & 19368, respectively.

15. Wizarat , *al-Mawsu'ah al-Fiqhiyyah*, vol. 5, 130–131, 142.

ibn al-Walid, while the Prophet was present, but that the Prophet himself did not take it when he was offered it. This is taken as the main authority for permissibility. Those who say it is reprehensible refer in authority to two Companions, namely 'Ali ibn Abi Talib and Jabir b. 'Abd Allah, who have considered lizard to be objectionable to eat. Since there is conflict of evidence on the matter, it is likely to fall under the normative principle of original permissibility (*ibahah*).[16]

According to al-Shatibi, the sin of direct indulgence in *makruh* and *haram* is greater than their indirect facilitation, for instance, of acts and conduct that serve as the means toward securing them, and which are not the ends or objectives in themselves. The degree of prohibition and repulsiveness of acts that serve as means toward a sinful act will accordingly be less than committing the acts that are the ends and objectives, and not merely the means. *Makruh* may in some cases serve and qualify as a means to *haram*.[17]

Certain organs of lawfully slaughtered and halal animals have also been declared to be non-halal. These include blood, the phallus, testicles, vagina, glands, gall bladder, and bile, which are considered by the Hanafis to be *makruh tahrimi* due to the fact that the prohibitory hadith text on them is a solitary hadith that is not entirely free of all doubt.[18] A reference is also made to the Qur'anic prohibition of *al-khaba'ith* (filthy stuffs) in sura al-A'raf, 7:157, and the said items are then subsumed by that expression. Besides, it is added that these are disliked and considered unclean by the people of sound nature. The hadith on this subject provides, on the authority of Mujahid that "the Prophet, pbuh, disliked (*kariha Rasul Allah*) of a sheep these organs (the same seven organs are then mentioned)."[19] The Shia Imamiyyah take identical position on these seven organs, despite some isolated reports that record ten organs. The preferred position is that the seven organs just mentioned are prohibited for consumption.[20]

The textual authority for *makruh* may consist of a reference to something that is specifically identified as *makruh*, or may be so identified by a word or words that convey an equivalent meaning thereof. The word *makruh* occurs

---

16. Wizarat, *al-Mawsu'ah al-Fiqhiyyah*, vol. 5, 142–143.

17. al-Shatibi, *al-Muwafaqat*, 152.

18. Cf. al-Zuhayli, *al-Fiqh al-Islami*, vol. 3, 667.

19. The hadith is recorded by al-Bayhaqi in *Sunan al-Bayhaqi*, also quoted in Wizarat, *al-Mawsu'ah al-Fiqhiyyah*, vol. 5, 152.

20. Fadlullah, *Fiqh al-At'imah*, 161.

in its literal sense, for instance, in the following verse of the Qur'an, which refers to certain aspects of human conduct, such as being less than accurate in giving weights and measurements, taking a position on matters on which one has no knowledge, walking the earth with a sense of arrogance, and failure to keep one's promise. The text then declares:

All of these are evil and abomination in the sight of your Lord. (al-Isra', 17:38)

In another Qur'anic passage, it is enjoined:

And seek not that which is bad to give in charity when you would not take it for yourselves save with closed eyes. (al-Baqarah, 2:267)

This last expression is held to convey a *makruh*. The subject (of *makruh*) is also looked at under the Qur'an text that "he (the Prophet) forbids to them (Muslims) all that which is unclean (*khaba'ith*)" (al-A'raf, 7:157). But this verse, which is a manifest text (*zahir*), is also quoted in respect of the seven above-mentioned organs and many other animals and objects. A manifest/ *zahir*, as opposed to a clear text (*nass*), in the language of *usul al-fiqh* conveys a probability only. It is not certain, in other words, that the seven items that were labeled as reprehensible were actually meant to be included under the *khaba'ith*. The prohibitive view also holds these organs to be abhorrent to people of sound nature (*al-taba'i' al-salimah*).[21] The other three schools (other than the Hanafi and Shia) are less restrictive, but their preferred position also considers the organs in question to be *makruh*.[22] As for the use of rennet (*minfahah*) from the stomach of cattle for use in the fermentation and processing of cheese, if it is taken from a lawfully slaughtered animal, it is held to be halal by consensus. If rennet is taken from carrion, it is non-halal according to the majority, but halal according to the Hanafis on the ground of an analogy they draw between this and the milk of such animals.[23]

Other instances of *makruh* to be noted in conjunction with the rituals of slaughter include rough handling (such as dragging the animal by its feet), abandoning the *tasmiyah* (i.e., reciting the name God) according to

---

21. Cf. Wizarat, *al-Mawsu'ah al-Fiqhiyyah*, vol. 5, 152.

22. Cf. Wizarat, *al-Mawsu'ah al-Fiqhiyyah*, vol. 5, 153.

23. Cf. Wizarat, *al-Mawsu'ah al-Fiqhiyyah*, vol. 5, 155.

the Shafi'is and Malikis, slaughter in front of another animal, the use of bones and stones as slaughtering tools, cutting or skinning the animal before the complete exit of life, not facing the *qiblah*, and citing the name of Muhammad next to that of Allah. The Malikis do not stipulate facing the *qiblah* as a requirement of slaughter due to the absence of textual evidence on this. The basis of this they say is a weak analogy that is drawn between the obligatory prayer (*salah*) and slaughter, which are altogether two different things.[24]

The question of tobacco and smoking, and whether the slaughterer should avoid it, is more complex. Smoking is undoubtedly widespread among Muslims, though not in slaughterhouses, yet scholars have different opinions about it. The majority hold smoking to be reprehensible. It is a waste of money and it has no nutritional value, nor does it have any medically proven benefit. Its health risks are almost certain in connection with such diseases as lung cancer, heart attack, and emphysema among the smokers. To abstain from smoking generally, and in the slaughtering environment in particular, is therefore highly recommended, and practicing it is therefore reprehensible. Smoking should in some circumstances be even banned altogether.[25] The risk of declaring smoking as *haram* is that by doing so, one is virtually declaring millions of smoking Muslims as sinners and transgressors, which is hardly advisable. More importantly perhaps is the absence of a textual injunction on the issue, and the juridical principle is that *haram* can only be created based on the authority of a clear text.

The textual authority for *makruh* may also be a hadith that conveys an equivalent meaning of *makruh*. There is a hadith, for example, in which the Prophet discouraged any prayers at midday until the decline of the sun, with the exception of Friday prayers. The actual words used in the hadith are that the Prophet disliked (*kariha al-nabiy*) prayers at that particular time.[26] An equivalent term to *makruh* also occurs in the hadith which says: "The most abominable of permissible things (*abghad al-halal*) in the sight of God is divorce."[27] *Makruh* may also be conveyed in the form of a prohibition but in a language that indicates only reprehensibility. An example of this is the

---

24. Cf. Ibn Rushd, *Bidayat al-Mujtahid*, vol. 1, 329; al-Zuhayli, *al-Fiqh al-Islami*, vol. 3, 663–664.

25. Cf. Douglas, "The Fabric of Muslim Daily Life," vol. 3, 17.

26. For details, see Kamali, *Principles*, 331.

27. al-Bayanuni, *al-Hukmu al-Taklifi fi al-Shari'ah al-Islamiyah*, 224–225.

Qur'anic text that states, in an address to the believers warning them against excessive questioning, "O ye who believe! Ask not questions about that which, if made plain to you, you may dislike it" (al-Ma'idah, 5:101). Another illustration of this is the saying of the Prophet to "[a]bandon that which you are doubtful about in favor of that which you do not doubt."[28]

28. Ibid., 225

# II

# *The Recommended (*Mandub*)*

*MANDUB* (ALSO KNOWN as *sunnah, mustahab, nafl*) denotes an act or conduct that the shariah has recommended, but which is not binding. To comply with the *mandub* earns one spiritual reward, but no punishment is imposed for its neglect. *Mandub* is the opposite of *makruh*, and this means that avoidance of *makruh* amounts to *mandub*. Handling the slaughtered animal with clemency and care is *mandub*, and rough handling of it is *makruh*. To set up a charitable endowment (*waqf*), to attend to the sick, to be kind to one's family and friends, to speak well to the people, and to honor one's neighbor and one's guest are all recommended.

If the *mandub* is an act that the Prophet has performed on some occasions but omitted on others, it is called *sunnah*, which is also of two types: It is emphatic *sunnah* (*sunnah mu'akkadah*, also known as *sunnat al-huda*) if the Prophet has performed it regularly, or has strongly recommended it, such as attending the mosque congregation for obligatory prayers (*salah*), and calling out the call for prayer (*adhan*) preceding it. To perform an act of merit, such as offering two units of *sunnah* prior to the obligatory early and late afternoon (*zuhr* or *'asr*) prayers, or being generous in charity above the level of the obligatory alms tax (*zakah*) are examples of supererogatory *sunnah*, or *sunnah ghayr mu'akkadah*. The schools of law have employed a variety of other expressions for *mandub*, such as *tatawwu', fadilah, ihsan*, and *ragha'ib*, all of which share the basic meaning of recommendable and praiseworthy, albeit with finer distinctions that often consist of sound advice and cultural refinement.[1]

---

1. For details, see Kamali, *Principles*, 419f.

*Shariah and The Halal Industry.* Mohammad Hashim Kamali, Oxford University Press. © Oxford University Press 2021.
DOI: 10.1093/oso/9780197538616.003.0012

The recommendable in dietary substances in Islam relates to some food items that are either mentioned in the Qur'an in a positive context or which were favored by the Prophet, pbuh, such as honey, figs, olives, dates, and milk. Most of these are mentioned in the Qur'an, and the Prophet is also known for his liking of certain foods, such dates and milk, hence Muslims generally prefer these as they were liked by the Prophet, but more specifically to open one's fast with dates is commonly practiced during Ramadan.[2] It is also recommendable for one to delay taking a predawn meal (*sahur*) during the fasting month to the latest segment of the night and to hasten one's breaking of the fast (*iftar*) as soon as the sun sets.[3]

Much of the *fiqh* information on the recommendable in foodstuffs and drinks also relate to mannerism, supplication and thanksgiving, and the use or otherwise of certain utensils. Thus, it is known that the Prophet usually started his meal with the supplication "All praise and thanks be to God who has satisfied our needs and quenched our thirst. His favors cannot be compensated for nor denied."[4] He recommended the same after eating, and advised those who forgot to say it at the outset to say it anytime during the meal. Whatever the Prophet has practiced or recommended would thus be *mandub*.

Reports indicate that the Prophet used to wash his hands before and after taking a meal, and that he took his meal while sitting and started taking food with his right hand. He has also instructed that one should take food which is nearest to where one is seated first, and that one who eats with the hand should also take food from the near side of the dish and not the middle. He has further advised against blowing on the food, as this could taint the food with traces of saliva and unpleasant breath. He used to drink while sitting, which is the recommended position, although he has on certain occasions been seen to drink water in the standing position. He has similarly advised against drinking directly from the pitcher, which would be reprehensible, for evidently hygienic reasons.

Hadith reports further indicate that the Prophet strongly discouraged the use of gold and silver utensils, in his quest, presumably, of modesty and

---

2. Hadith reports also mention a special variety of dates, known as *'ajwah*, that the Prophet liked most and spoke well of its nutritional value. For details of hadith reports on this and other food items, see Awang, "*Istihalah*," 72–73, also www.mdcpublishers.com.

3. Cf. Wizarat, *al-Mawsu'ah al-Fiqhiyyah*, vol. 6, 127.

4. Hadith reported by al-Bukhari on the authority of Abu Umaimah, quoted in Wizarat, *al-Mawsu'ah al-Fiqhiyyah*, vol. 6, 70.

avoidance of vainglory and extravagance. Gold and silver were declared units of value and were consequently used as currency in those days.[5]

Furthermore, the Prophet has advised on the etiquette of eating, stating that one who eats may say a word of praise about what is taken, but to restrain from making derogatory remarks such as "it is too salty," "sour," "not fresh," "not well cooked," and the like (this last may arguably not apply to commercially supplied food such as one takes in restaurants). Thus, it is reported on the authority of Abu Hurayrah that he never heard the Prophet making a derogatory remark about the food he ate. If he liked it, he took it, or else left it if he didn't, but that the context for all this was permissible food.

As for the forbidden food varieties, the Prophet has been heard on many occasions to have denounced it and discouraged others from eating it.[6] It is further recommendable, on the authority of hadith, for the host to take food together with his guests, and for the latter to take of the food that is presented, even if they had to open a supererogatory fast for the purpose. For the host goes into the effort of preparing food for the guests, and it is for the latter to show appreciation by eating from it.[7] Further, on the authority of hadith, it is recommendable for the host to treat all the guests present equally in serving them, even if some of them might be of a superior status than others. To do the opposite would thus be reprehensible (*makruh*).[8]

5. For details, see Wizarat, *al-Mawsuʿah al-Fiqhiyyah,* vol. 6, 70–71.

6. Wizarat, *al-Mawsuʿah al-Fiqhiyyah,* vol. 6, 123.

7. Wizarat, *al-Mawsuʿah al-Fiqhiyyah,* vol. 6, 117–118.

8. Wizarat, *al-Mawsuʿah al-Fiqhiyyah,* vol. 6, 122.

# 12

# Requirements of a Valid Slaughter

THE RITUALS OF a valid slaughter and its accompanying requirements of sanitation and cleanliness are fairly well known to the halal industry, and mostly correspond with the prevailing practices of many majority Muslim countries. Although some of these may be different in certain details, they are generally deemed to be compliant with the shariah guidelines. The scriptural rationale of slaughtering is that God Most High has permitted only pure and clean food (*al-tayyibat*; al-Ma'idah, 5:4) and animals do not become *tayyib* without the exit of blood which is shed forth in the way He has shown, that is by way of a valid slaughter (*dhabh*). From a scientific viewpoint also, it is often stated that draining of blood is necessary because blood carries pathogens that could harm human health. Theology and science would thus appear to stand in harmony on this aspect of halal slaughter.[1] This may also explain why death by strangulation of an animal, when it falls to its death from a great height, or when it is gored by other predatory animals it has been declared non-halal, due partly to uncertainty over the draining of blood. A valid slaughter begins with the recitation of God's name, which differentiates it from the way predatory animals treat their feed.[2]

What follows next expounds in some detail the shariah requirements of a valid slaughter, which is followed, in turn, by an attempt to identify that which is deemed recommendable (*mandub*), as opposed to what may constitute the reprehensible (*makruh*) in halal slaughter

---

1. Cf. Ahmed, "Understanding What Is Permissible," 20.

2. Cf. Wizarat, *al-Mawsu'ah al-Fiqhiyyah*, vol. 21, 177.

*Shariah and The Halal Industry.* Mohammad Hashim Kamali, Oxford University Press. © Oxford University Press 2021.
DOI: 10.1093/oso/9780197538616.003.0013

practices. To begin with, the basic requirements of a valid slaughter are as follows:

1. The element of intention (*niyyah*): The majority of Muslim jurists, including the Shia Imamiyyah, have held that a lawful slaughter occurs only when it is with the intention of a valid use, and not merely to kill an animal for the sake of killing or for fun. Intention as such is held to be an obligatory aspect of the halal slaughter. Hence, a slaughter without such an intention is non-halal. A minority view is also recorded to say that *niyyah* is not obligatory, on the analysis that slaughter is a rational act, not an act of worship, and the purpose is to kill an animal (not a fit subject for a *niyyah* as such), and that this purpose can also be achieved without the *niyyah*. The majority view that holds the *niyyah* to be obligatory is based on the view that slaughter is part of a devotional act, or *'ibadah*, and its validity is therefore contingent on a *niyyah*.[3] What *niyyah* means to the majority is a state of mind espoused by the belief that the slaughtered animal is made halal for eating through *tadhkiyah* (purification) by means of a valid slaughter. Those who maintain the view that the slaughter of the Ahl al-Kitab is not valid make the same point to say that they do not subscribe to this belief.[4] When a person slaughters an animal through forgetfulness or mistake concerning the identity of the animal, or had doubts about whether or not to slaughter it, if the person had cut the major veins without a *niyyah*, the slaughter is invalid. The same applies when someone drops a sharp knife by accident and cuts the veins of the animal without intending a ritual slaughter.[5] Whereas Imam Malik has proscribed slaughter by the drunk and the insane, Imam Shafi'i has permitted it, along with the majority. The difference of opinion on this matter relates to the question of *niyyah*. Those who maintain that *niyyah* is a precondition of a valid slaughter hold that the child, the insane, and the drunken are not capable of a valid *niyyah*; but those who say that *niyyah* is not a precondition of slaughter allow the same.[6]

2. Reciting the name of God Most High or *tasmiyah*[7] at the time of slaughter is obligatory (*wajib*) according to the majority of leading schools, including

---

3. al-Qurtubi, *Bidayat al-Mujtahid*, vol. 1, 329.

4. al-Qurtubi, *Bidayat al-Mujtahid*, vol. 1, 330–331.

5. al-Qurtubi, *Bidayat al-Mujtahid*, vol. 1, 328; al-Zuhayli, *al-Fiqh al-Islami*, vol. 3, 658–659; Fadlullah, *Islamic Rulings*, 294.

6. al-Qurtubi, *Bidayat al-Mujtahid*, vol. 1, 331. See also Ibn Qudamah, *al-Mughni*, vol. 13, 64.

7. *Tasmiyah* is the abbreviation of the Arabic phrase "*Bismillah al-Rahman al-Rahim*" (in the name of God, the beneficent, the merciful).

the Shia Imamiyyah and the Zahiris, whereas the Shafi'is consider it to be *sunnah mu'akkadah* (emphatic *sunnah*—that which the Prophet has regularly practiced), adherence to which is highly recommended and abandoning it is reprehensible. All schools would, on the other hand, exonerate from these requirements the case of genuine forgetfulness without intentional preclusion,[8] or when the person who slaughters is dumb and unable to recite, or acts under duress. The majority position is based on the authority of a clear Qur'anic verse addressing the believers to "eat not that on which God's name has not been mentioned" (al-An'am, 6:121; al-Ma'idah, 5:3). The Shia Imamiyyah are emphatic on the requirement of *tasmiyah*, but like the majority exonerate omission due to forgetfulness or ignorance, adding the proviso, however, that *tasmiyah* must be recited whenever the person remembers it or else it may be recited at the time of eating. If one who deliberately leaves out *tasmiyah*, the slaughter is non-halal.[9] *Tasmiyah* is also permissible, according to both the Sunni and Shia schools of law, for one who is in a state of impurity (*junub*—following sexual intercourse), and for a menstruating woman.[10] Recital of *tasmiyah* only once is sufficient when slaughtering a number of animals, mechanically for instance, at exactly the same time. However, if *tasmiyah* is left out deliberately or when the name of other deities is cited, the slaughter becomes invalid and forbidden to eat for Muslims. It is noteworthy that the Qur'an stipulated *tasmiyah* for slaughter, in contrast to the pre-Islamic Arabian practice of reciting the names of ancient deities. It is also instructive to note that humankind is not naturally entitled to take the life of an animal unless it is with the permission of the Creator, and *tasmiyah* is an affirmation and acknowledgement of that.[11]

*Tasmiyah* is accomplished, according to the majority of the leading schools, including the Shia Imamiyyah, by reciting the illustrious name of God, and it is recommendable to add a form of praise, such as "Allahu

---

8. The reason for this is the renowned hadith "my *ummah* is exonerated for [for what they do] duo to mistake, forgetfulness and duress." Also quoted by al-Qurtubi, *Bidayat al-Mujtahid*, vol. 1, 328.

9. al-Tabarsi, *Mustadrak*, vol. 16, 138–139.

10. Ibn Qudamah, *al-Sharh al-Kabir*, Cairo: Dar al-Hadith, 1425/2004, vol. 13, 69. This is because *tasmiyah* may be uttered by a person in a state of impurity, even by an unbeliever, and impurity (*janabah*) is not a greater enormity than disbelief. See also al-Tabarsi, *Mustadrak al-Wasa'il*, vol. 16, 139.

11. al-Zuhayli, *al-Fiqh al-Islami*, vol. 3, 659. Fadlullah, *Islamic Rulings*, 294.

Akbar" (God is Greatest) after *tasmiyah* and the like. That said, reciting the name of Allah is sufficient without any addition.[12] Reliable reports indicate that when slaughtering, the Prophet would utter the full phrase "*bismillah-i Allahu Akbar*." Arabic phrasing is recommended, but the purpose is to recite God's illustrious name, and Arabic equivalents in other languages are also acceptable.[13]

It is noted that the idolators of pre-Islamic Arabia used to recite the names of their idols, such as Al-lat, al-Manat, or al-'Uza, when they slaughtered. This was unacceptable to the monotheistic beliefs of Islam, where devotion and worship is to be for God the Most High alone. Hence the prohibition in Muslim slaughter of reciting any other name than that of God is on purely theological grounds, which is to preserve the integrity of *tawhid* (belief in divine oneness) and the purity of Islamic faith.[14] Similarly, slaughter that is carried out in the name of a king, a great leader, or an arriving traveler becomes non-halal unless it be by way of expression of gratitude to God for a particular favor and a clear *niyyah* to that effect. It is reported that the people of Bukhara have passed a *fatwa* that it is *haram* to slaughter an animal for a sultan in order to seek closeness to him.[15]

3. Animal slaughter by atheists who do not believe in God, and more specifically the associators (*mushrikun*) and idol worshippers (*'abadat al-awthan*), is invalid based on Qur'anic verses (al-Ma'idah 5:3; al-An'am, 6:121). This is also the position with regard to apostates who have renounced Islam, and non-Muslims who are not followers of a revealed scripture. Slaughter by an apostate who has renounced Islam is not recognized, even if the person converts to a monotheistic religion, such as Christianity or Judaism.[16]

There is general agreement on the foregoing, but Muslim schools and scholars have recorded divergent views on the validity of slaughter by

---

12. Fadlullah, *Islamic Rulings*, 294. See also Fadlullah, *Islamic Lanterns*, 315, 317.

13. However, if someone merely say "O Allah grant me blessing/forgiveness—Allahumma ighfir li" or merely mentions "salam" this is not enough. See Ibn Qudamah, *al-Mughni*, vol. 13, 68.

14. Cf. al-Qaradawi, *al-Halal wa'l-Haram*, 45.

15. Cf. Wizarat, *al-Mawsu'ah al-Fiqhiyyah*, vol. 21, 194. See also 'Assaf, *al-Halal wa'l-Haram*, 285.

16. al-Jaziri, *al-Fiqh 'ala'l-Madhahib*, 404; al-Qaradawi, *al-Halal wa'l-Haram*, 61–62; Fadlullah, *Islamic Rulings*, 294.

Magians and Sabians, as well as women, children, the insane, the drunken, thieves, and usurpers. Since theft and usurpation of an animal that belongs to another person is forbidden, does it then follow that the thief's slaughter is also *haram*? The majority have responded that valid ownership is not a precondition of halal slaughter/*tadhkiyah*. Ibn Wahab from the Maliki school has added the information, as recorded in al-Muwatta of Imam Malik, that it is *makruh* based on a hadith report in which the Prophet was asked about a sheep that was slaughtered without the permission of its owner, and the Prophet said in response to "feed the prisoners with it."[17]

The Shia Imamiyyah also maintain that attaining the age of majority is not a requirement so long as the person has reached the age of discernment (*mumayyiz*) and pronounces *tasmiyah*. Slaughter by women is also valid, although Imam Ja'far al-Sadiq has added it is preferable that when a man is available that he slaughters, but otherwise a woman's slaughter is valid. The same permissive position is extended to a eunuch and a blind person if the blind person is confident enough to handle the slaughter.[18]

4. Ritual slaughter is allowed by a person who is follower of a revealed scripture, including Christians and Jews. The Qur'an has affirmed in an address to the Muslims that "the food of the *ahl al-kitab* is halal for you (al-Ma'idah, 5:5).[19] The key word in this verse, namely *ta'am*, literally means food of all kind that sustains the body, and includes animal food as well as plant food, such as wheat, barley, dates, and rice. It is noted, however, that for the people of Hijaz (Mecca and Medina) and Iraq of earlier times, *ta'am* only meant types of wheat, despite the fact that the Qur'an applies it more widely to include seafood, as in the verse "permissible to you is the game of the sea and its food (*ta'amuh*)." Muslim jurists have used *ta'am*, and its plural *at'imah*, to mean all that is eaten or drunk, except for that which intoxicates. Drinks that intoxicate are referred to as *ashribah*. So, unlike the earlier specifications over the meaning of *ta'am*, Muslim jurists use the word in its generic sense—inclusive, that is, of plant and animal

17. al-Qurtubi, *Bidayat al-Mujtahid*, vol. 1, 331–332; Wizarat, *al-Mawsu'ah al-Fiqhiyyah*, vol. 21, 184.

18. al-Tabarsi, *Mustadrak*, vol.16, 144–145.

19. For details, see al-Qaradawi, *al-Halal wa'l-Haram*, 61; al-Zuhayli, *al-Fiqh al-Islami*, vol. 3, 659; al-Jaziri, *al-Fiqh 'ala'l-Madhahib*, 406.

food, rice, milk, etc.[20] The Ja'fari Shia have recorded the same information but also add a report that Imam Ja'far al-Sadiq has specified *ta'am* to grains and pulses (*al-hubub*), thus excluding slaughtered animals.[21] As our review elsewhere in this book shows, later juristic opinion does not confine *ta'am* to grains and pulses.

The renowned Companion Ibn 'Abbas has gone on record to say that *ta'amuhum* in reference to People of the Book in the foregoing verse means their slaughter, a meaning that is also upheld by many Companions as well as the imams Malik and Shafi'i. They also concur to the effect that the upright and the sinner (ones convicted of adultery, slander, and drinking) among Muslims and the Ahl al-Kitab are all equal in this regard. The same is said about the *dhimmi* (non-Muslim citizen) and the *harbi* (citizen of enemy state) of the People of the Book—that their slaughter is deemed valid.[22] It is further stated that "when a Christian slaughters in the name of Jesus, it is still lawful for us" to consume.[23] The food and slaughter of the Ahl al-Kitab is therefore halal to Muslims generally, even if they omit the *tasmiyah*, or even if they recite the name of Jesus or Moses. Some Muslim jurists have disputed this position, but since the Qur'anic permission is conveyed in unqualified terms, it is halal for Muslims to consume their food and their slaughter.

The Shafi'is are alone in their additional stipulation regarding the identity of Ahl al-Kitab: the Ahl al-Kitab status of Jews and Christians is confirmed only when it is not known that their ancestors converted after the abrogation of their scripture. Hence, if it is known that the ancestor of a Jew embraced Judaism after the advent of Christianity and Prophet Jesus, his slaughter is non-halal. Similarly, if it is known that the ancestor of a Christian embraced Christianity after the advent of Islam and Prophet Muhammad, his slaughter would be non-halal. For embracing those religions after their replacement by the subsequent revelation is equivalent to apostasy and unacceptable.

Ibn Taymiyyah has said, and rightly so perhaps, concerning the Shafi'i position, that the religious identity of a person, whether a person is a Kitabi or non-Kitabi, is determined by affirmation of the person himself, not by

20. For details, see Wizarat, *al-Mawsu'ah al-Fiqhiyyah*, vol. 13, 263–264.

21. al-Tabarsi, *Mustadrak*, vol. 16, 198.

22. Ibn Qudamah, *al-Mughni*, vol. 13, 57.

23. Ibn Qudamah, *al-Mughni*, vol. 13, 65.

reference to his ancestors. If a person follows Christianity or Judaism and confirms his status as such, that is sufficient to ascertain his status.[24]

While some authors have written that the Ja'fari Shia hold slaughter by the People of the Book to be forbidden, Fadlollah wrote the following: "[A]s for the People of the Book (Jews and Christians) are concerned, their slaughtered animals are allowed but with carrying out *tesmiyeh*, although avoiding it is better."[25] The majority position of the Shia on this is based on a report from their sixth Imam, Ja'far al-Sadiq, who said, with reference to the slaughter of the People of the Book, "do not eat their slaughter." The main reason given is that they do not mention the name of Allah on their slaughter, and that even if they do mention God's name, they probably mean their own deities. Reports further add that a man queried Ja'far al-Sadiq on this while reciting the above-quoted Qur'anic verse (al-Ma'idah, 5:5), which clearly permits the food (*ta'am*) of the People of the Book. "What would you say to this then?" asked the man, to which Ja'far al-Sadiq reportedly replied that "this is with regard to grains and pulses (*al-hubub*) and the like."[26] The Shia position is evidently divided on the subject.

Juristic disagreement has also arisen with regard to the offspring of a couple, one of whom is a Kitabi and the other a non-Kitabi, and over the question of whether the slaughter of such a person is halal. The Hanafi and Hanbali schools presume the person to be a Kitabi and that the slaughter is also halal, regardless as to which of the parents was a Kitabi. The Malikis have held that the status of the offspring is determined by the religion of his or her father through a valid marriage. The Shafi'is hold that the slaughter of a person of mixed parentage is non-halal.[27]

5. According to general consensus of the leading schools of Islamic law, severance is required of the four vital passages in the slaughter of animals, namely the trachea,[28] the esophagus,[29] and the carotid arteries and jugular

---

24. For details, see Wizarat, *al-Mawsu'ah al-Fiqhiyyah*, vol. 21, 184–185.

25. Fadlullah, *Fiqh al-At'imah*, 294.

26. For details, see al-Tabarsi, *Mustadrak al-Wasa'il*, vol. 16, 146–147; see also Burj, *Ahkam al-Dhabh*, 37f.

27. For a summary of the scholastic views, see Wizarat, *al-Mawsu'ah al-Fiqhiyyah*, vol. 21, 186.

28. The trachea (*halqum*, or respiratory tract) is a tube-like structure that connects the voice box (larynx) with the bronchial parts of the lungs.

29. The esophagus (*mari'*) is a tube like-structure that connects the throat (pharynx) with the stomach.

veins,[30] to hasten the bleeding and death of the slaughtered animal. Minor disagreements have arisen to the effect that slaughter occurs even if the esophagus is not cut, and even if the trachea is not cut, provided that the two main arteries are. Whereas Imam Abu Hanifah records the view that three of the four passages must be severed, inclusive always of the two main arteries, his disciple al-Shaybani holds that all four must be cut. The reason for such differences is the absence of a clear text on the subject, and the information in the hadith seems to be emphatic on the severance of the two main arteries but less than specific on the other two passages. It is recommended to sever the four passages all at once.[31] Slaughtering by hand is not a requirement, hence it may be by operating an instrument or machine that achieves the purpose swiftly, provided that the other requirements of a valid slaughter are duly fulfilled.[32]

When slaughter becomes confused with death by other means such that it becomes unknown whether the bird or animal died of slaughter or drowning, for instance, it becomes non-halal on the authority of a hadith narrated by 'Adi b. Hatam, which states that "if it (the bird) falls into water, do not eat it—*wa in waqa'at fi'l-ma' fala ta'kul*." The Prominent Companion 'Abd Allah Ibn Mas'ud has confirmed this and added that the combination presents a situation of halal and *haram* coming together, and that the latter prevails. Thus, if a bird is shot and falls into water and then dies there, it becomes non-halal. [33]

Except for the camel (which requires *nahr*, or stabbing with a weapon in the lower part of the throat closer to the chest in a standing position, with the front left leg tied up), all other animals should rest on the left side with their heads lifted upward. *Nahr* is authorized in the Qur'anic verse "so turn to thy Lord in prayer and sacrifice-*wa'n– har*," referring to a camel (al-Kawthar, 108:2). Muslim scholars have thus generally agreed that *nahr* is recommendable (*mandub*) in the case of camels, whereas slaughter is enjoined for all other animals. For it is provided in another verse, "And remember Moses said to his

---

30. Jugular veins (*wadajain*) refer to carotid arteries—blood vessels that carry oxygenated blood from the heart to the tissues, and jugular veins that carries de-oxygenated blood from tissues back to the heart.

31. al-Qurtubi, *Bidayat al-Mujtahid*, vol. 1, 326; al-Jaziri, *al-Fiqh 'ala'l-Madhahib*, 406; Ibn Qudamah, *al-Mughni*, vol. 13, 54.

32. 'Assaf, *al-Halal wa'l-Haram*, 283.

33. For details, and also the hadith at issue, see Ibn Qudamah, *al-Mughni*, vol. 13, 73.

people: God commands that you sacrifice [by slaughtering—*an tadhbahu*] a heifer" (al-Baqarah, 2:67), In yet another verse, the text refers to the slaughter of a sheep with the word *dhabh* (al-Saffat, 37:107). The first verse on the sacrifice of camels employ *nahr*, whereas the second verse, referring to the heifer, and the third, referring to sheep, clearly use *dhabh*.[34] The Imams Abu Hanifah, al-Shafi'i, Malik, and many prominent figures among the Companions have concluded from these verses (especially the phrase "God commands you— *innallaha ya'murukum*" in the second verse) that the camel's slaughter is permissible only by way of *nahr* and all other animals and birds by way of *dhabh*, and that this order may not be reversed so as to apply *dhabh* to camels and *nahr* to other animals. Then it is added that the Prophet has followed the Qur'anic specifications and changing them is not permissible—although a minority opinion maintains that reversing the order is *makruh* but does not make the animal non-halal for consumption.[35] This view also quotes in support the general import of a generally agreed upon hadith (*muttafaqun 'alayh*), wherein the Prophet is quoted to have said that "when the blood (of an animal) is shed forth and God's name is mentioned, you may eat it."[36] It is not a valid slaughter to drain the blood of an animal separately with an instrument and then slaughter it without knowing whether it was actually alive. Hence, it would be non-halal.[37]

6. Immediacy and swiftness are requirements of slaughter, according to the majority opinion. If the slaughterer lifts his hand before completing the slaughter but returns immediately to complete it, it is still valid, but not if the interval is longer. This is the majority view. Among the Maliki

---

34. Ibn Qudamah, *al-Mughni*, vol. 13, 54; Burj, *Ahkam al-Dhabh*, 11. More specifically, *nahr* is done by inserting a sharp tool in the place called *lobbeh*, which is the hollow space at the top of the chest attached to the neck, regardless as to whether the camel (and also giraffe) are in a standing position, kneeling, or lying on its side, although it is better when done in the standing position. Cf. Fadlullah, *Islamic Rulings*, 295.

35. Ibn Qudamah, *al-Mughni*, vol. 13, 56; al-Qurtubi, *Bidayat al-Mujtahid*, vol. 1, 325. The minority view also cites a hadith, as Ibn Qudamah quotes it on the same page, from Aishah that the Prophet did *nahr* on a bull on the occasion of Farewell Pilgrimage (this is labeled as actual hadith, or sunnah *fi'liyyah*, that ranks below verbal hadith, or Sunnah *qawliyyah*). Hence, *nahr* of an animal other than the camel does not make it unlawful for consumption, but goes against mainstream practice and precedent, and according to some is *makruh* to eat, although it is permissible when necessity dictates such.

36. al-Bukhari, vol. 7, 92, hadith no. 5503—and quoted in al-Qurtubi, vol. 1, 325; and Ibn Qudamah, *al-Mughni*, vol. 13, 14.

37. al-Zuhayli, *al-Fiqh al-Islami*, vol. 3, 680.

scholars, Sahnun (d. 240/845) has held that any disruption in the act of slaughter makes the it unlawful for consumption. Ibn Habib (d. 238H/ 853), another Maliki jurist is critical of Sahnun's view and thinks that it would have been best to say that any disruption in the immediacy of slaughter is reprehensible. If the slaughterer lifts his hand thinking that he has finished the slaughter but only then realizes that it is not so and returns to finish it, it is still lawful. The Hanafis consider immediacy in cutting the vital passages recommendable and delay in it reprehensible.[38]

7. Women are qualified to carry out a valid slaughter in the same way as men. This is the majority (jumhur) position, including that of Imam Malik, based on the authority of a hadith reviewed below. Contrary to some claims that it is makruh in the Maliki school, the leading Maliki scholar Ibn Rushd al-Qurtubi writes that it is not makruh and that this is also the position of Imam Malik. The majority position on this is based on two separate hadith reports, one narrated by Mu'adh bin Saeed and the other by Jabir bin 'Abdullah, to the effect that the Prophet validated slaughter by a woman and by a [discerning] child (sabi mumayyiz) when they uttered the tasmiyah. Additionally, since the Prophet has not qualified the woman as such, she may be Muslim, Christian, or Jewish—all are qualified. Ibn Qudamah has concurred and also quoted two hadith reports on the subject, one of which is generally agreed upon (mutta-faqun 'alayh) to the effect that a woman, a slave girl of Ka'b bin Malik, was tending to a flock of cattle and noted that one of the sheep had fallen, and that she rushed to slaughter it with a sharp stone. The Prophet was asked about it and he said "you may eat it." Ibn Qudamah has drawn several conclusions from this hadith, including (1) a woman's slaughter is valid; (2) the woman may be a freewoman or slave; (3) her slaughter is valid even if she is in the state of menstruation, as the Prophet did not specify the permissive position in any way; (4) the permissibility of slaughter with a stone; (5) the slaughter of an animal feared to die; and (6) permissibility of slaughter by one who does not own the animal.[39] The man or the woman who slaughters may furthermore be in a state of impurity (jenabah or menstruation). To this it is further added by way

---

38. al-Qurtubi, Bidayat al-Mujtahid, vol. 1, 327; al-Jaziri, al-Fiqh 'ala'l-Madhahib, 406; al-Zuhayli, al-Fiqh al-Islami, vol. 3, 658; Burj, Ahkam al-Dhabh, 118.

39. Ibn Qudamah, al-Mughni, vol. 13, 65–66, al-Qurtubi, Bidayat al-Mujtahid, vol. 1, 331.

of recommendation that the said person may, however, wash his or her hands and face just before the slaughter, although this is not strictly a requirement.[40]

The slaughtered animal must also fulfill the following four conditions:

a. it is alive at the time of slaughter;
b. it died as a direct result of the slaughter;
c. it is not a hunted game in the precinct of the sacred mosque of Kaʿbah; and finally, which is a Maliki stipulation;
d. that slaughter (*dhabh*) and stabbing (*nahr*) are not confused with one another.

As for the first condition, the Shafiʿi and Hanbali schools stipulate that the animal is alive prior to slaughter with a degree of certainty, termed as "ascertained life" (*al-hayat al-mustaqirrah*). This is said to exist when, upon slaughtering, the animal moves violently or blood spurts out of it. This is especially important in cases of animals that might have suffered severe blows, strangulation, and the like, which render them lifeless and it becomes uncertain whether they died of these causes or from slaughtering. Abu Yusuf of the Hanafi school has stated in this connection that if it is certain that the animal will live if not slaughtered, and it is not in the actual process of dying, then *hayat mustaqirrah* exists. But if the animal is on its last breath, as it were, and it is then slaughtered, it would be non-halal. The Maliki school maintains similar views as those of Abu Yusuf.[41] Imam Abu Hanifah himself has held, however, that so long as the animal is alive and life is ascertained in any measure, weak or strong, it is sufficient and the slaughter is valid. When the animal is known to be alive prior to slaughter, in other words, it is not necessary to establish whether it moves violently after slaughter or blood spurts out of it, provided it is not known that the animal had suffered from lethal causes (strangulation and the like). Abu Hanifah added further that movement which is indicative of life is one that is noted prior to slaughter, not necessarily after it, and so long as the slaughter leads to a normal flow of

---

40. al-Qurtubi, *Bidayat al-Mujtahid*, vol. 1, 331; Abu Zayd, *Al-Intifaʾ bil Aʿyan al-Muharramah*, 52–53; Burj, *Ahkam al-Dhabh*, 57–58. Al-Bukhari cites the hadith (in *kitab al-Dhabaʾih waʾl-sayd, bab zabihat al-marʾah*), and so does al-Qurtubi, and Abu Zayd Jumanah.

41. Wizarat, *al-Mawsuʿah al-Fiqhiyyah*, vol. 21, 180.

blood—that should also be sufficient.[42] The substance of these views tends to be particularly relevant in the context of electrical stunning, which tends to give rise to questions regarding the existence or otherwise of *hayat mustaqir-rah*. This is the subject of a separate section of this volume in the chapter on "Islam and Science."

There is little disagreement on the second condition that the animal dies due to slaughter and not another cause. Thus, if someone cuts an animal in two and another person slaughters it, it is non-halal.[43]

As for the third condition that the slaughtered animal is not a game animal in the actual precinct of the sacred mosque of Ka'bah, this is due to the clear text where God Most High says in the Qur'an that He has made the mosque of Ka'bah "a sacred sanctuary," and that no hunting is permitted and no blood is shed thereby (al-'Ankabut, 29:68), and then says in another address, "O believers! Kill not the game while in the Sacred Precinct or in the pilgrims' garb" (al-Ma'idah, 5:95).[44] Hence hunting and the slaughter of animals and birds in the sacred mosque of Ka'bah is non-halal and equivalent to carrion regardless of whether the slaughterer is performing the haj or otherwise.[45] As for the fourth condition that slaughter (*dhabh*) is not substituted by stabbing (*nahr*), this is a Maliki stipulation. The other leading schools consider this to be reprehensible (*makruh*) and the slaughter is therefore still valid.[46]

The following slaughter practices are recommended (*mandub*):

- Recitation of both *tasmiyah* and the phrase "God is Greatest"—that is, *Allahu Akbar*—the latter of which is known for short as *takbir*, especially according to the Shafi'i school. The majority hold that *tasmiyah* is obligatory (*wajib*).
- Completion of slaughter in daylight so as to prevent error in its correct procedures, especially as the four passages that need to be cut may not be as visible during the night. Added to this is the point that nighttime is for

42. al-Kasani, *Bada'i' al-Sana'i'*, vol. 5, 50; Muhammad Amin, *Hashiyah Radd al-Mukhtar*, vol. 5, 187; Wizarat, *al-Mawsu'ah al-Fiqhiyyah*, vol. 21, 181–182.

43. Wizarat, *al-Mawsu'ah al-Fiqhiyyah*, vol. 21, 182.

44. These verses are specific on hunting in the precincts of Ka'bah. Outside this context a person in a state of *ihram* for *hajj* is therefore allowed to slaughter domestic birds and animals and there is general consensus on this. For details, see Wizarat, *al-Mawsu'ah al-Fiqhiyyah*, vol. 21, 189.

45. Wizarat, *al-Mawsu'ah al-Fiqhiyyah*, vol. 5, 183.

46. Wizarat, *al-Mawsu'ah al-Fiqhiyyah*, vol. 5, 183.

tranquility and rest, and slaughter may be even more painful to the animal at night.

- Facing the *qiblah* toward Mecca is generally recommended, although the issue has invoked different views. Some have gone on record to say that facing the *qiblah* is permissible (*mubah*) only, still others maintain that it is obligatory. According to yet another opinion, facing the *qiblah* for slaughter is reprehensible (*makruh*). Al-Qurtubi, who records all these views, comments that this is rather a rare situation in that one hardly finds contrasting positions of this type in the shariah. The normative position under the Maliki school is that of permissibility (*ibahah*), on the analysis that except for the ritual prayer/*salah*, facing the *qiblah* is not a requirement even in some forms of worship (*ibadat*), except for *salah*, and drawing a parallel between slaughter and *salah* is rather far-fetched—and so is drawing an analogy between this and the position of a deceased person during the funeral prayer. The majority position on this is based on reports that when the Prophet offered animal sacrifice (*adhiyah*), he would face the *qiblah*, and that the Companions followed suit.[47]

For the Shia Imamiyyah, facing the Ka'bah at the time of slaughter is mandatory. However, when a Sunni follower who does not believe that it is a necessary condition to face the animal toward the Ka'bah, and "carries out the slaughter without directing the animal, with neither its slaughtering point (the neck) nor its front (facing toward the Ka'bah), it is [still] allowed for us to eat from this animal."[48] In a report from Imam Ja'far, he is quoted to have said, "When you decide to slaughter an animal, then avoid torturing it, and avoid slashing or cutting any part [of its body]; sharpen the blade you use, and face the *qiblah* until it dies." In another question he was asked whether it was permissible to slaughter the animal while it is standing; he replied, "This is not acceptable. The Sunnah is to lie the animal on one side while also facing the *qiblah*."[49] If an animal is slaughtered not facing the *qiblah* due to ignorance or forgetfulness, the slaughter is still halal for consumption. If not facing the *qiblah* is deliberate, the person has

---

47. al-Qurtubi, *Bidayat al-Mujtahid*, vol. 1, 329; Burj, *Ahkam al-Dhabh*, 119.

48. Fadlullah, *Islamic Lanterns*, 316.

49. As quoted in al-Tabarsi, *Mustadrak al-Wasa'il*, vol. 16, 132.

sinned, and it is preferable not to consume that slaughter, provided that violating the Sunnah is intentional.[50]

Regarding clemency to the animal and avoidance of rough handling,[51] according to a hadith Muslim al-Nishapuri has recorded on the subject, the Prophet has said:

> God has prescribed the doing of good (al-ihsan) in all things. So when you have to kill, do it in a good way, and when you slaughter, do it in a good way. You must sharpen the tool of slaughter and make the slaughter animal comfortable.[52]

The ihsan in slaughter also means that one animal does not see another being slaughtered; and then again that the slaughter knife should not be sharpened in front of the animal, and also that the animal is not handled roughly. When selecting animals for slaughter, it is advisable not to select productive animals that give much milk and other useful yields. This is also the subject of a hadith, wherein the Prophet instructed his Ansari host who praised God for being honored with hosting the Prophet. The host was about to slaughter a sheep of his to make a meal for the Prophet, and the Prophet told him to "avoid the milky ones—iyyaka wa'l-halub."[53] Al-Qaradawi, who quoted this hadith, comments that the public interest aspect is also a consideration in animal husbandry and choice of livestock for slaughter, in the event, that is, when less productive animals are also available.[54] Care for animal health is also the subject of another hadith instruction wherein the Prophet is reported to have said, in a hadith that all major hadith collections have recorded, that animal owners and those in charge of their upkeep "do not make the healthy livestock [drink] the leftover [water] of a sick one—la yuridanna mumrid 'ala musih."

> This was particularly addressed to camel owners when taking the animals for watering—that a sick animal should not be positioned such

---

50. As quoted in al-Tabarsi, Mustadrak al-Wasa'il, vol. 16, 118.

51. al-Qurtubi, Bidayat al-Mujtahid, vol. 1, 325f; al-Zuhayli, al-Fiqh al-Islami, vol. 3, 661–663.

52. Hadith on the authority of Shaddad bin Aws. Also cited in Ibn Qudamah, al-Mughni, vol. 13, 54; al-Qaradawi, al-Halal wa'l-Haram, 59. Fadlullah, Islamic Rulings, 294.

53. al-Mundhiri, Mukhtasar Sahih Muslim, 350–351, hadith no. 1306.

54. al-Qaradawi, Dawr al-Qiyam, 165.

that the healthy one drinks water that comes from the direction of the sick one. They should instead be separated for fear of spreading disease.[55]

It is further reported in this connection that the second caliph 'Umar b. al-Khattab saw a person dragging an animal he was about to slaughter. The caliph scolded him and asked him to treat the animal well. According to another report, 'Umar saw a person mistreating a sheep he was about to slaughter; the person put his foot on the face of the animal while he was sharpening the knife. The caliph punished him for this with lashes of the whip.[56] Al-Tirmidhi and al-Hakim have also recorded the report that pre-Islamic Arabs practiced mutilation of the hump of the camel and the fat tail of the sheep while alive. The Prophet emphatically prohibited this cruel practice and said, "There is to be no mutilation of animals while still alive; anyone who consumes a mutilated part is like taking a non-halal carcass."[57] The Shia Imamiyyah is in agreement with the majority position on the principles of clemency and *ihsan* to animals. Thus it is recommended that before slaughtering, the animal is treated in a way that saves it from harm and torture, mutilation of body parts, and also that it does not see the blade being sharpened, nor should the animal be exposed to other acts that discomfort it.[58] It is further stated that the tool of slaughter should be sharp but that it be lawfully owned—a stolen knife or one that is acquired through usurpation would thus not meet the requirements of a valid slaughter.[59] Al-Tabarsi has recorded a directive from Imam 'Ali ibn Abi Talib, who said, "Be gentle with the animal you slaughter, and avoid rough handling before and after the slaughter."[60]

Offering drinking water to the animal prior to slaughtering is also recommended.

Richard Foltz draws the following conclusions from his own review of the evidence on slaughter done the Islamic way: "First, the tradition

---

55. Hadith also quoted in al-Qaradawi, *Dawr al-Qiyam*, 165.

56. Hadith recorded by al-Bayhaqi and cited in al-Zuhayli, *al-Fiqh al-Islami*, vol. 3, 663.

57. Cited in al-Qaradawi, *al-Halal wa'l-Haram*, 59.

58. Fadlullah, *Islamic Rulings*, 298; Fadlullah, *Islamic Lanterns*, 250.

59. Ibn Qudamah, *al-Mughni*, vol. 13, 61.

60. al-Tabarsi, *Mustadrak al-Wasa'il*, vol. 16, 132, sec. 19371.

takes the relationship between humans and other animal species quite seriously. Second, animals are seen as having feelings and interests of their own. And third, the overriding ethos enjoined upon humans is one of compassionate consideration."[61]

The following are considered reprehensible (*makruh*) in the slaughter rituals:

- Slaughter by a disabled person.
- Abandoning the *tasmiyah* according to those who do not consider it obligatory, namely the Shafi'is and some Malikis. It is then added that if someone says "in the name of God and in the Name of Muhammad," and what is meant is association with God, the slaughter is *haram*, but if the intention is slaughter in God's name and seeking blessings in the name of Muhammad, the slaughter is *makruh*.[62]
- Facing the animal in a direction other than the *qiblah*.
- *Nahr* of the cattle and *dhabh* of the camel; the normal method is in the reverse order.
- Inflicting pain on the animal, such as by severing the head completely or breaking the skull, dragging the animal, and slaughter from the back of the neck.
- Slaughter by a dull or a small and unsuitable knife. It is also reprehensible to use other tools such as stone, bone, etc., when a sharp metallic knife may be available.[63]
- The majority of jurists consider slaughter from the top or side of the neck as reprehensible (*makruh*), but if the cut and severance of vital veins is swift, the slaughter is considered valid.[64]
- Slaughter at nighttime when daytime is also possible. The Shia Imamiyyah records the same position by stating that slaughter at night is reprehensible until the daybreak, except in emergency situations or imminent fear of destruction.[65]

---

61. Wizarat, *al-Mawsu'ah al-Fiqhiyyah*, vol. 21, 197–198. See also Foltz, *Animals in Islamic Tradition*, 27.

62. Wizarat, *al-Mawsu'ah al-Fiqhiyyah*, vol. 21, 193.

63. al-Qurtubi, *Bidayat al-Mujtahid*, vol. 1, 327–328; al-Zuhayli, *al-Fiqh al-Islami*, vol. 3, 663–664; al-Qaradawi, *al-Halal wa'l-Haram*, 55f; Wizarat, *al-Mawsu'ah al-Fiqhiyyah*, vol. 5, 196.

64. al-Zuhayli, *al-Fiqh al-Islami*, vol. 3, 657; Fadlullah, *Islamic Rulings*, 294–295.

65. al-Tabarsi, *Mustadrak al-Wasa'il*, vol. 16, 143, sec.19413.

- Severing of some and not all of the vital passages, as this is likely to torture the animal and slow down the slaughter.
- Sharpening the slaughter knife in front of the animal.
- Slaughter by the left hand unless the person is naturally left-handed.[66]
- Time should be given for the animal to cool before it is skinned; for instance, it can be chopped and mutilated, or placed on fire and the like. It is reprehensible to do otherwise, and there is general agreement of the leading schools of Islamic law on this.[67]
- Mental competence is a requirement of valid slaughter, and this applies to everyone—man, woman, and a discerning child (competence is a prerequisite especially of *tasmiyah*). This is the majority view, which maintains that slaughter is non-halal if done by a drunken person, an insane person, or a child without mental capacity. The Shafi'is maintain that it is halal but reprehensible (*makruh*).[68]
- To this list the Shia Imamiyyah add that slaughter is reprehensible on Friday before the decline of the midday sun (*zawal*). It is also reprehensible to skin the slaughtered animal before its spirit leaves, or to carry out slaughter in front of another animal of the same type, as well as to slaughter an animal that the slaughterer has himself reared.[69]
- It is reprehensible to skin the animal, break its bones, or sever a limb immediately after slaughter and prior to cooling down and complete exit of life. For this too tortures the animal.[70] The Shia Imamiyyah confirm this and record a statement from Imam Ja'far, who proscribed breaking the neck bone of the animal during slaughter. Furthermore, in a report from Imam 'Ali ibn Abi Talib, it is stated that he entered the butchers' quarter of the Kufan market while riding a mule he had borrowed from the Prophet, and 'Ali said in a very loud voice, addressing the butchers, "Do not break the neck of the animal you slaughter, and avoid hastening the death of the animal such that interferes with its natural course."[71] Further emphasis is laid on clemency to the slaughter animal in that at all times the butcher must avoid severe killing (*al-nakha'*) that inflicts cruelty.

---

66. Cf. al-Qurtubi, *Bidayat al-Mujtahid*, vol. 1, 325–326; Burj, *Ahkam al-Dhabh*, 123.

67. Wizarat, *al-Mawsu'ah al-Fiqhiyyah*, vol. 21, 198.

68. Ibid., 184.

69. Fadlullah, *Islamic Rulings*, 298.

70. Cf. Ibn Qudamah, *al-Mughni*, vol.13, 72; al-Qurtubi, *Bidayat al-Mujtahid*, vol. 1, 328f.

71. al-Tabarsi, *Mustadrak al-Masa'il*, vol. 16, 134, secs. 19381 & 19382, respectively.

Abandonment of what is *mandub* in slaughter, or committing what is *makruh*, still does not render the slaughter non-halal. Yet observing the *mandub* in slaughter is regarded as the hallmark of purity and *tayyib*, that which is wholesome and praiseworthy.

Certain aspects of the distinction between the *makruh* and *haram* are not always known by common folk or even industry practitioners. There is a need, therefore, for raising awareness of the *makruh* and *mandub* in slaughtering practices. The Malaysian Halal Standards also do not articulate what is *mandub* or *makruh* in slaughtering practices. Some individual speakers and writers, moreover, tend to haphazardly label as *haram* that which may actually amount to no more than *makruh*. *Haram* is sometimes pronounced all too readily, sometimes for greater emphasis and attention, not just in food matters but more generally. This should be avoided as per the clear textual warning of the Qur'an, as follows:

> And let not your tongues describe in falsehood that "This is lawful and this is forbidden," for this is tantamount to ascribing lies to God. (al-Nahl, 16:116)

Yusuf al-Qaradawi discusses this in some detail to say that the leading imams of jurisprudence were extremely reluctant to declare anything as *haram*. When they had occasion to proscribe something in a *fatwa* they often chose to declare it as *makruh*. This is not an issue, but declaring something *haram* is truly a serious one.[72]

Some of the halal procedural guidelines also stipulate the ritual cleansing of animal hides that have not undergone halal slaughtering. This is evidently not a requirement according to a renowned hadith, recorded by Muslim and Abu Dawud, which provides that "when any hide is tanned, it is purified."[73] The ruling of this hadith is general (*'aam*) and unqualified, hence it includes "all hides even of the dog and pig. This is the position of the Zahiri school, also endorsed by Abu Yusuf, the disciple of Abu Hanifah, Sahnun, and Ibn 'Abd al-Hakam (d. 870/1228) from the Maliki school, and it is preferred by al-Shawkani."[74] According to yet another hadith narrated by all the major hadith

---

72. al-Qaradawi, *al-Halal wa'l-Haram*, 27.

73. Abu Dawud, *Sunan Abu Dawud*, vol. 2:1149, hadith no. 411. The hadith is also recorded by al-Tirmidhi, al-Nasa'I, and al-Darimi. See for a discussion also, Kamali, *Principles*, 153.

74. al-Qaradawi, *al-Halal wa'l-Haram*, 51–52.

collections, except for Ibn Majah, and also quoted by al-Qaradawi, Ibn 'Abbas has narrated that a sheep that belonged to Maymunah, the Prophet's wife, had died, and when it came to the Prophet's attention, he asked, "Did you take its skin, which could be tanned and then used?" The Companions responded that it had died (without slaughter), to which the Prophet commented, "It is only forbidden for eating [not for other uses]."[75] Furthermore, it is quite obvious from our perusal of the relevant rules that the shariah prohibition of carrion is confined to eating and does not extend to the use of the animal's hide, horns, bones, and hair, all of which are permitted. They are valuable assets, or *mal*, as they often carry a market value, and if they could be put to a good use, they should not be wasted.[76]

The second view on this is held by the majority of Hanafi, Shafi'i, Maliki, and Hanbali schools, which maintain that the pig hide and inherently *najis* object (*najis al-'ayn*) are not cleansed by tanning. Having quoted both these views, Nazih Hammad prefers the first and says that tanning does purify all hides, and there is no objection from the shariah viewpoint to the use of tanned hide from all animals directly or in the manufacture of other products.[77]

A valid slaughter under the Malaysian Standards is described as one that is in accordance with shariah law; that is, when it involves severing the trachea (*halqum*), esophagus (*mari'*), and both the carotid arteries and jugular veins (*wadajain*) to hasten the bleeding and death of the animal.[78] It is required that the slaughtering process takes into account animal welfare in accordance with shariah law. This process must fulfill the following requirements:

a. Slaughtering is to be performed only by a practicing Muslim who is in full possession of his faculties and understands the rules of animal slaughter in Islam.

b. The slaughterer shall have a valid certificate for halal slaughter issued by a competent authority.

c. The act of slaughter is done with *niyyah* (intention) in the name of Allah and not for other purposes, and the slaughterer is well aware of his or her action.

---

75. al-Qaradawi, *al-Halal wa'l-Haram*, 48.

76. al-Qaradawi, *al-Halal wa'l-Haram*, 51.

77. Hammad, *al-Mawad al-Muharramah*, 80–81. Hammad refers for the majority view to Ibn Qudamah, *al-Mughni*, vol. 1, 89; and al-Sarakhsi, *al-Mabsut*, vol. 1, 202.

78. MS 1500-2009 (Clause 2.5)

d. The animal to be slaughtered is alive or deemed to be alive with a degree of certainty (i.e., ascertained life, or *hayat al-mustaqirrah*), and in good health at the time of slaughter.[79]

It is further provided that the act of halal slaughter begins with an incision on the neck at some point just below the glottis (Adam's apple), and after the glottis for long-necked animals, and it must sever the trachea, esophagus, and both the carotid arteries and jugular veins to hasten the bleeding and death of the animal. *Tasmiyah* is immediately cited before slaughtering, and the slaughterer is also recommended to be facing the *qiblah*.[80] The slaughter knife or blade should be sharp, and slaughtering is done only once. The "sawing action" of the slaughter is permitted as long as the slaughter knife or blade is not lifted off the animal during the slaughtering. Bones, nails, and teeth must not be used as slaughtering tools. A trained Muslim inspector is, furthermore, appointed to check that the animals are properly slaughtered according to shariah law. With regard to poultry, it is provided that scalding should only be carried out on birds that are deemed dead as a result of halal slaughter.[81]

As for the processing, handling, distribution, and serving of halal food, the Malaysian Standard (MS 1500-2009) lays down the following requirements: The processing of food or its ingredients must preclude using any components or products of animals that are non-halal or *najis* under shariah law. All the equipment and facilities used must also be free from contamination with *najis*. The processed food, or its ingredients, is safe for consumption, non-poisonous, and non-intoxicating.[82]

It is further provided that following the due fulfillment of the requirements of valid slaughter, "the halal certificate shall be issued by the competent authority in Malaysia." From that point onward, each product may be marked with "the halal certification mark of that authority provided the product conforms to the requirements of this standard."[83] Thus, it is understood

---

79. The animals are deemed to be alive or possess *hayat al-mustaqirah* when blood gushes out during slaughtering and there is movement of the animals after slaughtering.

80. The phrases to be uttered in *tasmiyah* are *bismillah allahu akbar*, or simply *bismillahir rahman arrahim*.

81. MS 1500-2009 (Clause 3.5.2).

82. MS 1500-2009 (Clause 3.5.3).

83. Ibid., Clauses 5–6.

that a certificate is needed for every new product and not, as it were, a blank standard for an organization or producer that can then issue many new products under one cover. For purposes of clarity, it is also provided that halal food and halal artificial flavor may not be named nor synonymously named after non-halal products such as ham, bacon, beer, rum, and other such names that might create confusion.[84]

---

84. Ibid., Clause 3.7.4.

# 13

# Gray Areas and Doubtful Matters
# (al-Shubhat, Mashbuh, Mashkuk)

THE TERM "GRAY areas" refers to certain intervening (and often unde-
termined) matters that fall between the halal and *haram*. Doubts may arise
mainly because of two factors: either the source evidence of the shariah is not
free from doubt in respect of meaning or authenticity, or its application to a
particular subject or case is uncertain.

The Qur'an (al-ʿImran, 3:7) confirms that some parts of the Qur'an are inherently doubtful, and refers to them as *mutashabihat*. The precise meaning
of certain expressions, words, or phrases of the Qur'an under the category
of *mutashabihat* is, however, not known to anyone but God Himself. For
instance, a number of suras—nineteen, to be precise—of the Qur'an begin
with abbreviated letters, known as *muqatta'at*, which have no clear meaning
and remain a mystery, and are thus inherently ambiguous—although some
commentators say that the Prophet knew their meaning. The Prophet has
acknowledged this in a long hadith to the effect that halal and *haram* had
been made clear from one another, but that "in between them there are the
doubtful matters which are not known to most people whether they are halal
or *haram*. One who avoids them for the purity of one's religion and honor
would have saved oneself."[1] To avoid doubt, and to make an effort to stay
clear of it, is thus conducive to piety and one's good name and reputation for
good practices. This much is indicated in the wording of this hadith, which
evidently speaks of requital and absolvence (*istibra'*), and the course of action
recommend concerning it is to take caution over doubtful matters.

---

1. al-Mundhiri, *Mukhtasar Sahih Muslim*, 253, hadith no. 956.

*Shariah and The Halal Industry.* Mohammad Hashim Kamali, Oxford University Press. © Oxford University Press 2021.
DOI: 10.1093/oso/9780197538616.003.0014

The advice so conveyed in this hadith is, in al-Qaradawi's view, one of "obstructing the means to an evil end (*sadd al-dhara'i'*), which is informed by a certain insight into the health of one's personality and character."[2] Indulgence in *mashbuhat* can, in other words, lead to *haram*, and the advice is to block the means that lead to *haram*. In yet another hadith, Muslims are instructed to "abandon that which is doubtful to you in favor of that which is clear of doubt. For the truth brings assurance and falsehood brings doubt."[3]

The possibilities of indulgence in doubt have undoubtedly increased in our times. Today, doubts arise, for instance, about factory farming, where animal remains are fed to other animals, and the use of hormones and antibiotics also present difficulties in verifying whether the meat one buys or consumes is doubtful/*mashbuh* or halal. Factory practices may also fail the test of compatibility with the Islamic principle of compassion to animals. Definitive answers to these questions need to be informed by expert opinion and scientific evidence. The frequent incidence of BSE (mad-cow disease) in some countries[4] has also raised questions about their feeding and rearing methods and the wholesomeness of the meat of such animals. These are genuine doubts that merit further investigation and research.

Some commentators have advanced the view that in their choice of food and meat for consumption, Muslims should aim not only at that which is halal, but also at what is *tayyib* (pure and naturally appealing), which is a step beyond halal. This is basically sound advice, but it is often inaccurately conveyed. One commentator, for instance, wrote that "Muslims are required to eat meat that is not only halal but also *tayyib* (pure)."[5] The question posed here—whether Muslims are required as such to go a step beyond halal in their choice of food—is something that the *fiqh* tradition does not stipulate, as will presently be elaborated.

In the event of doubt over meat and whether or not it has been duly slaughtered, and when there is no information as to whether it was in the possession of a Muslim with the knowledge of ritual slaughter, it is best to

---

2. al-Qaradawi, *al-Halal wa'l-Haram*, 37.

3. al-Tabrizi, *Mishkat*, vol. 2, 845, hadith no. 4046.

4. BSE stands for bovine spongiform encephalopathy. See more on this in Foltz, *Animals in Islamic Tradition*, 118. Foltz informs us that "Middle Eastern countries now import much of their meat from places such as New Zealand and that factory farming presents considerable difficulties in verifying whether meat is halal."

5. The view is attributed to Mazhar Hussaini, director of the North American Halal Foundation, quoted in Foltz, *Animals in Islamic Tradition*, 118.

avoid consuming it. This is by reference to the normative position regarding doubtful meat, which is the lack of purification (*tadhkiyah*), which means that it is non-halal. The halal status of meat is not a matter of presumption but of positive knowledge. In situations of dire necessity, it is permissible, however, to consume it to save oneself from starvation. However, if the doubt concerns whether it is from a halal animal or a non-halal animal, but it is known that it has been duly slaughtered, the principle of original permissibility is applied and it is presumed halal, unless there be evidence to suggest otherwise.[6]

Other subjects that may be looked at under "doubtful matters" are gelatin, insulin, pig skin and hair. Removing doubt regarding these objects, and indeed all doubtful matters, is done by ascertaining the nature of the object and any specialized know-how concerning it. Some of these may also involve recourse to the principle of necessity (*darurah*)—as in the case of insulin for a diabetic patient, whereas others may not present a case of recourse to necessity.

## Gelatin

Gelatin is an insoluble soft glutinous substance, a protein similar to hemoglobin, insulin, and eggs. It is derived from acid- or alkaline-treated collagen (a primary protein component of animal connective tissue), which includes skin, bone, and tendon. Crude gelatin is separated from the skin or bones of fish, camels, cattle, sheep, and pigs. It is used in and incorporated into numerous synthetic foods, medicines, and nonfood products. It is applied, for instance, in cakes, cheeses, desserts, pancakes, beverages, juices, and some instant foods as powder (jelly or puddings), and in all kinds of yogurt, gums, and sticky confections. It is likewise utilized as a part of the production of medicine—in capsules, for example—and is also used in the manufacture of toothpaste, moisturizers, and creams, and in the formation of suppositories or pessaries. Gelatin derived from swine, dairy cattle, poultry, and fish is also used as a food ingredient for gelling, stabilizing, foaming, and emulsifying. Gelatin is, moreover, applied in nonfood products such as those used in photography, cosmetics, and carbonless paper.[7]

There is no issue with regard to extracting gelatin from the skin, ligaments, and bones of animals that are halal for consumption and have been

---

6. Fadlullah, *Fiqh al-Atʿimah*, 191.

7. Cf. Awang, "Istihalah," 64.

slaughtered in a shariah-compliant manner. This kind of gelatin is noncontroversial and may be used and consumed as a part of food or medication. [8]

The basic issue over gelatin that has come under scrutiny is whether it is actually transformed well enough to have lost all of its original properties during the process of food manufacture. Gelatin that has been so transformed in the process of manufacture and treatment, and has changed into another substance totally different from the *haram* substance from which it was extracted, also poses no major issue regarding its permissibility for consumption. But if the gelatin has not been changed completely and still retains some of the attributes of the *haram* substance from which it was taken, then it is doubtful and most likely impermissible for consumption.

Expert opinion is, however, divided over the matter. Some say that complete change of the original gelatin substance is possible, while others maintain that this is not always the case. A few researchers have expressed the view that gelatin which is obtained from the bone and skin of cows and pigs undergoes a complete change and is not the same as the substance from which it was extracted, and that it has obtained synthetic properties that vary from those of the original substance; hence it is properly subsumed under the rubric of the *fiqh* principle of substance transformation (*istihalah*). From the *fiqh* perspective, *istihalah* transforms the unclean or prohibited substance to create another substance that is different in name, properties, and attributes. *Istihalah* may likewise be characterized as a complete change that happens both physically and synthetically, as already explained. The transformed substance must have a new name and all its characteristics must be different from the original substance.

Some researchers have maintained, however, that the synthetic procedures to which the skin and bones of pigs are subjected in order to extract gelatin do not bring about a complete change, and that it is rather an incomplete change, because gelatin still holds some of the attributes of the impure substance from which it was taken. According to Wafeeq ash-Sharqawi, administrative president of the committee of the Arabian Company for Gelatin Products in Egypt, the skin and bones of pigs do not undergo a complete change, and by testing it is possible to trace the origin of the gelatin that is derived from the skin and bones of pigs after they are subjected to the synthetic process. It is further stated that the availability of a few properties in this gelatin makes it

---

8. al-Zuhayli, *al-Fiqh al-Islami*, vol. 4, 329.

possible to determine its source. So one cannot say that the parts of the pig that are transformed into gelatin have undergone a complete change.[9]

Mohammad Aizat Jamaludin's study on this issue also suggests that the chemical composition of gelatin still remains.[10] He concludes from his research that the amino acid in gelatin stays intact and does not experience any synthetic change, despite the fact that the procedure of gelatin extraction involves extreme chemical treatment. Denaturation of protein, which includes heat treatment, alcohol, acid, alkaline, or heavy metals, could break up only the tertiary and auxiliary protein structure, but the peptide bonds and amino acids remain intact. Therefore, it is argued that gelatin changes only physically and does not undergo a complete chemical transformation. It is concluded, therefore, that *istihalah* in gelatin cannot be applied, as there is no complete transformation.[11]

Nazih Hammad does not agree with this, and holds that gelatin, whether from porcine, bovine, or ovine animal sources, undergoes a transformation that fulfills the Islamic law requirements of *istihalah*, and as such it is not prohibited for consumption. This is because gelatin no longer possesses the original attributes of the skin and bone of swine or carrion from which it was derived. Since it no longer has the form, taste, smell, or chemical structure of its original source, it falls under the basic shariah norm of permissibility.[12]

This is also the decision of the Islamic Fiqh Academy of the Muslim League (held in Mecca, December 13-17, 2003) with the proviso that transformation is complete and that none of the original properties of the porcine substance are known to have survived. A partial transformation that causes only a change of form leaving the substance totally or partially unaffected would fail to render the substance in question permissible.[13]

---

9. Wafeeq ash-Sharqawi's views appear in Nafsiyah, "*Risalah fi Fiqh as-Siyam*," 28.

10. Jamaludin et al., "Istihalah: Analysis on the Utilization of Gelatin," 174–178.

11. Jamaludin et al., "Istihalah: Analysis on the Utilization of Gelatin," 174–178.

12. Hammad, "Dieting the Islamic Way"; also quoted by Awang, "Istihalah," 60. Dr. Nazih Hammad is a shariah specialist who taught in Faculty of Shari'a at Um Alqura University, Makkah for 17 years. He is a member of the Islamic Fiqh Academy, Auditing and Accounting Organisation for Islamic Financial Institutions (AAOIFI), and Fiqh Islamic Council of North America.

13. The Fiqh Academy decision was carried in *al-Sharq al-Awsat* (London), no. 9173, July 9, 2004, 14; also quoted by Awang, "Istihalah," 60.

The majority of Muslim jurists have agreed that the use of *istihalah* is applicable only when a complete physical and chemical change takes place during the process. Gelatin becomes halal if it has been transformed into something else. It merits a mention that *istihalah* is also not a unidirectional process but can occur in two ways: that which is clean and permissible has changed so that it becomes unclean, impure, and *haram*, and that which is impure becomes clean and halal as a result of *istihalah*.

The following conclusions have been drawn from the foregoing analysis:

- Gelatin derived from the bones, skin, and tendons of prohibited animals and sources is permissible for consumption only if a complete *istihalah* has taken place.
- Soap produced by treating and changing pig or dead animal fat turns into a clean substance by the process of *istihalah*, and therefore using this soap is permissible.
- Cheese processed with rennet, obtained from animals that are dead, is clean and permissible to eat.
- Ointments, creams, and cosmetics that contain pig fat are all unclean. Their use is impermissible in shariah except when *istihalah* or transformation (of the material into one with totally different properties) is ensured.[14]

A general advisory note is inserted, however, that one should try to avoid doubtful substances when other options are easily available and there is no compelling necessity to resort to using that which is doubtful. If a Muslim is certain or knows on a balance of probability that meat, fat, or ground bones of an unlawful animal have been mixed or added to any food, drink, or medicine, then it is not permissible to consume it on grounds of caution. This conclusion is based on what the Prophet has been quoted as saying, in an evidently advisory rather than mandatory language addressing the faithful: "Leave that which makes you doubt for that which you do not doubt."[15] Two other widely used items that have given rise to extensive juristic debates are lard and insulin, which are discussed next.

---

14. Kamali, *The Parameters*, 21.

15. Hadith No. 11, the *Forty Hadith* by Imam Al-Nawawi.

# Lard

With regard to the use of pig fat, or lard, the Eighth Fiqh-Medical Seminar of 1996, organized by IOMS and held in Kuwait, concluded that foodstuffs containing lard that do not undergo denaturation, such as some varieties of cheese, vegetable oil, skin moisturizing oil, lubricants, butter, cream, biscuits, chocolates, and ice cream, are prohibited due to the impermissibility of the pig and its derivatives. The same prohibitive stance is taken regarding body lotions and cosmetics that contain pig fat unless the substances from which they are derived undergo a transformation that eliminates their original properties.[16] Nazih Hammad concurs with the Fiqh-Medical Seminar ruling.

The Islamic Organization for Medical Sciences (IOMS), in its eighth session in Kuwait (May 1995), held that food items that utilize lard, such as certain varieties of cheese, biscuits, chocolates, and ice cream, are forbidden for consumption, based on the general consensus of Muslim scholars on the prohibition of pig fat, and also that cases of necessity are not likely to arise concerning these. The resolution further added that creams, lotions, and cosmetics that utilize pig fat are also impermissible unless it is ascertained that they have undergone a process of complete transformation by way of *istihalah*.[17] Nazih Hammad wrote that toothpaste involves the use of some pig fat, but that the chemical process of its manufacture is such that no trace of the original pig fat is left, so it is lawful to use.[18]

It is further noted that the extensive use of lard by Western food and pharmaceutical producers is due to its much reduced price over the years, mainly on account of a general awareness of its health hazards. The use of pig fat in products such as soap is generally not an issue among Muslim scholars, as it is understood to be a typical case of complete transformation (*istihalah*), and the use of all soap varieties is generally held to be permissible. As for the use of pig fat for medicinal purposes, especially uses that do not involve eating, this too is allowed on grounds of either necessity (*darurah*) or need (*hajah*). In this regard, Hammad has quoted Ibn Taymiyyah, who was asked about a certain skin disease that someone was afflicted with, and whether the use of pig fat was permissible for him. In response, Ibn Taymiyyah said that medication that involved eating pig fat was impermissible. As for medication that

---

16. As quoted in Hammad, *al-Mawad al-Muharramah*, 70.

17. As quoted in Hammad, *al-Mawad al-Muharramah*, 70; also in Abu Zayd, *Al-Intifa' bil A'yan al-Muharramah*, 83.

18. Hammad, *al-Mawad al-Muharramah*, 84.

involved external application of pig fat, that is allowed, but should be washed away afterward, and should preferably be at times that do not involve performance of ritual prayer (*salah*). The issue has been debated by other Muslim scholars too, and the correct position is that of permissibility, on the grounds both of necessity (*darurah*) and need (*hajah*) under the stipulations just mentioned. This is because the external uses of pig fat rank a degree less on the scale of shariah prohibitions. This may resemble poison, which may not be swallowed but may be externally applied on medical advice.[19]

## Insulin

Insulin is a medicine that is often obtained from pig body parts. It is a hormone used to treat diabetes, a condition where the patient's pancreas does not properly respond to insulin. When insulin is absent or lacking in the body, glucose is not taken up by body cells and emerges instead in blood and urine, posing a threat to the patient's health.[20]

There are several treatment options for diabetics, including drugs that restore a normal sugar ratio in the bloodstream or stimulate insulin secretion. In some cases, however, the available drugs fail to be effective, in which case the physician resorts to the use of insulin, which is mostly derived from pig pancreas. While there are insulin treatments made from genetically engineered human cells, they are in short supply and exceedingly expensive.[21]

According to the 8th Fiqh Medical Seminar recommendations, diabetics are permitted to take insulin obtained from pigs, based on the shariah principle of necessity (*darurah*). Nazih Hammad, however, has arrived at the conclusion that the principle of necessity need not be invoked, and instead suggests that the matter falls under *istihalah*, for the production of insulin from pig pancreas involves a detailed and complex chemical process that transforms the pig tissue into a substance devoid of its original attributes. He adds that, without any doubt, insulin obtained from the pig pancreas juridically fulfills the requirements of the Islamic principle of *istihalah*, and diabetic patients may use it for their needs.[22]

---

19. As recounted in Hammad, *al-Mawad al-Muharramah*, 84–85, quoting also Ibn Taymiyyah's *al-Fatawa al-Kubra*, vol. 3,7, and adds in passing that Ibn Taymiyyah's views concur with those of Imam Malik as mentioned in al-Baji, *Al-Muntaqa Sharh al-Muwatta'*, vol. 7, 262.

20. Hammad, *al-Mawad al-Muharramah*, 78.

21. Hammad, *al-Mawad al-Muharramah*, 78.

22. Hammad, *al-Mawad al-Muharramah*, 78.

The difference between the two positions is that *istihalah* allows an unrestricted recourse, whereas necessity is a narrower juridical principle that can only be employed when several conditions are met, as are expounded in a separate section on necessity (*darurah*) in this volume.

In a monographic study on the medicinal uses of pig body parts and pig-based pharmaceuticals, Abdul Halim Ihsan and other members of his team[23] present a detailed and insightful account of the various applications and uses of pig body parts for medicinal and pharmaceutical purposes, of which a brief account is presented here, notwithstanding some technical terminology and input.

Glucagon, which is derived from pig pancreas, is used in the treatment of beta-blocker overdose and also in the treatment of severe hypoglycemia. Another derivative of pig pancreas, kallirein, is used in the treatment of male infertility and some peripheral vascular diseases. Pig pancreas is also added to several preparations of digestive enzymes. Some of these can also be obtained, the same authors add, from the human and bovine pancreas.[24]

Pig intestinal mucose (PIM) is used in the preparation of Ardeparin to prevent deep vein thrombosis. PIM also possess anticoagulant properties and is used to prevent blood clotting—just as it is also used in the preparation of Dalteparin for the management of unstable angina. A PIM equivalent can, however, be derived from the lungs of bovine.[25]

Pig brain is used in BNP (brain natriuretic peptide) as a diagnostic aid for heart failure by measuring the plasma concentration in individuals. Pig brain is also used in gangliosides to treat damage to the nervous system. Equivalent alternatives are also found and can be extracted from other mammalian brains.[26]

Pig pituitary gland is used to treat disorders such as spasms and multiple sclerosis. Pig thyroid gland is also used to treat an array of disorders that come about with old age, such as Paget's bone disease and post-menopausal osteoporosis. Alternatives for the former are obtained from the bovine pituitary gland, and for the latter from salmon and human equivalents.[27]

---

23. Ihsan, Ahmad, et al., *Halal Index*, 2011.

24. Ihsan, Ahmad, et al., *Halal Index*, 4, 44, 54, 90.

25. Ihsan, Ahmad, et al., *Halal Index*, 8, 28, 34.

26. Ihsan, Ahmad, et al., *Halal Index*, 8, 40.

27. Ihsan, Ahmad, et al., *Halal Index*, 2, 14.

Pig bile is used in the preparation of Chenodiol, which dissolves cholesterol gallstones. It is also used as dietary supplement in newborn infants and children with inborn bile acid disorders. Therapeutically, it is employed to stimulate the liver into producing bile. Alternative equivalents can be obtained from the bile of bovine and other vertebrates.[28]

Pig cartilage is used in the preparation of chondroitin sulfate, which is an anti-inflammatory and anti-rheumatic agent. Alternative equivalents are obtained from bovine and shark cartilage.[29] Glycerol is obtained from pig adipose tissue and has multiple applications in the reduction of intracranial pressure, the management of constipation, and the production of sweeteners, plasticizers, and preservatives. Glycerol can also be produced synthetically from propylene and other sugars.[30]

It would fall beyond our scope here to provide further details, but we note that Halim Ihsan and his team have in no less than 110 pages written on the various applications of pig bone marrow, abdominal fat, lungs, liver, etc., which are all being employed in the manufacture of drugs that are currently in use. Yet the authors have also identified equivalent non-porcine alternatives that do exist. That said, no further information is provided as to the extent of reliance on these available alternatives, and whether or not the information on these medicines, be it from non-halal sources or their available halal alternatives, inform the readers as to the sources from which they are derived.

One also wonders whether Muslim countries and clients have made any credible efforts and investments to access or make the permissible alternatives available for general use. We know that the halal industry has made inroads into the pharmaceutical sector, and also halal cosmetics, but halal medicine may still be awaiting greater and more penetrating research and investment initiatives to bring about significant changes to the wide-ranging applications of pig body parts in the manufacturing of so many drugs and pharmaceutical products.

From the Islamic viewpoint, most of the medicines derived from pig body parts would fail to qualify the test of Islamic permissibility if and when suitable permissible alternatives can be easily obtained. This is also a decisive factor, theoretically at least, in one's recourse to the principle of necessity (*darurah*). Necessity would still play a role, especially in cases where the

---

28. Ihsan, Ahmad, et al., *Halal Index*, 20–21.

29. Ihsan, Ahmad, et al., *Halal Index*, 24.

30. Ihsan, Ahmad, et al., *Halal Index*, 46.

known permissible alternatives that may well exist but which may not be accessible or even produced/marketed by the Muslim country where the need arises. Complete transformation under the rubric of *istihalah* and extreme dilution under the principle of *istihlak* are also relevant, in addition to the principle of necessity. But more shariah insights on some of these questions can perhaps be gained from our discussions below. Some relevant points are taken up in the context of the discussion that follows on the uses of pig hair and skin.

## Pig Hair

Muslim jurists have disagreed regarding the permissibility or otherwise of utilizing pig's hair for manufacturing and trading purposes. According to one view attributed to Imam Abu Hanifah, his disciple Muhammad b. Hasan al-Shaybani, Imam Ahmad ibn Hanbal, and Abu 'Amr al-Awza'i, it is permissible to use swine hair for weaving, but not for sale and purchase. For the basic position is one of impermissibility: when the Qur'an prohibits pig meat, that prohibition also applies to all other parts and products obtained from the animal. The Qur'an merely specifies the flesh of the swine simply because that is the main part for human consumption. This is the position also of the Qur'an commentators Shihab al-Din al-Alusi (d. 1854) and Muhammad Rashid Rida (d. 1935). The exceptional permission for weaving is also said to be by way of juristic preference (*istihsan*).[31]

The second view is one of permissibility of utilizing the pig hair generally, as it is clean (*tahir*), regardless of whether the animal is alive or dead. This is the view of Imam Malik, Abu Yusuf of the Hanafi school, (another view of) Imam Ahmad ibn Hanbal, and also that of Ibn Taymiyyah from the Hanbali school. Ibn Taymiyyah, who gave a *fatwa* on the subject, has said the following: "The preferred view is that hair is clean generally of all animals, including dogs and pigs. . . . This is because the norm of shariah in regards to objects (*al-a'yan*) is cleanliness. Hence nothing is to be regarded unclean unless there is clear evidence to the contrary."[32]

---

31. al-Kasani, *Badai'u al-Sanai'fi*, vol. 5, 143; Ibn Qudamah, *al-Mughni*, vol. 1, 9; Hammad, *al-Mawad al-Muharramah*, 81. Qur'an commentators, al-Alusi and Rida are both quoted in Wizarat, *al-Mawsu'ah al-Fiqhiyyah* (Kuwait), vol. 5, 140.

32. Ibn Taymiyyah, *Majmu'a Fatawa*, vol. 21, 617 as quoted in Hammad, *al-Mawad al-Muharramah*, 82. See also Al-Sarakhsi, Shams al-Din. *Al-Mabsut*. Beirut: Dar al-Ma'rifah, 1989.

The third view on the use of pig hair is one of total prohibition, for pig is inherently unclean (*najis al-'ayn*), all of it, including its flesh, fat, and every other part. This is the view of the Shafi'i and Hanbali schools, and also that of Ibn Hazm al-Zahiri. Ibn Hazm even wrote that there is general consensus (*ijma'*) to the effect that nothing of the pig is permissible, and that includes its flesh, fat, skin, nerve, cartilage, bone, head and limbs, milk, and hair, not even for weaving or anything else, male and female, old and young of the animal are all included. Yet the author of *Mawsu'ah Fiqhiyyah* who has quoted Ibn Hazm makes the point that the claim of consensus is not credible, simply because of the differences of opinion that evidently exist.[33] Having quoted all three views on the subject, Nazih Hammad prefers the second view, which is generally permissive on the cleanliness of all animal hair. Hence there is no objection, from the shariah viewpoint, to all useful applications of pig hair, whether wholly or partially, and when it is mixed with other hair or their synthetic equivalents.[34]

## Doubtful Ingredients and Additives

While many additives and ingredients can be clearly identified to be halal or *haram*, there are others which are not so clear. Substances of this kind are questionable and doubtful, and more information may be needed to categorize them as either halal, recommendable (*mandub*), forbidden, or reprehensible. Food falling under the category of doubtful (*mashbuh*) should preferably be avoided on grounds of purity and integrity of one's faith. It is advisable perhaps to place the doubtful substances under the category of *mashbuh* until further information becomes available to clarify the position. This includes ingredients such as gelatin, emulsifiers, fat, and enzymes of doubtful origins. All of these are doubtful. Many of them do in fact have alternatives that are either halal or are vegetarian products that can just as easily be used in their place.[35]

Imported meats may also be put in the "doubtful foodstuffs" category. Questions as to the origin of the imported foods have led Muslim scholars to a binary classification of the imported meats according to their place of

---

33. Ibn Hazm, *al-Muhalla*, vol.7, 388. See also Wizarat, *al-Mawsu'ah al-Fiqhiyyah*, vol. 5, 140 at footnote 2.

34. Hammad, *al-Mawad al-Muharramah*, 82.

35. Cf. Kamali, "Principles of Halal and Haram," 38f.

origin, whether from Christian or Jewish countries or outside this category, as explained below:

a. Muslim jurists are in agreement to the effect that meats and other food-stuffs imported from non-Muslim countries, such as Europe and America, where the majority are either Christians or Jews, are lawful provided they are not derived from forbidden sources and animals. It is not recommended to investigate whether the meats were slaughtered according to Islamic rituals or not. This is because permissibility is the basic principle that applies to slaughter and foodstuffs of the People of Scripture, as confirmed by a clear text of the Qur'an (al-Ma'idah, 5:5), except where there is a proof to the contrary. Muslims are not, however, permitted to eat meat over which an invocation is made to a deity other than Allah.[36] Therefore, unfounded doubts that advise abstinence are of no account and permissibility prevails. If it is known that pronouncing the name of God on an animal is deliberately avoided, the flesh of that animal is not halal according the majority of jurists.[37]

b. Meat and meat products imported from Zoroastrian (*Majusi*) origins and others whose residents do not believe in the concept of ritual slaughter are also forbidden for Muslims, according to the majority of the Muslim jurists, who hold that most of these people are polytheists and disbelievers. Another opinion holds that they are also counted among the People of Scripture (Ahl al-Kitab); hence, their slaughter becomes halal by analogy. It is reported that Ibn Hazm al-Zahiri (d. 456/1064) considered the Zoroastrians to be included among the People of Scripture and consequently applied the same rules that apply to the Ahl al-Kitab also to Zoroastrians.[38]

c. The doubtful varieties of meat products can include meat products mistakenly labeled as halal when these are in fact not halal. It makes no difference whether the mislabeling is intentional or otherwise. It is also possible that purely sales and marketing factors drive these decisions in total disregard of their relevant shariah rules. When a meat product is labeled as halal with no reference to the certifying authority, the chances are that the meat

---

36. Cf. Qur'an, al-Nahl, 16:115. See also Douglas, "The Fabric of Muslim Daily Life," vol. 3, 16–17.

37. Cf. Kamali, "Principles of Halal and Haram," 42f.

38. al-Qaradawi, *al-Halal wa al-Haram*, 63.

in question is mislabeled and therefore falls under the doubtful category. Research findings also caution that a producer looking for halal meat as an ingredient must not assume that a meat item labeled as halal is authentically so. To be certain, a halal certificate should be requested for every lot of meat to be used. Since meat is the most critical ingredient, the supervising authority should evaluate the status of its supplier, and in case of doubt recommend another supplier. Market surveys have also noted Muslim customer responses to the effect that they will not buy minced meat from non-halal stores. Several large and small food chains are also known to mix pork with beef. Even in Malaysia, according to a report, a factory producing dried tofu, apparently with halal certification, was operating next to a pig farm in the Cheras district of Kuala Lumpur. The product was found to be made in doubtful conditions, with only a thin wall separating the pig farm and the factory. Several stray dogs were also seen roaming the place, and a wood-processing factory in the area produced massive amounts of dust in a small space. Thus, "[i]t is believed the halal logo by JAKIM that is used by the company for its product packaging is fake."[39] It is noted as well that it took some time for JAKIM to take action. The director general of JAKIM at the time, Othman Mustapha, announced that starting January 1, 2013, the use of "halal" logos, symbols, and words such as "Muslim food" and "Ramadan buffet" that confuse Muslim consumers, will be banned. Any organization found guilty may face fines up to RM200,000 for the first offense and up to RM500,000 for the second and subsequent offences. It was further announced that all imported food items to be declared halal should also have the halal logo and certification issued by the authorities in the producing countries that are recognized by JAKIM.[40]

Some doubt in the halal identification process also emanates from the fact that non-Muslims tend to dominate the industry in so many ways. With the exception of the act of slaughtering that must be done by a Muslim person, according to the applied halal regulatory requirements, the other segments of the industry remain open for non-Muslims. The supply chain elements such as farming, food manufacturing, commodity trading, logistics, restaurants, hotels, and retail chains are also dominated by non-Muslim countries and

---

39. See Hamdan and Raman, " 'Halal' Food Factory," n43.

40. Report in *New Straits Times*, December 29, 2012, 10.

businesses. Muslim countries and companies have, in fact, only a limited role in the halal food value chain in most Muslim countries.[41]

A team of researchers from two US universities reported that in North America, some small companies have used halal symbols. The word "halal," or just the letter "H," is used to signify that the food is halal, but such symbols are not widely accepted. Many other halal logos have started to appear on North American packages, usually on imported foods. Indonesia, Malaysia, Singapore, and Thailand have central halal bodies, each with their unique logos. However, as the volume of halal products, both local and international, offered in the marketplace grows, it is expected that determining the standards for reliable halal certification will become more complex.[42] Other aspects of doubtful (*mashbuh*) in food substances that merit attention are food enhancers, ingredients, and additives.

According to official Malaysian Standards, fresh fruits and vegetables are all halal. Processed fruits and vegetables may be unacceptable if they are produced in processing plants using non-halal oil, fats, preservatives, flavoring, coloring, etc. Additionally, if the procedures used in producing these items do not involve on-site Muslim supervision, it would be prudent for the producer to obtain halal certification for its products and services.

Bakery goods give rise to particular halal concerns. Production processes for bakery goods must not use hidden ingredients, fillers, and alcohol-based or animal-based ingredients that may render the product questionable and doubtful. It is important to assure that the additives, colorants, and preservatives are from halal sources and are processed according to approved procedures without the usage of alcohol-based or porcine ingredients.

Halal food shall be processed, packed, and distributed under hygienic conditions in premises licensed in accordance with good hygiene practices, good manufacturing practices, or what may have been specified in the *Garispanduan amalan pengilangan yang baik* (Practical guidelines to good manufacturing) of the Ministry of Health Malaysia, MS 1514 or MS 1480, and public health legislation currently in force by the competent authority in Malaysia.

---

41. Tieman, "Control of Halal Food Chains," 538–542.

42. Regenstein, Chaudry, and Regenstein, "Kosher and Halal in the Biotechnology Era," 104–105.

## *Food Additives*

As a general rule, the principles that apply to foodstuffs, such as meats and bever-ages, are also applicable to food ingredients, enhancers, and additives. Muslims are consequently under obligation to abide by the injunctions of shariah con-cerning foodstuffs, additives, cosmetics, and medicine, which could be either harmful or subject to doubt as to whether they are good for their health and well-being. However, in situations of necessity, which are often stipulated and carefully identified in the Islamic law literature, the legal maxim that "necessities make the unlawful lawful," may apply. While this maxim contemplates situations of necessity (*darurah*), another maxim-cum-hadith articulates the general prin-ciple of shariah pertaining to harm and prejudice in such terms that "harm may neither be inflicted nor reciprocated in [the name of] Islam." As already noted, the normative shariah position on cleanliness spells out the basic position that all things are juridically clean, except for those that are declared otherwise. To ascertain the rulings of shariah on a certain ingredient or additive, the nature and known effects of these substances must naturally be taken into consideration.

Any food ingredient and additive derived from a halal source is also deemed to be halal, provided it is good and wholesome and also clear of impurities and harmful elements. It is safe to say that food ingredients and additives derived from plants and other sources that are known to be clear of doubt, such as halal synthetic food, eggs, fish, and duly slaughtered meats, are all halal. All deriva-tives of fish and vegetables are also halal, and all that is derived from cows, sheep, goats, and other halal animals are lawful for consumption provided they are not from dead animals or added to or mixed with that which is *haram* by itself.

Some ingredients and additives are added to food to preserve it from spoilage, or else to improve its color, flavor, and texture for consumption, and indeed, to extend its freshness. Some of these additives are natural, such as sugar, salt, and honey, while others are synthetic, such as sodium bicarbonate, sodium nitrate, and synthetic vitamins. However, in light of the rules and regulations that protect human health and the lives of the consumers, a good number of incidents have been specified and recorded to enable further scru-tiny that may lead to scientific conclusions. Some of the chemicals used in food processing have in fact proven to be injurious and harmful to health and are therefore doubtful and questionable. A number of food additives are known to be carcinogenic and contain toxic substances that may affect human sexual behavior and other aspects of normal health.[43] If such ingredients and

---

43. Cf. Kamali, "Principles of Halal and Haram," 24f.

additives prove, through reliable testing, not to be injurious, but are helpful for human health and well-being, they may be consumed and classified as halal. However, if they prove harmful to health, they may be considered as either *makruh* or *makruh tahrimi*, and even *haram* if there is definitive proof to justify such a determination. A ready recourse to the original principle of permissibility (*ibahah*) and the assumption that all things are permissible unless proven otherwise may not be always justified. Permissibility is valid and applicable when there is no suspicion of any possible harm concerning a food or beverage item. However, in terms of human health and safety and in instances where the possibility of harm, be it immediate or long term, still exists, one ought to advise caution and refer to reliable evidence, or advise suspension (*tawaqquf*) until such evidence obtains.

It merits attention, furthermore, that recourse to legal stratagems (*hiyal*) that seek to procure *haram* under a different guise or name is forbidden in shariah. This includes ingredients that originate in *haram*, such as pork, pork byproducts, and meats that are not ritually purified. Using substances derived from forbidden animals, or derivatives that have undergone chemical transformation, such as gelatin used in the production of medicine, including tablets and capsules, derived from the organs or tissues of pigs, the majority of Islamic scholars and researchers have issued *fatwas* and held them to be forbidden. Foodstuffs containing pig fat that do not undergo denaturation, such as some varieties of cheese, vegetable oil, butter, cream, biscuits, chocolate, and ice cream, are also declared prohibited. All of this must be avoided, barring a situation that may warrant an exception due to "necessity." Necessity is, admittedly, not always predictable. But with regard to food additives, barring highly exceptional situations, one would normally expect that cases of pressing necessity or public interest to warrant their consumption would be rare. This is because people's lives do not depend on them, and avoiding them normally does not lead to disruption and chaos of normal order in society. Thus, to avoid them becomes the obvious option.

The shariah prohibition of alcohol applies to all alcoholic beverages, including wine, beer, whiskey, and brandy, but also to all things that intoxicate and negatively affect one's rational faculty and judgment. As for an alcohol-based ingredient or additive in medicine, Muslim jurists would be expected to follow the guideline of hadith in their issuance of *fatwas* that medicine with alcoholic ingredients is generally forbidden. Exceptions to this rule are made for situations in which there is no other alternative and no alcohol-free medicine is available to cure an ailment. As for medicines currently in production that contain a very small measure of alcohol for the purpose of non-sedating preservatives or solvent, until suitable alternatives are found, they may be used. All narcotic drugs and substances are generally prohibited, and under no circumstances are they permissible except on specific medical grounds that may be determined by qualified physicians. The shariah grounds for some of the foregoing are explained in the earlier discussion of *haram*.

Foods containing even a small amount of wine that exceed 1 percent alcohol should be avoided according to available *fatwas* on the subject. This would include chocolates, drinks, deserts, or other foods that have a high alcohol content. Exceptions to such items that contain very small amounts of alcohol have been made by professional *fatwa* organizations based on the shariah principles of extreme dilution (*istihlak*) and substance transformation (*istihalah*). Intoxicants, alcohol, and hard drugs are forbidden in any quantity, large amounts or small, as per explicit *fatwas* issued on the subject. The rules of exceptional permissibility on the basis of *darurah* are also not expected to be applicable here due to the absence of the necessity factor and the availability of permissible alternatives. [44]

Many medical issues have arisen in connection with the rules of necessity. For instance, some medicines and mouthwashes contain alcohol. If a nonalcoholic alternative can be found for them, that would be preferable. It should be noted, however, that only ethyl alcohol (such as methylated spirits and ethanol—the alcohol found in alcoholic drinks) are intoxicating and are therefore *haram*.[45] There is no problem in using perfumes or scents (e.g., eau de cologne) in which alcohol is used as a solvent for manufacturing of fragrances or aromatic liquids, or in using body lotions that contain alcohol, as none of these are fit for consumption. There is no objection, on the other hand, to personal preferences when nonalcoholic alternatives may not be of equally good quality, or when a company, a country, or individual only select to buy or import the nonalcoholic alternatives. These nonalcoholic varieties are increasingly becoming available, especially in the halal pharmaceutical sector.

In contrast, small quantities of alcohol can be found in certain halal foods, such as bread and soy sauce. These may sometimes contain minute amounts of alcohol as a result of a natural reactions between certain chemicals during the manufacturing process (as opposed to alcohol being deliberately added to food to add flavor), and so could not be classified as *haram*.

---

44. al-Qaradawi, *al-Halal wa'l-Haram,* 72. See also al-Harithi, *al-Nawazil fi'l-At'imah,* vol. 2, 921.

45. al-Qaradawi, *al-Halal wa'l-Haram,* 53; Uwais, *Mawsu'ah al-Fiqh al-Islami,* vol. 1, 174.

## Food Ingredients (Halal E-Codes)

E-numbers represent specific food additives that are used by the food industry in the manufacture of various food products. These E-numbers have mainly been formulated by the European Economic Community (EEC) and are adopted by the food industry worldwide.

The E-numbering system was developed in order to keep track of the massive amounts of additives available in the market, and it became a legal requirement on packaging in the 1980s. E stands for European and denotes that additives tagged with an E-number has passed the safety tests and has been granted clearance for use in the European Union.

In order to standardize products and avoid confusion, each additive is assigned its own unique number. At a later stage, the numbering system was adapted for international use by the Codex Alimentarius Commission, hence the International Numbering System (INS) was born. INS maintains the same number for each additive, but without the letter E.[46]

Food additives can be divided into several groups, although there is some overlap between them. The list below gives a brief description of the relevant categories of additives.

Acids—food acids are added to make flavors "sharper," and also act as preservatives and antioxidants. Common food acids include vinegar, citric acid, tartaric acid, malic acid, fumaric acid, and lactic acid.

Acidity regulators—acidity regulators are used to change or otherwise control the acidity and alkalinity of foods. Anti-caking agents keep powders such as milk powder flowing freely and prevent it from solidification in one mass.

Antifoaming agents—antifoaming agents reduce or prevent foaming in foods.

Antioxidants—antioxidants such as vitamin C act as preservatives by inhibiting the effects of oxygen on food, and are generally beneficial to health.

Bulking agents—bulking agents, such as starch, are additives that increase the bulk of food without affecting its nutritional value.

Food colorings—colorings are added to food to replace colors lost during preparation, or to make food look more attractive.

---

46. JAKIM, "Halal E-Codes."

**Color retention**—in contrast to colorings, color retention agents are used to preserve the existing color of food.

**Emulsifiers**—emulsifiers allow water and oils to remain mixed together in an emulsion, as in mayonnaise, ice cream, and homogenized milk.

**Flavors**—flavors are additives that give food a particular taste or smell, and may be derived from natural ingredients or created artificially.

**Flavor enhancers**—flavor enhancers enhance a food's existing flavors.

**Flour treatment agents**—flour treatment agents are added to flour to improve its color or its use in baking.

**Humectants**—humectants prevent foods from drying out; they preserve humidity.

**Preservatives**—preservatives prevent or inhibit spoilage of food due to fungi, bacteria, and other microorganisms.

Preservatives have a longer history compared to many other food additives. Among the well-known preservatives traditionally known is salt, which kills many corrupting micro-organisms, especially in meats. Sugar is also used in jams and other sweets and is known to lengthen their usual durability for months, even in hot climates. Vinegar is also used, as is the smoking method, as well as nitrogen and air evacuation methods. Historically, the number of such methods began to increase with improved scientific knowledge of the chemical effects of acids, alkalines, and other combinations for preserving various types of foods. Gradually, the harm some of these caused to human health also became better known, and Muslim scholars began, in turn, to add their input into these developments. Many *fatwas* were issued as a result, some of which were in response to new demands for assurance by the halal industry operators.[47]

**Propellants**—propellants are pressurized gases used to expel food from its container.

**Stabilizers**—stabilizers, thickeners, and gelling agents, like agar or pectin (used in jam, for example) give foods a firmer texture. While they are not true emulsifiers, they help to stabilize emulsions.

**Sweeteners**—sweeteners are added to foods for flavoring. Sweeteners other than sugar are added to keep the food energy (calories) low, or because they have beneficial effects for diabetes mellitus and tooth decay.

---

47. For details, see al-Harithi, *al-Nawazil fi'l-At'imah*, vol.2, 929f.

**Thickeners**—thickeners are substances that, when added to a mixture, increase its viscosity without substantially modifying its other properties.[48]

In response to a question on the permissibility or otherwise of food additives, the European Council for Fatwa and Research issued the following *fatwa*:

The items that carry the letter "E" and a string of numbers are additives. Additives comprise more than 350 compounds, including preservatives, coloring, flavorings, and sweeteners. These are divided into four groups according to their origin:

1. Compounds of artificial chemical origin.
2. Compounds of vegetal origin.
3. Compounds of animal origin.
4. Compounds dissolved in alcohol.

The ruling on all these compounds is that most of them do not affect the status of these foods being halal, for the following reasons:

The first and second groups are halal because they originate in permissible substances and no harm is deemed to come from using these items from the shariah perspective, or else that the harm is negligible and the known benefits are predominant. The position would be the opposite in the event that the items in question endangered human safety and health. The same line of argument also applies to a large extent to animals and plants.

The third group, comprising items of animal origin, is also mostly halal, especially if the items concerned have undergone substance transformation during the process of manufacturing. This is the case especially when the additive or doubtful ingredient is transformed radically from its original form into a new clean and pure form through a process of chemical transformation.

As for the fourth group, these items are usually colorings and are normally used in extremely small quantities that dissolve in the final product through the process of extreme dilution (*istihlak*), which consequently renders it into an excused matter.

---

48. JAKIM, "Halal E-Codes." The halal additives list was established by The Halal Technical Committee of JAKIM in 2006 and it has been improvised to match with current EU approved additives.

Therefore, foods or drinks that contain any of these ingredients remain halal and permissible for the Muslim consumption. One must also remember that Islam, by its own affirmation, is a religion of ease, and Muslims are therefore strongly discouraged from making matters inconvenient and difficult, especially over matters that concern the general public and represent public need (*hajah*) for them.[49]

Al-Qaradawi wrote that he was sent a long list of enzymes, preservative agents, and food additives, some of which originated in the swine bone or fat, and his views were solicited in regard to their permissibility or otherwise. He specified some of the E-code items, such as "E153, E422, and many others" in that list. He then added that he looked into the permissibility of consuming these food items, which included enzymes, and drew some conclusions, which are summarized below.

Al-Qaradawi begins by saying that, unlike some commentators who thought otherwise, not all enzymes can be said to be forbidden, even if they originate in swine bones and fat. For the majority of Muslim jurists (*jumhur al-fuqaha'*) have held that substance transformation (*istihalah*) leads to a change in their shariah ruling, such that a forbidden item may become permissible, and vice versa. Thus, when wine changes into vinegar, or when filth is burnt and turned into ashes, or when an animal, including pig or dog, dies in salt and is consumed by it such that it turns into salt, it is no longer what it was, neither dog nor pig, as those original substances can no longer be said to exist. Their properties, their names, and their shariah rulings also undergo a complete transformation. For the rules of shariah stand on effective causes that may no longer obtain, and their rulings change likewise.[50]

Al-Qaradawi further adds that "we therefore do not base our judgment on the origin of things." For the origin of wine may be grapes or another permissible substance, but when it becomes wine and acquires intoxicating property, it becomes *haram*, and it becomes halal again when the same changes into vinegar. In a similar vein, substances that may have originated in pig, such as gelatin that is made from pig bones, and has then undergone substance transformation, its chemical composition has changed and it is no longer forbidden. Al-Qaradawi then adds that expert opinion also confirmed substance transformation that occurs in products such as soaps and

---

49. Cf. al-Harithi, *al-Nawazil fi'l-At'imah*, vol. 2, 937f.

50. al-Qaradawi, *Fi Fiqh al-Aqaliyyat al-Muslimah*, 141.

toothpaste that originate in the swine but have then undergone a complete transformation such that they no longer relate to their origin and are therefore halal.[51]

Othman Mustapha, Malaysia's Islamic Development Department (JAKIM) director general at the time, announced in May 2014 that food products with the E-code or number on the label were not necessarily processed through *haram* or prohibited sources.

He said the E-code referred to additives and commonly used by European Union countries, Australia, New Zealand, North America (particularly Canada), and Israel. He stated that "the numbering scheme is based on the International Numbering System set by the Codex Alimentarius Committee."[52] In addition, "it is a collection of various standards, codes of practice, recognized international guidelines related to food, food processing and food safety aimed at safeguarding public health and to ensure compliance with the ethical trading code of conduct."
Additives are labelled as follows:

E100–E199: color
E200–E299: preservatives
E300–E399: oxidants, phosphates, antioxidants, and acid inhibitors
E400–E499: thickeners, moisturizers, stabilizers, and emulsifiers
E500–E599: salt, acidity regulators, and anti-caking agents
E600–E699: flavor enhancers
E900–E999: sweeteners and glazing agents
E1000–E1999: additional chemicals

"Not all additives with the E serial number to make food products are from non-halal sources. The sources of the additives could be plants, synthetic, microbes, natural, chemicals and animals," said Othman. However, he added that E471, a mono- and diglyceride emulsifier, had been the most queried additive. "It is synthetic fat derived from glycerol and natural fatty acids found in plants such as palm oil or animal fat. It is generally a compound of various edible substances similar to natural fat."

---

51. al-Qaradawi, *Fi Fiqh al-Aqaliyyat al-Muslimah*, 142.

52. https://www.astroawani.com/berita-malaysia/local-products-with-e-code-halal-for-muslims-jakim-36652.

Othman urged food industry players to clearly define the additives in their products so as to leave no room for doubts among Muslim consumers as to the food's status. JAKIM, through its Halal Hub division, would also require companies that apply for the halal certificate to fully declare the contents of their products, including additives, he said.[53]

---

53. Ibid.

## 14

# The Role of Custom ('Urf)

GENERAL CUSTOM ('*URF*, '*adah*) is a recognized source of law and judgment in Islamic jurisprudence. It is defined as "recurrent practices that are acceptable to people of sound nature."[1] To constitute a valid basis of judgment,
custom must be sound and reasonable and must not contravene a clear text
or principle of the shariah. Custom is rejected if it is in conflict with a clear
injunction of shariah, such as some tribal practices that deny women their
rights of inheritance, or local communities that consume the flesh of snakes
and monkeys. In the event, however, of a partial conflict between a text and
custom, the latter may qualify or specify the former. A valid ruling of custom
often takes precedence over the normal rules, or the ruling of analogy (*qiyas*).
This is because custom represents the people's convenience, and adopting it
is often tantamount to removal of hardship, which is one of the expressed
purposes of shariah. It is commonly acknowledged that a great deal of the
*fiqh* rules and the rulings of *ijtihad* have taken their cues from the prevailing
practices of their time.

The role of custom is evidently recognized in the evaluation of the *mandub* and *makruh* in foodstuffs, which often correspond with what is approved
or disapproved by the people of sound nature (often referred to as the *ahl
al-'urf*). The law may recognize some food as halal, but that food may not be
liked by the people and may thus, for all intents and purposes, be relegated to
the category of *makruh*, or else a *mubah* may be elevated to the level of *mandub* by the people's preference for it. For instance, all seafood is declared to
be clean and edible by the clear text of a hadith, and there is little doubt that
this would include such items as prawn and shark. But prawn is not taken, for

1. Cf. Kamali, *Principles*, 369; Shabbir, *al-Qawa'id al-Kulliyyah*, 244f.

*Shariah and The Halal Industry.* Mohammad Hashim Kamali, Oxford University Press. © Oxford University Press 2021.
DOI: 10.1093/oso/9780197538616.003.0015

instance, by the Hanafi Muslims of Pakistan, and many people have similar reservations about shark. There is in principle no shariah objection to customary practices of this kind. When people of sound nature approve of such practices, then, according to a leading maxim of *fiqh*: "Custom is the basis of judgment (العادة محكمة)."[2] Custom also determines the question, for instance, of whether or not an object is regarded as valuable property, or *mal*, that carries market value. For instance, honey bees and silk worms were at one time not regarded to be valuable assets, but were later determined to qualify as *mal* by the people's usage and acceptance of them as such, and a *fatwa* was accordingly issued in its support.

It should be noted, however, that custom is changeable with the advancement of science and technology, which often set in place new practices that may soon gain wide recognition and acceptance. People's tastes regarding foodstuffs are also affected by media advertisements and so forth. New practices take hold among people as and when they prove to be convenient, and are often adopted and then reflected in their lifestyle and food varieties. All of this is likely to carry the seal of shariah approval if none of its basic principles have been contravened. Furthermore, people's approval and disapproval also play a role in the determination of what may be regarded as a compelling necessity (*darurah*), or what may not so qualify.

Many commentators and philologists have gone on record to say that the customary and linguistic usage of Arabs at the time of the Qur'anic revelation constituted the basic framework of understanding the text. For instance, when the Qur'an referred to clean and pure food in the phrase that refers to what the Prophet teaches his followers—*wa yahillu lahum al-tayyibat* (and makes permissible *to them* clean and pure food)—the pronoun here referred to the Arabs who were the audience of this revelation at the time. Then, in the same verse, follows the phrase '*wa-yuharrimu 'alayhim al-khaba'ith* (and made *haram to them* the filthy substances), where the reference is again to the Arabs who lived in the Hijaz, for they were the recipients of the Qur'an and the main constituents and audience also of the Sunnah. Hence the unqualified words and pronouns of the Qur'an refer to their customary practices, especially those among them who lived in urban and settled communities. Their linguistic usage also constituted the basic framework of textual interpretation.[3]

---

2. Tyser et al., *The Mejelle*, Art. 36. The *Mejelle* records several other legal maxims on custom, including: "the use of men is evidence according to which it is necessary to act" (Art. 37). For further details, see Kamali, *Principles*, 371.

3. Cf. Ibn Qudamah, *al-Mughni*, vol. 13, 83.

With regard to animals and life forms that were unfamiliar to the Arabs at the time, questions were asked as to whether the animal in question resembled any of the varieties familiar to them, and if it did, an analogy was likely to be attempted. But if no resemblance was found, the likely position would still tilt toward permissibility by reference to the general guidelines found in the Qur'anic verse cited earlier (al-An'am, 6:145). That verse begins with the declaration that nothing that God Most High has revealed to the people is *haram* unless it be one of the ten varieties of forbidden items stated therein. For the Shafi'is and Hanbalis, regarding an unknown animal on which there is no guideline in the scripture nor general consensus, whether it is permissible or otherwise, reference is to be made to the people of sound nature (*ahl al-tab' al-salimah*) among the generality of Arabs, be it urban or rural and under normal conditions, although the Hanbalis prefer the urban populations (*ahl al-amsar*) among them. Bedouins, poor people, and those who are in need or on the verge of starvation should not be asked, it is said, as they may eat whatever they find, and hence their views do not establish guidelines.[4] The only exception of note here is the Maliki school, which, even though accepting the role of general custom as a source of law and judgment, still did not attach the same degree of credibility to the Arab custom and relied mainly on the scripture in the determination of *tayyib* and *khabith*. Two other verses of the Qur'an that the Maliki school have cited in this connection, in addition to the one just mentioned, where God Most High declared:

He created for you (your benefit) all that is in the earth. (al-Baqarah, 2:29)

He has explained to you in detail that which has been forbidden to you. (al-An'am, 6:119)

Reading these and other Qur'anic verses together led Muslim jurists and commentators in the leading schools of Islamic law, especially those of the Maliki school, to the conclusion that nothing was forbidden for human consumption and benefit unless the scripture clearly identified and determined it as such.[5]

---

4. al-Zuhayli, *al-Fiqh al-Islami*, vol. 3, 513–514. The traditional view that prefers Arab and affluent people may be adjusted in Muslim countries with non-Arab populations; their customary practice and general preference would, in the present writer's opinion, hold a similar shariah validity in matters of interpretation that could be so contextualized.

5. Ibn Qudamah, *al-Mughni*, vol. 13, 75–76; al-Zuhayli, *al-Fiqh al-Islami*, vol. 3, 507–508; Wizarat, *al-Mawsu'ah al-Fiqhiyyah*, vol. 5, 146–147.

## 15

# Meat, Poultry, Seafood, and Dairy Products

GENERALLY, GOATS, SHEEP, cows, buffaloes, deers, camels, gazelles, zebras, giraffes, and all wild animals that do not have canine teeth are halal for slaughter and consumption, and all schools of Islamic law, including the Ja'fari Shia, are in agreement on this. Excluded from the halal category are beasts of prey having canine teeth, claws, and fangs, such as lions, wolves, dogs, tigers, leopards, and cats, as they feed on meat including carrion.

The Qur'anic references to cattle (*al-an'am*) and their permissibility for human benefit and consumption has raised questions as to the precise meaning of *al-an'am*—what it includes and what it does not. The word also occurs in several verses, including:

> Lawful unto you (for food) are all four-footed animals (*bahimat al-an'am*), with exceptions that are named otherwise. (al-Ma'idah, 5:1)
>
> It is God who made cattle for you (*ja 'ala lakum al-an'ama*) that you may use for riding and some for food. And in them there are other advantages for you. (Ghafir, 40:79–80)
>
> And cattle He has created for you (*wa'l-an'ama khalaqaha lakum*) to derive from them warmth and numerous (other) benefits, and of their (meat) you eat. And you have a sense of pride and beauty in them when you ride them home in the evening. They carry your heavy loads . . . and He created horses, mules and donkeys for you to ride and for beauty. (al-Nahl, 16:5–8).

Commentators have differed on the precise meaning of *al-an'am* in these verses. The first view, which is attributed to Ahmad b. Yahya al-Nahwi (d.

*Shariah and The Halal Industry.* Mohammad Hashim Kamali, Oxford University Press. © Oxford University Press 2021.
DOI: 10.1093/oso/9780197538616.003.0016

291H/904) of Baghdad and author of *Ma 'ani al-Qur'an wa I'rab al-Qur'an* (Meanings and pronunciation—desinential inflection of the Qur'an) maintains that *al-an'am* refers to all grazing livestock that God Most High has created, without any specification. This wider meaning is implied in the first of the three verses above, which mentions all four-footed animals and is not confined to cattle as such, but also includes all that which resemble the familiar varieties. The second meaning, which is recorded in *Tafsir al-Razi*, is that it refers to camels only. This is the meaning Ibn Manzur has recorded in *Lisan al-'Arab* for *al-an'am*. To confine *al-an'am* to camels only is a weak position. For one thing, Ibn Manzur has used the singular *al-n'am*, whereas the Qur'an pluralizes it to give it a wider application, but even if one agrees that it meant camels to some Arab communities, that still does not preclude the inclusion of cows and sheep, or indeed all four-footed animals. The third view is attributed to many Companions and Successors, and also to some early scholars, including al-Hasan and Qatadah, and recorded by al-Tabari (d. 310/923), which maintains that *al-an'am* means camels, cows, and sheep. It is then added that this last meaning is prevalent among the Arabs. This is perhaps supported further by how the Qur'an uses *al-an'am* in the third verse, which refers to the many uses of *al-an'am*, then followed by a reference to three animals—horses, mules, and donkeys—in a way that distinguishes these from the *bahimat al-an'am* variety of the familiar edible cattle (camels, cows, sheep, and goats). This is the preferred position also recorded in *Tafsir Ibn Kathir* (vol. 2, p. 5), but Ibn Kathir widens it a little by adding that animals similar to camels and cows, such as the wild varieties of the same and gazelles, etc., are also included in the meaning of *al-an'am*, which is inclined to support the first or the wider interpretation.[1] Abdullah Yusuf Ali also relies on the wider meaning of *al-an'am*, and his comments on the many uses thereof include their uses for riding, beauty, and comfort as well as for food. The many other uses of *al-an'am* include their uses for ploughing, and for their milk, wool, or hair; from their carcasses, too, people derive bones and horns for many industrial uses and so forth.[2]

*Haram* meat and meat products include pig meat of all kind, and pork and porcine products and ingredients. All Muslims are forbidden from consuming pork, without exception. It is also *haram* to raise, transport, or trade in swine and porcine products and derivatives. The Malikis have held predatory

---

1. For details on all these views, see al-Harithi, *al-Nawazil fi'l-At'imah*, vol. 2, 517–520.

2. Ali, *Meaning of the Holy Qur'an*, 1023, note 4456.

animals to be reprehensible or *makruh* for human consumption, but have held some, such as fox, hyena, and elephants, to be halal. It is reported that the two leading disciples of Imam Abu Hanifah, Abu Yusuf and Muhammad al-Shaybani, have concurred. The majority of schools and leading Imams, including Abu Hanifah, Malik, al-Thawri, the renowned Madinese scholar and Successor Saʿid ibn al-Musayyib, and the Jaʿfari Shia have held them to be *haram*, as they are subsumed under the hadith *"dhi nab min al-siba"* that include predatory animals with canine teeth, fangs, and tusk, be they small, such as mice and other rodents, or large, such as lions, tigers, and bears, regardless of whether they are carnivores or herbivores, and whether domestic (such as cats), or wild (such as hyenas and wolves).[3] Animals that qualify as one or both of these (i.e., predatory, and having canine teeth and tusks) are subsumed under the hadith and therefore non-halal. There is some discussion and odd reports from the Companions that suggest the permissibility of hyenas, yet the majority position on hyenas and cats, both wild and domesticated, is that they are forbidden. As for zebras, wild camels, and gazelles, they are halal by general consensus. The ruling on domesticated donkeys is that they are non-halal; zebra is a wild donkey, but when a zebra is domesticated, it also takes the ruling of domesticated donkey and becomes non-halal—based on the clear terms of the hadith that proscribe the flesh of domesticated donkeys. The hadith of Jabir bin ʿAbd Allah quoted above is also quoted in authority on the prohibition of donkeys. Then again, if a domesticated zebra returns to the wild, it becomes halal again.[4]

Horse meat is halal regardless of its type and breed, whether Arabian or otherwise. This is on the authority of a hadith reported by Jabir ibn ʿAbd Allah that "the Prophet, pbuh, prohibited the flesh of domesticated donkeys, but gave permission concerning the horsemeat."[5] According to the Hanafis, and also a minority opinion in the Maliki school, horsemeat is halal, but both these schools have held them to be reprehensible (*makruh*), as horses are used for *jihad*. This is also the position of the Shia Imamiyyah. There is no question over the permissibility of the leftover of a horse, and its milk, which are halal. Those who hold horsemeat to be strongly reprehensible (*makruh*

---

3. Cf. Ibn Qudamah, *al-Mughni*, vol. 13, 104. There are some reports, even in the hadith, on the permissibility of *hyenas*, as Ibn Qudamah explains, but which are disputed as *hyenas* are predatory and do have canine teeth.

4. Wizarat, *al-Mawsuʿah al-Fiqhiyyah*, vol. 5, 134–135.

5. Hadith reported by both al-Bukhari and Muslim; see Ibn Qudamah, *al-Mughni*, vol. 13, 77; Wizarat, *al-Mawsuʿah al-Fiqhiyyah*, vol. 5, 138.

*tahrimi*), which includes the Hanafi scholar Hasan ibn Ziyad, and Ibn Khalil of the Maliki school, refer to the Qur'anic verse, quoted above, especially the portion that states, "And (He created) horses, mules and donkeys for you to ride and beautify [your lives] with" (al-Nahl, 16:8), which evidently precludes their use for food. But then it is added that these readings are in the nature of interpretation, as neither the verse itself nor the evidence in hadith are specific enough to warrant definitive conclusions. This last verse clearly refers to mule and donkey side by side with the horse. We know from evidence in the hadith that donkeys and mules are non-halal, which would leave the horse as an exception—hence a degree of ambiguity is still present. Yet it is fairly clear from the general tenor of the existing evidence, especially the evidence in hadith, that horsemeat is halal but the donkey and mule are non-halal.[6]

In a hadith the renowned Companion Khalid ibn al-Walid has reported, he has stated that "the Prophet, pbuh, prohibited the flesh of donkey, horse and mule—*naha rasul Allah 'an luhum al-humur wa'l-khayl wa'l-bighal.*" Yet a different version of this hadith has been recorded on the authority of Jabir b. 'Abd Allah, and cited by al-Bukhari and Muslim, provides that "the Prophet, pbuh, prohibited, on the day of [the battle of] Khaybar the flesh of domesticated donkeys but permitted the flesh of horse." Due to the mixed nature of the evidence on these animals, most scholars of the Hanafi and Hanbali schools are inclined to place donkey and mule under the category of *makruh*, based on caution, although the Shafi'is consider them to be *haram*.[7]

The permissibility or otherwise of four animals—giraffe, rabbit, desert lizard (*al-dabb*), and gerbil (*al-yarbu'*)—has aroused disagreement among Muslim scholars from early times due to the mixed nature of the evidence concerning them. Badriyyah al-Harithi has listed only these four as among animals on which the scholars are in disagreement, and then scrutinizes the evidence on all of them in about fourteen pages. We shall not examine the details, but review only the conclusions she has arrived at. She notes that the evidence she has examined is mostly in the nature of probability and preference, but it is generally affirmative on all four, saying that they are all halal,

---

6. Cf. Ibn Qudamah, *al-Mughni*, vol. 13, 77; Wizarat, *al-Mawsu'ah al-Fiqhiyyah*, vol. 5, 138–139; al-Qurtubi, *Bidayat al-Mujtahid*, vol. 1, 344; Fadlullah, *Islamic Rulings*, 290.

7. Cf. Ibn Qudamah, *al-Mughni*, vol. 13, 77; Wizarat, *al-Mawsu'ah al-Fiqhiyyah*, vol. 5, 138–139; al-Qurtubi, *Bidayat al-Mujtahid*, vol. 1, 344; Fadlullah, *Islamic Rulings*, 290. See also al-Zuhayli, *al-Fiqh al-Islami*, vol. 3, 675–676.

notwithstanding some differences of opinion that may still obtain in the leading schools of law.[8]

According to the Malaysian Halal Standards, aquatic animals are those which live in water and cannot survive outside it, such as fish. All aquatic animals are halal except for those that are poisonous, intoxicating, or hazardous to health. Animals that live both on land and water, such as crocodiles, turtles, and frogs, are not halal. Aquatic animals which live in *najis* waters or continually fed with *najis* are also not halal.

The Malaysian Halal Standard (MS 1500-2009) includes, under "sources of halal food and drinks," three main sources, namely animals, plants, and chemical and there are separate sections also for minerals, drinks, and genetically modified food (GMF).

Animals are, under MS 1500-2009, divided into two categories: land animals and aquatic animals. It is then declared at the outset that "all land animals are halal as food" except the following: (a) animals that are not slaughtered according to shariah law; (b) *najis mughallazah* (intensely unclean) animals, namely pigs and dogs and their descendants; (c) animals with long pointed teeth or tusks that are used to kill prey, such as tigers, bears, elephants, cats, monkeys, etc.; (d) predator birds such as eagles, owls, etc.; (e) pests and/or poisonous animals such as rats, cockroaches, centipedes, scorpions, snakes, wasps and other similar animals; (f) animals that are forbidden to be killed in Islam, such as bees (*al-nahlah*), woodpeckers (*hudhud*), etc.; (g) creatures that are considered repulsive, such as lice, flies, etc.; (h) farmed halal animals that are intentionally and continually fed with filth/*najis*; and (i) other animals forbidden to be eaten in accordance to shariah law, such as donkeys and mules.[9]

## Birds

Birds are generally held to be permitted, especially those with flowing blood in their bodies (*dhi dam sa'il*) that also have feathers, do not have strong claws with which they could hunt, and do not predominantly live on consuming carrion and filth. It is also understood that not all birds with strong claws fit for hunting do actually hunt, and what they may consume is also not always carrion and filth, in which case they would qualify as halal. An example of

---

8. al-Harithi, *al-Nawazil fi'l-At'imah*, vol. 2, 525–541.

9. MS 1500-2009 (Clause 3.5.1.1.1).

this is ostrich, which is halal. The halal poultry include chicken, fowl, quails, turkey, hens, geese, doves, barn sparrow, partridge, stork, crane, sand grouse, starling, and duck, and most likely also those that resemble these in looks, habit, and lifestyle. Textbook writers have quoted hadith reports on most of these, stating that they are halal, and are therefore included in the meaning of the Qur'anic verse that "He (Prophet) makes lawful to them (Muslims) the *tayyibat*" (al-A'raf, 7:157).[10]

Non-halal birds include those that prey on carcasses, such as vultures, crows, eagles, falcons, peregrine falcons, sparrow hawks, owls, and other scavenger birds. Bats of all types are also forbidden. Parrot and peacock are non-halal according to the Shafi'is, due to their abominable flesh, but halal according to the Hanbalis, whereas the Hanafis have held many of these, excepting bats and vultures (which are *haram*), to be *makruh tahrimi*, or reprehensible close to *haram*. They are *haram* according to the majority, but not according to the Maliki school. Yet there is some disagreement among the Maliki jurists themselves on this. A minority of the Maliki jurists have held these birds to be *makruh* near to *makruh tahrimi*. The main evidence on this is the hadith of Ibn 'Abbas, cited earlier, wherein the Prophet declared birds with claws (*dhi makhlab*) prohibited for human consumption. Some disagreement has arisen on the meaning of this term. The Arabs tend to use *dhi makhlab* in reference to birds that always hunt with their claws, which would preclude some birds that do have claws, such as cockerel, doves, and sparrows, but do not hunt with them; they are therefore not included in the hadith expression of *dhi makhlab*. These latter birds use their claws for other purposes, such as holding and digging, but not for predatory activities.[11] The permissive Maliki opinion on these birds is based on their reading of the Qur'anic verse cited above (al-An'am, 6:145), which specifies the prohibited varieties of substances and then declares that nothing beyond the mentioned items is *haram* for consumption. All other animals and birds are therefore presumed to be lawful unless there be specific evidence on them in the Sunnah to say otherwise.

The Hanafi, Shafi'i, and Hanbali schools, as well as the Shia Imamiyyah, are in agreement that birds which always or most of the times feed on carrion and filth are prohibited, and this include the large black and speckled

---

10. Cf. Ibn Qudamah, *al-Mughni*, vol. 13, 88–89; al-Zuhayli, *al-Fiqh al-Islami*, vol. 3, 677; al-Harithi, *al-Nawazil fi'l-At'imah*, vol. 2, 520–521.

11. Ibn Hazm, *al-Muhalla*, vol. 4, 405; see also Fadlullah, *Islamic Rulings*, 292.

crows, although the Hanafis say these are *makruh tahrimi*, since the evidence on their prohibition is less than decisive. Included in this is the vulture, which always feed on carcasses, even though it does not actually hunt with its claws, the smaller field crow, which has a red beak and feet, and also the raven. The magpie is held to be *haram* according to the majority, but *makruh tahrimi* according to the Hanafis, for it feeds on both grains and carcasses. The Malikis, on the other hand, have held all types of crows to be halal, although a group of the Maliki jurists preclude from this the ones that feed on filth and carcasses. Basic authority on the prohibition of crows is found in a hadith on the authority of 'Aishah that the Prophet has said: "Five *fawasiq*—obnoxious creature—are to be killed [regardless as to] whether one is within or outside the state of sanctity (i.e., *ihram* for the haj): snake (in some reports it is rat), Black Kite (*al-hadʾat*), crow, rabby dog (*al-kalb al-ʿaqur*), and scorpion."[12]

With the minor exception of hunted birds and animals that may be out of reach for ritual slaughter, in all other cases, animals that are not properly slaughtered are non-halal. This includes improperly slaughtered animals as well as ones that die naturally from disease, altercations with other animals, or cruelty by humans. The milk and eggs of prohibited animals and birds are also forbidden for consumption.

Hunting of permitted animals like deer, and birds like dove, pheasants, and quails, is permitted for the purpose of eating but not for pleasure. Hunting by any means and with any tools (like guns, arrows, spears, and trapping) is permitted. Trained dogs and birds may also be used for catching or retrieving the quarry. The name of God may be pronounced at the time of ejecting, firing, or launching the hunting tool. The dying bird should be slaughtered by slitting its throat as soon as it is caught. If the *tasmiyah* is uttered at the time of pulling the trigger and the bird or animal dies before the hunter reaches it, it would still be considered halal.[13]

## Fish and Marine Life

Fish and seafood, including shellfish and all fish that have hard scales on their exterior surface, are halal. Included in this are also "sea locusts," or prawns. Fish and seafood may be hunted or caught by any reasonable means available,

---

12. Hadith recorded by both al-Bukhari and Muslim; see also Wizarat, *al-Mawsuʿah al-Fiqhiyyah*, vol. 5, 136; al-Qurtubi, *Bidayat al-Mujtahid*, vol. 1, 344; and Ibn Qudamah, *al-Mughni*, vol. 13, 83.

13. Cf. Wizarat, *al-Mawsuʿah al-Fiqhiyyah*, vol. 5, 138–142.

as long as it is done humanely, and need not be ritually slaughtered. The dead of the sea are halal on the authority of a clear hadith, as earlier cited. This hadith also sustains the conclusion that all marine creatures are clean, whether caught alive or dead, including those found floating in the water, and that no ritual slaughter or other form of purification is necessary. It is further concluded that the floating carcass of the sea is clean, regardless of whether it died naturally or due to an accident or other cause, provided in all cases that no obvious evidence of disease or decay is noticeable. However, no fish must be made to suffer in the name of slaughter. Thus, it is unlawful to bludgeon a live fish or marine creature, nor may they be cut open while alive. It must not be cooked alive either, but should be left to die naturally. There is no special method of killing the sea locust either. Hunting of all kind is strictly prohibited during the haj pilgrimage to Ka'bah and within the defined boundaries of the city of Mecca. Amphibians, such as frogs, alligators, turtles, and seahorses, are forbidden. As for the eggs of fish and sea animals, they follow the same ruling as the fish or animal themselves. In the event of decay or signs of disease, it is likely to fall under the rubric of that which is naturally objectionable and filthy (*khaba'ith*). And lastly, neither the Qur'an nor the hadith evidence specify the religion of the person who might have caught, hunted, or found the dead of the sea. Muslims and non-Muslims therefore all stand on the same footing.[14]

The *fiqh* scholars do not include sea birds under marine life, for the simple reason that they do not live under the water but immerse therein temporarily or on occasions when they try to catch something. Hence the rules of ritual slaughter would be applicable to them as to other birds in general. Geese and ducks are not included in marine animals either—they are halal without any doubt, but are subject to ritual purification by slaughter. There is disagreement over the permissibility of snails. Those who consider snails to be halal also consider lobster to be halal, and those who consider lobster to be non-halal also maintain the same about snails. This is based on the analysis that lobster originates in snails, and the ruling of the one therefore applies to the other.[15]

The permissive position of the majority of schools of Islamic law, excepting the Hanafi, on marine creatures is extended, as already noted, to

---

14. Cf. Wizarat, *al-Mawsu'ah al-Fiqhiyyah*, vol. 5, 132. See also Fadlullah, *Islamic Rulings*, 291, 297.

15. al-Haitami, *Tuhfat al-Muhtaj*, vol. 9, 378.

amphibians, or marine animals that can live on land for a fair amount of time, such as turtles, frogs, lobsters, and even crocodiles. The Hanafis are more restrictive, subscribing to the view that all sea animals, except for fish, are non-halal. Some early Hanafi scholars, such as Ibn Abi Layla (d. 83/702) and al-Layth b. Sa'd (d. 791/1389), have excepted frogs, lobsters, sea snakes, otter, and shark to be halal, but with slaughter or *tadhkiyah*. The majority position of the Hanafi school maintains that all of these are non-halal, and that frogs, lobsters, and sea snakes are subsumed by the Qur'anic prohibition of *al-khaba'ith* (filthy) and forbidden. Al-Kasani has to this effect cited a hadith wherein the Prophet was asked about the fat of frog which was used in a medicine, but the Prophet merely prohibited the killing of frogs, and this is deemed to include consuming its flesh too.[16] The Shafi'i school considers amphibians that can live permanently in sea or on land to be non-halal if they have no equivalent on land. Included in this are frogs, turtles, and crocodiles. Al-Rafi'i, al-Nawawi, and al-Ramli, among key Shafi'i jurists, have concurred with this. However, it is noted that the correct Shafi'i position on this is that of al-Nawawi, which is articulated in al-Majmu'. Thus it is held that all animals that actually live in the sea are halal even if it is possible for them to survive on land, except for the frog and poisonous animals.[17] This they say is the purport of the renowned hadith that "the sea water is clean and so is the dead of the sea which is halal—*Huwa al-tahuru ma'uhu al-hillu maytatuh*."[18] As for marine animals other than fish, they are also clean except for beaver and bear (in Arabic: *khinzir al-maa' wa kalb al-maa'*), as they cannot be subsumed under fish (*al-samak*), and also that their equivalents on land are non-halal. As for sea animals that resemble halal animals on land, they are halal even if they can live on land.

Names such as "snake fish" (*marmahi*), and "water pig" (*khinzir al-maa*) do apparently matter. This can be seen, for instance, with reference to lobsters (*'aqrab al-maa'*, lit. "water scorpion") and snake fish, which are juxtaposed to their equivalents on land and then subsumed under the same ruling (i.e., non-halal). It is further added that crocodiles and turtles are non-halal, as they are subsumed under the *khaba'ith*. That said, some of these additions have

---

16. al-Kasani, *Bada'i' al-Sana'i'*, vol. 5, 35, as also quoted in Uwais, *Mawsu'ah al-Fiqh al-Islami*, vol. 14, 264.

17. Cf. Wizarat, *al-Mawsu'ah al-Fiqhiyyah*, vol. 5, 130.

18. Hadith quoted in Wizarat, *al-Mawsu'ah al-Fiqhiyyah*, vol. 5, 131; also quoted by al-Zuhayli, *al-Fiqh al-Islami*, vol. 1, 114.

invoked differences of opinion in the Shafi'i school.[19] The Hanbali position concerning amphibians such as the otter, turtle, and lobster is that they are halal, subject to ritual slaughter.[20] As for the crocodile, they hold that they are subsumed under the category of predatory animals and therefore non-halal. The same applies to the sea snake, which is non-halal and falls under either the category of poisonous mammals or that which is abominable/*khabith*, as is the frog, which is non-halal, but on a different ground: the juridical prohibition of frogs is based on hadith that only proscribes the killing of frogs. With regard to shark, the Hanbali school is of the view that it is halal, even if predatory, as it is a variety of fish. The Shafi'i school subsumes crocodiles under predatory animals. Ibn Qudamah has recorded the Hanbali position to say that all sea game is permissible except for frogs. In support of this is also quoted a statement of Abu Bakr al-Siddiq that God Most High has purified all that which is in the sea, and then quoted to that effect the verse that "halal to you are the game of the sea and its foodstuff" (al-Ma'idah, 5:96).[21]

The majority position on marine creatures is that they are generally halal for human consumption, but that this applies to marine animals that live in deep sea and cannot live outside it. Quoted in authority for this are two verses from the Qur'an, as follows:

> Nor are the two bodies of flowing water alike—the one palatable, sweet and pleasant to drink, and the other salty and bitter. Yet from each you eat fresh and tender meat. (Fatir, 35:12)

> But forbidden to you is the pursuit of land game as long as you are in the Sacred Precincts (of the Holy Mosque in Mecca) or in pilgrim garb. (al-Ma'idah, 5:96)

It is stated that the text in both of these verses is general (*'aam*), in that they do not mention fish or any other animal by name—hence all game of the sea is included. It is on this basis that the Maliki school has applied the presumption of permissibility (*ibahah*) so widely as to include bear, otter, and monkey among the permissible animals, which the majority do not consider to be halal. However, a minority among the Maliki jurists maintain these to

---

19. For details, see Uwais, *Mawsu'ah al-Fiqh al-Islami*, vol. 14, 266–267.

20. Ritual slaughter of a lobster may consist of incision or piercing any part of its body.

21. Ibn Qudamah, *al-Mughni*, vol. 3, 529; Wizarat, *al-Mawsu'ah al-Fiqhiyyah*, vol. 5, 131.

be reprehensible, or *makruh tanzihi*, which is closer to *mubah*. The Shafiʿis consider it recommendable to slaughter sea creatures that are very large in size and live long lives, such as large fish and whales. This kind of fish is slaughtered horizontally in line with the tail that consist of a slit near the head whereas land animals are slaughtered by the neck.[22]

A great deal of the differences of opinion between the leading schools of law, especially when the Hanafis take a different view than that of the majority, depend on their differential approaches to textual interpretation. With reference to the general proclamations (*ʿaam*) of the Qurʾan, for instance, the majority consider the general of the Qurʾan and hadith to be speculative (*zanni*), and open therefore to interpretation and qualification, whereas the Hanafis maintain that the *ʿaam* of the Qurʾan is definitive (*qatʿi*), on the analysis that this is the nature of the language. Words normally convey their general and all-inclusive meaning, and they must be understood as such, unless there is evidence to specify or qualify them in some ways. The majority (*jumhur*) view on this may be illustrated as follows: When the Qurʾan delivers a ruling on fish, for instance, without specifying or qualifying the fish varieties, the word "fish" is too general to preclude some qualification, for instance, regarding poisonous fish, predatory fish, snake-like fish, small and large fish, and so forth, and whether it also includes the whale. The word "fish" is therefore open to interpretation, which may be attempted by the Sunnah, or by way of *ijtihad* in line with the methodology of interpretation found in *usul al-fiqh*.[23] This can also be said with reference to the hadith just quoted, when it says that "the dead of the sea is clean"—this too is a general and speculative proclamation and is, according to the majority (*jumhur*), open to interpretation. That said, the Hanafis are also known for their pragmatism and often tend to make suitable exceptions to the general when deemed necessary and appropriate. Somewhat like the Shafiʿi school, the Hanafis maintain as a rough guide to interpretation in the present context that marine animals which look like halal cattle and similar other land animals are presumed to be halal, but *haram* if they look like the prohibited land varieties.[24]

Fish gelatin is fully halal and acceptable to almost all mainstream religious bodies. Milk and dairy products such as cheese, ice cream, and yogurt

---

22. Wizarat, *al-Mawsuʿah al-Fiqhiyyah*, vol. 5, 130.

23. For details on the rules of interpretation Kamali, see *Principles of Islamic Jurisprudence*, chapter 4, "Rules of Interpretation I: Deducing the Law from Its Sources," 117–167 (see for *ʿaam* and *khass* 140–155).

24. Wizarat al-Awqaf, *al-Mawsuʿah al-Fiqhiyyah*, vol. 5, 130.

must not contain gelatin unless that gelatin is known to be from halal sources. Many cheeses contain rennet and other enzymes that are derived from animals. It is important to assure that these are derived from halal animals or from microbial or plant sources. Halal-certified hard and soft gelatin capsules are also available, and so are vegetarian capsules made with starch, cellulose, or other vegetable ingredients.

## Insects and Worms

Schools and scholars of Islamic law have differed on the permissibility or otherwise of insects for human consumption. Only the locust is mentioned in the clear text of hadith, and all schools concur on its permissibility. There is also evidence in hadith, as already noted, on the permissibility of desert lizard (*al-dabb*), and although the hadith on this subject does not convey a decisive ruling, it is understood to incline toward permissibility. The Shafi'is and Hanbalis have held permissible the consumption of worms that are born in food such as cheese and fruit on two conditions: (1) that it is eaten together with the food that carries it, whether alive or dead, but not if it is separated. This ruling is based on the *fiqh* principle-cum-legal maxim that "the follower follows—*al-tabi'u tabi*" If the carrier food, be it fruit, vegetables, or a dairy product, is halal, so is its worm. However, if the worm is taken out and separated, it is no longer subsumed by that principle. (2) That the food variety, be it solid or liquid, that carries the worm has not decayed or changed its color and taste; otherwise it will fall under the *khaba'ith* (unclean) and therefore non-permissible. This analysis is extended to situations where a worm, mothworm, or ant falls into food, such as oil or honey and the like, whether cooked or uncooked; here the presumption of permissibility continues if the taste and color remain unaffected and no decay is detectable, but not if they have been so infected. It is recommendable in all cases, however, to take out the visible insect or doubtful segment of the foodstuff before it is consumed.[25] Muslim jurists have, on a broader note, held three different views concerning the insects as follows:

1. That all types of insects fall under the category of abominable (*khaba'ith*), as they are deemed so by people of sound nature. The Hanafi school is more

---

25. Ibn Qudamah, *al-Mughni*, vol. 8, 605; Wizarat, *al-Mawsu'ah al-Fiqhiyyah*, vol. 5, 43; Fadlullah, *Islamic Rulings*, 290.

inclined toward taking this position than the other schools. The Ja'fari Shia also maintain that all insects, crawling or flying, except for the locusts, are forbidden for human consumption. The same position is maintained with regard to lizards, snakes, scorpions, and rats.[26]

2. Insects that are not harmful or evidently filthy are halal, and this is the position mainly of the Maliki school, but subject to ritual purification as follows: If the insect in question is of a type with no flowing blood in its body, such as snails, beetles, or wasps, it is purified in the same manner as the locust. As for those with flowing blood in their bodies, they are subject to ritual purification in the same way as specified for other animals.[27] The Malikis also maintain the view concerning mice and rats that they are *makruh* if it is known that they have come into contact with filth, but are *mubah* otherwise. This is perhaps where one can distinguish between *mubah*/halal, which is merely tolerated but repulsive otherwise, and *tayyib*, pure and wholesome that is clean and naturally appealing.

3. The third position on insects has it that no general ruling can be advanced over all insect varieties. So the best position is that which looks into each of them according to their individual particularities and characteristics.[28]

---

26. Wizarat, *al-Mawsu'ah al-Fiqhiyyah*, vol. 14, 277.

27. This distinction between insects with or without fluid blood in their bodies is often used as a pointer with regard to the cleanliness or otherwise of their dead. The dead of the animals with fluid blood is unclean, and is made unclean also if they fall into liquid food—unlike the ones without flowing blood in their bodies, which do not have the same effect. That said, *fiqh* manuals tend to discuss various types of insects individually, each according to their own characteristics. Cf. Wizarat, *al-Mawsu'ah al-Fiqhiyyah*, vol. 5, 141.

28. Wizarat al-Awqaf, *al-Mawsu'ah al-Fiqhiyyah*, vol. 5, 144; Uwais, *Mawsu'ah al-Fiqh al-Islami*, vol. 14, 272–274.

# 16

## Fatwa *Issuance in Shariah*

MANY ASPECTS OF the lawful and unlawful in food, medicine, and other areas have been regulated through legislation and expert guidelines, and when that is the case, there may be no need for separate *fatwas*. This is because a law duly passed by the people's elected assembly and head of state, while not contrary to any of the shariah principles, becomes the ruling (*hukm*) of the lawful authority (*ulil-amr*) and commands obedience—hence there remains no room for a separate *fatwa* on a matter that is regulated by that law. Yet *fatwa* would still have a role, either to elucidate those positions, suggest the best methods for their implementation under new conditions, or address questions posed by people, Muslims and non-Muslims, who ask for greater clarity and guidance, especially pertaining to Islam.

This chapter begins with an overview of *fatwa* in shariah, its history of development, and its role in bringing the shariah closer to the realities of people's lives. This is followed by brief information on *fatwa*-related developments in Malaysia, although a fuller picture of this is provided in Part II, under "*Fatwa* Issuance in Malaysia," which deals with halal-related *fatwa*s issued by the Malaysian authorities.

Literally meaning "a response," *fatwa* (pl. *fatawa*) is defined as a response given by a qualified scholar (i.e, a mufti) to a particular issue put to him by a person or a group of persons or organization. The mufti expounds the Islamic position on the issue and conveys it to the questioner. It is not a requirement, although recommended, for a *fatwa* to explain the evidence on which it is founded, which is, however, a requirement of *ijtihad*. A *fatwa* issued by a competent scholar, who explains the evidential basis of his or her *fatwa*, and also includes an element of originality and research, may well be equivalent to

*Shariah and The Halal Industry.* Mohammad Hashim Kamali, Oxford University Press. © Oxford University Press 2021. DOI: 10.1093/oso/9780197538616.003.0017

*ijtihad.*[1] Whereas a *fatwa* consists essentially of conveying (*ikhbar*) the ruling/ *hukm* of shariah in response to a question, *ijtihad* consists of the extraction and formulation of such a ruling from the sources of shariah, in the event where the relevant answer is not available in the existing sources. This would mean that *ijtihad* has a stronger elements of originality and research compared to *fatwa*.[2] It is advisable for the mufti, however, to explain the rationale of the *fatwa* as well as its supportive evidence for purposes of educating and enlightening the questioner. *Fatwa* and *ijtihad* consist mainly of an opinion that does not bind the person or persons to whom they are addressed. The recipient of a *fatwa* is consequently free to refer the matter to another mufti and obtain a second, or even a third, *fatwa* on the same matter, none of which would be binding, and it is that person's choice whether or not to comply with any of them. The key Hanbali scholar Ibn Qayyim al-Jawziyyah (d. 751/ 1350), has warned against ascribing finality to the *fatwa* and *ijtihad* of anyone, including the *mujtahidun* of the past, for that would ignore the basic rule that *fatwa* and *ijtihad* are changeable with the change of times.[3]

Historically, *fatwa* began as a private activity independent of state intervention and control. The ulema who acted as muftis often responded to people's questions over issues and gave *fatwa* as a service to the community; they themselves usually set their professional standards without government intervention. They provided advice about questions of Islamic law and religion that people posed to them, and provided their assistance in court cases or for personal guidance.[4]

*Fatwa* is not permissible if it goes against the clear text or general consensus (*ijma'*), nor should a *fatwa* that is given be based on mere speculation and conjecture without a valid basis. Should there be conflicting views and interpretations in the sources, the mufti should not simply select an

---

1. Cf. Wizarat, *al-Mawsu'ah al-Fiqhiyyah,* "Fatwa," vol. 32, 25.

2. Examples of brief questions put to a mufti may be when someone asks him: "Is it an obligation for me to support may parents; or can I give a blind animal in sacrifice for *'Id al-Adha*?" Whereas the *fiqh* books usually record questions of this nature, in our times, muftis and scholars of shariah are often confronted with a wider mix of socioreligious, financial, and political issues and questions, which means that no ready answers may be available and the mufti may be called upon to explore and research the source evidence more often now than might have been the case in earlier times.

3. Ibn Qayyim, *I'lam al Muwaqqi'in,* vol. 4, 309.

4. Cf. Kamali, "The Johor Fatwa," 111f.

undigested position, but should try to verify and attempt, if possible, prefer-ence (*al-tarjih*) in order to establish a better and clearer response.[5]

A *fatwa* must be informed by the nature of the issue or incident it is addressing, and also verify correct application of the relevant rules, for real-life situations and issues that are hardly identical and may well involve new and unprecedented elements that require careful consideration. To give an example, A asks a mufti whether he has to support his father. The obvious answer to this found in shariah sources is the general obligation of an affluent son to support his indigent father. Then it has to also be ascertained whether or not the son is indebted, and his level of affluence and debt, which may barely be enough to support his wife and children, and also whether anyone among his immediate dependents happens to be ill and in need of special care and so forth—and only then should a *fatwa* be issued.[6]

Scriptural authority for *fatwa* is found in several verses of the Qur'an, in-cluding al-Nisa' 4:127 and 176, where God Most High gives direction to the Prophet by way of *fatwa*. In the former verse, it is provided: "They ask you for instruction (*yastaftunaka*) concerning the women. Say God does instruct you about them." The latter of the two verses provides guidance concerning a question of inheritance, known as *kalalah*:

> They ask thee for a juridical decision. Say: God directs you (*yuftikum*)
> about persons who leave no descendants or ascendants.[7]

It is further added that the Prophet, pbuh, also acted as mufti to his followers in the sense of explaining the guidelines of the Qur'an to them. A mufti thus becomes successor to the Prophet in the sense of explaining God's ordinances and their application to the people regarding the issues they encounter.[8]

In the event that the petitioner asks for evidence, and the evidence is a verse from the Qur'an or a hadith and can be understood with a simple ex-planation, the mufti must give it. Muftis who adhere to a particular school of law, and who are unable to derive rulings directly from the primary sources, would be likely to cite an earlier reference work from within the school of

---

5. Wizarat, *al-Mawsu'ah al-Fiqhiyyah*, "Fatwa," vol. 32, 33–34.

6. Wizarat, *al-Mawsu'ah al-Fiqhiyyah*, "Fatwa," vol. 32, 26.

7. A reference to *fatwa* also occurs in sura Yusuf (12:43), and then the explanatory function of *fatwa* is further mentioned in al-Nahl (16:44).

8. For details, see Wizarat, *al-Mawsu'ah al-Fiqhiyyah*, "Fatwa," vol. 32, 23.

his persuasion. Over the past centuries, however, several reform movements arose in different parts of the Muslim world that sought to reduce the influence of imitation (*taqlid*) of prior works that consisted mainly of the views and interpretations of medieval scholars.[9] The position is all the more so in contemporary times, mainly due to the accelerated pace of socioeconomic change and the fact that the nature of issues faced may well relate to new and unprecedented developments in science and civilization.

When a mufti gives an erroneous *fatwa*, he falls into sin if he does so without having the necessary knowledge and qualification, or if he is qualified but neglects to investigate and look into the issue carefully. He is not committing a sin, however, if he is qualified and applies himself well but still makes an honest error of judgment. He may revoke his own *fatwa* if his error becomes known to him, and may rectify it as soon as possible without causing greater damage. For it is preferable to stop falsehood at an early opportunity rather than allowing it to perpetuate and cause greater harm. The second caliph 'Umar ibn al-Khattab's precedent is often quoted in support of the position that a mufti may change his *fatwa* if upon further reflection it appears to him that he had fallen into error, or when there is a change of circumstances calling for a review. The substance of that advice applies equally to adjudication and *fatwa*.[10] Further confirmation for this comes from the precedent of Imam Shafi'i, who developed his juristic thoughts in two separate phases. He changed many of the *fatwas* he had issued in Baghdad after his arrival in Egypt during the last five years of his life, because of the differences of culture and custom of Egyptian society that had bearings on his earlier *fatwas*.[11] These changes became so voluminous over the course of time that they became known, as a result, to have established two *madhhabs*, an Old *madhhab* (*al-qadim*) and a New *madhhab* (*al-jadid*).

Subsequent changes in a *fatwa* are also likely to involve preference for that which secures the higher purposes (*maqasid*) of shariah in a better way. For *fatwa* and *ijtihad* are the means by which the *fiqh* secures the higher purposes, or *maqasid*, of shariah. The changeability of *fatwa* and *ijtihad* and their openness to subsequent rectification and amendment also equip Islamic law with the tools to accommodate the changing conditions of society and to better

---

9. Cf. Furber, "Elements of a Fatwa," 2.

10. al-Jawziyyah, *I'lam al Muwaqqi'in*, vol. 1, 86.

11. See, for a discussion, al-Tamawi, *al-Sulatat al-Thalath*, 305 ff.

align with the *maqasid* of shariah.[12] Ibn Qayyim al-Jawziyyah has further observed that a *fatwa* is not only liable to change with the change of time and considerations of public interest, but also by reference to the peculiarities of the issue with which the mufti may be faced—what is referred to in Arabic as *munasabah* (appropriate) or *mula'amah* (harmonious). Examples that Ibn Qayyim has given in this connection include suspension of the prescribed penalties (*hudud*) during the year of drought in the time of 'Umar b. al-Khattab, and also the *fatwa* that allowed the testimony of one witness plus a solemn oath (the standard being two witnesses) during the time of 'Umar ibn 'Abd al-'Aziz (d. 101/721)—for reasons mainly of alleviation of hardship, which is a higher purpose (*maqsad*) of the shariah.[13]

The prominent Shafi'i jurist 'Izz al-Din 'Abd al-Salam al-Sulami observed that real life situations are mixed most of the time. When there is a conflict of two benefits (*maslahatayn*) and both cannot be obtained, or when a similar conflict exists between two harms and both of them cannot be avoided, or when a conflict is encountered between securing a benefit and preventing a harm—credibility in all of these is to be attached to that which is greater and graver, even if it means loss of a minor benefit or toleration of a lesser harm.[14] Al-Sulami continued, stating that in the event of a combination of benefits and harms, if obtaining the former and preventing the latter is possible, this should be done, as per guidelines of the Qur'an.[15] But if this is not possible, then if the harm is greater than the benefit, preventing a harm is given priority over the loss of benefit, but if the benefit in question is greater than the harm one is trying to avoid, the benefit should be secured and the harm is tolerated.[16] It is further added that the public interest takes priority over the private interest, and that the normal rules of law may be suspended by virtue of a pressing necessity—as in the legal maxim of *fiqh* that "necessities make the unlawful lawful."[17]

Among the etiquettes of *fatwa* (*adab al-fatwa*) that the *fiqh* blueprint underlines, one is that *fatwa* should be succinct, address the question, and

---

12. Cf. al-Bishry, "al-Jama'ah al-Wataniyyah," 138.

13. al-Jawziyyah, *I'lam al Muwaqqi'in,* vol. 3, 10, 14; al-Bishry, "al-Jama'ah al-Wataniyyah," 139.

14. 'Abd al-Salam, *al-Qawa'id al-Ahkam,* vol. 1, 5.

15. The Qur'anic verse al-Sulami has more specifically quoted is: "So fear God to the extent of your ability," (al-Taghabun, 64: 16);

16. 'Abd al-Salam, *al-Qawa'id al-Ahkam,* vol. 1, 110.

17. 'Abd al-Salam, *al-Qawa'id al-Ahkam,* vol. 1, 188.

avoid unnecessary expatiation, unless additional details are deemed necessary because of the gravity of the issue and in order to avoid misunderstanding. It is reported from 'Abd Allah ibn 'Umar, and Imams Malik and Ahmad ibn Hanbal, that the mufti should only attempt a *fatwa* in its proper context, avoid expatiation, and, if unsure of the response, should refer the matter to a more knowledgeable person.[18] The normative position for the mufti is not to refuse giving a *fatwa*, but he may exceptionally refuse to give it, if the subject happens to be too complex for the questioner to understand, or when he fears greater misunderstanding is likely to arise.

The *fatwa* issuance function is nowadays entrusted mainly to learned shariah academies and councils, although individual scholars also give *fatwas* in their private capacities and in response to questions they are asked, for public information and guidance, just as they also compile and publish their collection of *fatwas*, often in large volumes for academic purposes. What is now seen is thus a mixed pattern of the old and the new: collective and individual *fatwas* issued by muftis and scholars in their official and non-official capacities. Collective *fatwas* and *ijtihads* are becoming mainstream and usually attempted by learned Fiqh academies and institutions of research with specialized knowledge on issues of public concern.

What follows next are two *fatwa*-related themes, namely selection, and piecing together.

---

18. Due mainly to a hadith, although thought to be a *Mursal* (disconnected) in which it is reported from the Prophet to have said: "The most prompting of you in *fatwa* is most promoting on (hell) fire—*ajra'ukum 'ala'l-futya ajra'ukum 'alan-naar.*" The advice of this hadith is evidently a sense of restraint on the part of scholar and mufti to avoid facile and frequent issuance of *fatwas*. Recorded by al-Darimi on the authority of 'Ubaydullah b. Abi Ja'far. See Wizarat, *al-Mawsu'ah al-Fiqhiyyah,* vol. 32, 23.

# 17

# *Selection (*Takhayyur, *also* Takhyir)

SELECTION (*TAKHAYYUR*) ENABLES the follower of one of the four
Sunni schools or *madhhabs* to opt for the ruling of another in situations
where this alternative ruling offers a preferable option. *Takhayyur* also
applies within the one and the same school when an individual, be it a
scholar-jurist or a commoner, opts for a minority or less preferred position
that may be available within his or her own school of following. It is often
noted that leading figures within the same school have offered different
interpretations, or else have changed an earlier ruling of their own school
on a subsequent occasion, when the earlier position had fallen out of date
due to advancement in knowledge or a change of times or even the customary practices of people.

*Takhayyur* is also an integral part of Islam. The faithful are given the
choice, for instance, in the performance of the daily prayers (*salah*), to perform it within the appointed time segments, at the beginning of that time,
at the end, or indeed at any point of time in between, although early performance is recommended. The person who observes belated fasting of Ramadan
is also granted the choice to do it any time in the year that follows until the
next fasting month, although early performance is advised here too. The obligation of haj is once in a lifetime, and the faithful have the option regarding
when to do it. *Takhayyur* also relates to a holistic understanding of the shariah
scale of Five Values, in that only the *wajib* and the *haram* in them are in principle mandatory. All the other three intervening value points, namely the recommendable (*mandub*), permissible (*mubah*), and reprehensible (*makruh*),
are optional, giving the faithful the choice of whether or not to act on them,
and if one does act, in what way, and so forth. The option in question may
change, however, when the lawful authority decides to elevate a permissible

*Shariah and The Halal Industry.* Mohammad Hashim Kamali, Oxford University Press. © Oxford University Press 2021.
DOI: 10.1093/oso/9780197538616.003.0018

or a recommended shariah position into an obligation, in which case it would require compliance.[1]

The permissibility of *takhayyur* is based on the premise that the four leading schools have accepted each other as valid interpretations of Islam, notwithstanding certain reservations some commentators have expressed over a measure of "opportunism" or "forum shopping" that such eclecticism may involve.

The leading schools of law tend to concur regarding the essential principles of law and religion, but have also differed over many details and offered different interpretations to a certain text of the Qur'an or hadith that was open to interpretation. *Takhayyur* naturally takes its origins in scholastic plurality and differentiation. Seen in a positive light, it offers flexibility and expedience in the choice of available options. We explore these points further, but also the uses, if any, of *takhayyur* over the prospects of standardization. Can takhayyur be used to advance the prospects of uniformity and standardization in the theory and practice of halal?

Two other related expressions to *takhayyur* should be mentioned, namely *tatabbu' al-rukhas* (lit. "chasing concessions") and *tarjih* (preference). The former is often associated with crossing school boundaries in search of concessions, whereas *tarjih* (similar to *takhayyur*) facilitates the preference of one positions amid available options, often for expediency and convenience, and to some extent for adaptation to changing times. The scholar-*mujtahid*, or a number of them collectively who deliberate over an issue, resort to selection if a choice of positions exists, and would simply opt for one among the leading schools of law. In *tarjih*, the jurist selects one of the two or more positions through an assessment of the existing evidence.

Textual authority for *takhayyur*, *talfiq*, and even *tatabbu' al-rukhas* is sought in several Qur'anic verses that favor facility and ease for the people. The following three are often quoted in support:

God intends for you ease and does not intend hardship for you. (al-Baqarah, 2:185)

God does wish to lighten your (burden): for man was created weak. (al-Nisa', 4:28)

---

1. See, for details, Wizarat, *al-Mawsu'ah al-Fiqhiyyah*, "Takhyir," vol. 11, 67–81. See also, on the Scale of Five Values and the element of option that obtains in a *wajib* and other value points, Kamali, *Principles*, 413–416 ff.

He (God) has not meant to impose hardship in religion on you (al-Haj, 22:78).

Also quoted in support is the hadith wherein the Prophet is quoted to have said "I have been sent to [facilitate] tolerance and ease—*bu'ithtu bi'l-hanifiyyat al-samhah*."[2] In another hadith the Prophet instructed two of his prominent Companions, Mu'adh b. Jabal and Abu Musa al-Ash'ari, upon being sent as judges to the Yemen with specific instructions:

> Make matters easy for people and do not make them difficult. Give glad tidings to people and do not repel them.[3]

The Qur'an and hadith evidently provide encouragement for the judge, jurist, and mujtahid, indeed for all Muslims, to opt for easier positions whenever available and avoid imposing hardship on people, without, however, compromising on principles. *Takhayyur, talfiq, tarjih*, and *tatabbu' al-rukhas* can therefore be utilized in the construction of suitable responses to people's needs and pursuit of valid benefits (*maslahah*), but not when they are employed as instruments of distortion and escape from basic principles.[4]

The Hanafi jurist Ibn 'Abidin (d. 1258/1842) used *takhayyur* on occasions, but held in the meantime that it should be based on an assessment of evidence, and done only by judges and jurists who are fully qualified *mujtahids*; if they are imitators (*muqllids*), they should follow the opinion of more knowledgeable jurists. *Takhayyur* was, as such, used in more or less the same way as *tarjih*—both required careful examination of evidence.

A certain shift of opinion occurred during the first half of twentieth century in favor of *takhayyur* away from the derogatory overtones that were attached to *tatabbu' al-rukhas*. For instance, when the then rector of al-Azhar, Mustafa al-Maraghi, eulogized Muhammad Rashid Rida (d. 1935) on the occasion of the latter's death, he said that "he was a man of learning who selected rules that were beneficial to people and suitable for their age" (*takhayyar al-ahkam al-munasibah li'l-zaman wa'l-nafi'ah li'l-umam*).[5]

---

2. Ibn Hanbal, *Musnad*, vol. 36, 623–624, hadith no. 22291.

3. al-Bukhari, vol. 1, p. 25, hadith no. 69; Abu Dawud, *Sunan Abu Dawud*, vol. 1, 145, hadith 380.

4. Cf. al-Ghafur, *al-Taqlid wa'l-Talfiq*, 26.

5. al-Maraghi, as quoted in Ibrahim, *Pragmatism in Islamic Law*, 180.

When the choice of juristic opinion is based on good evidence, be it in *takhayyur* or preference (*tarjih*), it would generally imply that the different opinions partake in reasonable disagreement (*ikhtilaf*) and cannot be regarded as arbitrary or false. This evidence-based departure from one school's doctrine in favor of another, whether made by jurists or laity, was permitted by most jurists. Rather it was the activity of choosing juristic opinions to derive questionable outcomes that generated controversy. In the exercise of *tarjih*, the jurist is not expected to depart, in any significant way, from the largely predetermined juristic options established by the schools' leading authorities. That said, *tarjih* sometimes contained ad hoc reasoning designed to privilege the result that a given jurist may have desired. While *tarjih* is located in between the *ijtihad-taqlid* continuum, *takhayyur, talfiq*, and *tatabbuʿ al-rukhas* fall under the rubric of *taqlid* (imitation) simply because existing juristic views are selected based on their utility.[6]

*Takhayyur* has been used in many of the twentieth-century statutory reforms of Islamic family law and inheritance, although instances of its application to the halal industry are somewhat rare. To give an example of *takhayyur* in marriage legislation, many non-Hanafi countries of the Middle East and Asia have opted for the Hanafi law position that entitles an adult girl to contract her own marriage, even in the absence of her guardian (*wali*), whereas the majority position on this requires the guardian's consent. Similarly, the adoption in statutory law reform of judicial separation/divorce based on prejudice/*darar*, which the Maliki law validates but the other schools do not permit, is another instance of *takhayyur*. Twentieth-century family law reform legislation has generally selected the Hanafi law position on the marriage contract and that of the Maliki law position on divorce.[7]

One can perhaps give examples of a form of *takhayyur* in the halal industry regulatory regime, as earlier noted, with regard to that of *tasmiyah*, which is recommendable (*mandub*) under Shafiʿi law, but which the other schools of law tend to regard as obligatory. The halal industry regulations in Malaysia and many other countries have opted for the majority position, even though Malaysia is a Shafiʿi country. Another example may be for a Shafiʿi country to select the position of the Maliki school, if so desired or when shortages of meat supplies or other conditions so dictate, with regard to the permissibility,

---

6. Cf. Ibrahim, *Pragmatism in Islamic Law*, 12.

7. A detailed account of Islamic law reform of the mid-twentieth century in the Middle East and North Africa, and some of the earlier ones in Egypt and elsewhere, can be found in Anderson, *Law Reform in the Muslim World*, 38–60 and *passim*.

say, of polar bear and otter, and that of the majority, except for the Hanafis, of amphibians, such as turtle, except for the crocodile, which is regarded a predatory animal. These scholastic positions offer scope for *takhayyur*, but there is scope also for the prevailing custom of particular countries and communities. The Maliki school is more liberal than most, and the differences in most cases relate to their respective understanding of the relevant passages of the Qur'an and hadith.

As already noted, slaughter by the Jews and Christians is halal for Muslims, an option that is not taken in the applied halal guidelines of Malaysia, and probably most other Muslim-majority countries. This would be an expedient option, of course, for Muslim minorities who reside in the West. Many of them may be uninformed of the available options and convenience in shariah in this respect, but one notices the increasing trend that they often search for halal slaughter according to mainstream Islamic rules. This is undoubtedly recommended, but for those who may find searching for halal meat particularly inconvenient, they may opt for the concession that the shariah provides with regard to slaughter by the followers of revealed scriptures (*Ahl al-Kitab*). This may be a more relevant example of *takhayyur* perhaps for the Shia Muslims who reside in the West, as the Shia Imamiyyah tend to be more restrictive, even prohibitive, over slaughter by the *Ahl al-Kitab*, notwithstanding some differences of opinions that exist over this among the Shia jurists themselves. The Shia would have, in this case, opted for a Sunni law position.

This last example may be seen as an unprecedented application of *takhayyur*, in view of the fact that the existing doctrine on this subject confines the range of selection to the four Sunni schools. Yet in light of the change of time and conditions, large-scale migration of Muslims to the West, and, more specifically, the Amman Message of 2005, which was the outcome of the largest-ever gathering of Sunni and Shia scholars in Amman to consider the challenge of intra-scholastic Muslim unity in the greater interest of all, and barring some instances of differences, they extended recognition to the Shia as a valid *madhhab*. The halal industry, too, has seen standardization and uniformity to be in the interest of developing customer and market confidence in its products and services worldwide, and may recognize and manifest available options within both the Sunni and Shia schools of jurisprudence.

A more objectionable instance of selection could perhaps be to opt for Imam Abu Hanifah's famous permission of drinking date wine (*nabidh*), so long as it does not lead to intoxication. Two renowned jurists, Uthman b 'Amr al-Hajib (d. 646/1240) and Shams al-Din al-Isfahani (d. 740/1340), of the Maliki and Shafi'i schools, respectively, have acknowledged this and recorded the view that a person who drinks date wine does not become a sinner *(fasiq)*.[8] Abu Hanifah's view in this regard is based on the analysis that the Qur'anic text that mentions *khamr*, a variety of wine that is obtained from grapes. The Muslims of Kufa, including some Companions, were reported also to have consumed *nabidh*. Yet this is not a good *takhayyur*, simply because of the clear hadith proclamation that "every intoxicant is *khamr* and all *khamr* is *haram*."

Modern legal reform and codifications of Islamic law have drawn on the resources of *takhayyur*, *tarjih*, and *talfiq*, yet the twentieth century also witnessed a renewed focus on training and operating in a specific school of law rather than shifting between the schools. Yet twentieth-century Islamic law reform also relied on a measure of selection among the schools. It would be correct to say, therefore, as one observer has noted, that "objections to eclecticism *(takhayyur)* in choosing among the schools of law have consequently declined."[9]

Responding to a question as to whether *takhayyur* and *talfiq* were largely the byproducts of modernity, Fekry Ibrahim commented that "pragmatic eclecticism (whether in the form of *takhayyur*, *tatabbu' al-rukhas* or *talfiq*) was hardly novel . . . as pragmatic eclecticism was indeed practiced throughout Islamic history."[10] And practiced by the Mamluk and Ottoman jurists, and subsequently also in nineteenth-century Egypt.

Al-Qaradawi contends that it is important for the jurisprudence of Muslim minorities living in non-Muslim countries *(fiqh al-aqaliyyat)*, and for modern jurisprudence generally, that the scholar-*mufti* does not restrict himself to one *madhab*. A modern jurist and *mufti* should, therefore, draw upon the four surviving schools and even the opinions of jurists whose scholastic affiliation is unknown, as well as upon the views of the Companions. Al-Qaradawi adds that diversity of stringent and lenient juristic views offers the opportunity to compare them and exercise careful weighing and preference *(al-muwazanah wa'l-tarjih)*.[11] As already noted, *tarjih* means giving preference to one opinion over others by weighing the different pieces of evidence. Social needs and context were rarely explicitly articulated among the criteria on which preference

8. al-Isfahani, *Bayan al-Mukhtasar Sharh Mukhtasar Ibn al-Hajib*, vol. 1, 694, as quoted in Ibrahim, *Pragmatism*, 121.

9. Brown, "Shari'a and State in the Modern Muslim Middle East," 359. See also https://financial-dictionary.thefreedictionary.com/Takhayyur (accessed on February 23, 2018).

10. Ibrahim, *Pragmatism*, 7–8.

11. al-Qaradawi, *Fi Fiqh al-Aqaliyyat*, 46.

was based, even though these needs were often behind the reviews leading to *tarjih*. Such references to social needs and context were, however, articulated under the rubric of *tatabbuʿ al-rukhas*. What al-Qaradawi referred to here is preference for a juristic view that is more suited to the change of times in the context of modernity, which he also termed differently as *al-muazanah waʾl-tarjih*, but also "selective *ijtihad*," instead of either *tarjih* or *tatabbuʿ al-rukhas*.

# 18

# *Piecing Together (*Talfiq*)*

IN *TALFIQ* (LIT. "joining together," or "piecing together") the jurist combines certain parts of the opinion of one school or jurist with parts of one or more views of another school or jurist in order to obtain a certain outcome. None of these segmented positions would individually validate the outcome so obtained, but when pieced together a permissive ruling is arrived at. For these reasons, and the complexity that *talfiq* may entail, it is viewed with a degree of circumspection.[1]

*Talfiq* may consist of merging the opinions of several schools of thought, or individual scholars, into one position that is often dissimilar to all the others, and that did not exist before. The novelty aspects of *talfiq* strike a closer note with *ijtihad* more than with *taqlid*. It is indeed "a jurisprudential principle suggesting that a jurist adhering to a particular school of law should abandon the jurisprudence of that school on a particular matter and adopt a competing point of view offered by another school if the latter is more practical and responds most to the need of the time."[2]

*Talfiq*, like all of its allied principles mentioned thus far, namely *tarjih*, *tatabbu' al-rukhas*, and *takhayyur*, take their origin in the recognition that the four major Sunni schools of thought represent a common heritage; thus, opinions are freely selected when doing so may serve the higher purposes of shariah in a better way, and may even facilitate beneficial choices akin to *maslahah* or public interest.

We have not seen instances of *talfiq* in the sphere of halal slaughter, food, and beverage, but one can hardly overrule its application in light of

---

1. Cf. Wizarat, *al-Mawsu'ah al-Fiqhiyyah*, "Talfiq," vol. 13, 294.

2. IslamicMarkets. "Talfiq." https://islamicmarkets.com/education/talfiq (accessed on February 23, 2018).

*Shariah and The Halal Industry.* Mohammad Hashim Kamali, Oxford University Press. © Oxford University Press 2021. DOI: 10.1093/oso/9780197538616.003.0019

unprecedented and yet ongoing developments of the halal industry. One notices, after all, so many scholastic differences on the permissibility or otherwise of certain animal and bird varieties, as well as amphibians, between the Maliki school and the majority, and to some extent between the other schools jurisprudence as well. Then came the more recent *fatwas* over issues, as well as rulings introduced by the regulatory authorities, that often transcended scholastic positions in an attempt to combine those positions with new scientific knowledge. Hence a certain openness to new possibilities has been in the picture, and might also generally be seen as advisable. Some illustrations of *talfiq* pertaining to worship matters, witnesses, and sale of property are given here.

An example of *talfiq* is whether a judge may admit the testimony of a sinful (*fasiq*) witness who testifies against an absent person. He may do so by way of *talfiq*: the Shafi'is do not accept the testimony of a *fasiq*, but allow ruling in absentia, whereas the Hanafis do not allow the ruling in absentia but allow the testimony of a *fasiq*. Combining the two positions, the judge may allow the testimony.[3]

An objectionable form of *talfiq* (and also concession chasing—*tatabbu' al-rukhas*) would be for a Muslim to marry a woman without the consent of her guardian, and without the presence of witnesses, and also without a dower, on the analysis that the Hanafi school did not require the guardian's consent of an adult woman, and that both Imams al-Shafi'i and Ibn Hanbal validate a marriage without the dower, and also that Imam Malik allowed a marriage without the witnesses—thus combining, by way of patching up or *talfiq*, all these concessionary positions in one permissive ruling. Yet the end result so derived is unacceptable, as it goes against general consensus (*ijma'*) and is therefore impermissible. It is generally held that none of those learned Imams would accept the kind of outcome obtained through the somewhat twisted combination of their respective views.[4] Imam Ahmad Ibn Hanbal has similarly been quoted to have said that "a man who follows the people of Kufa in [the drinking of] *nabidh*, and the people of Madinah in music and singing (*al-sama'*), and the people of Macca in [the practice of] temporary marriage (*mut'ah*) is a profligate (*fasiq*)."[5]

---

3. Ibrahim, *Pragmatism*, 113, citing Ibn Biri, Ibrahim bin Husayn, al-Kashf wa'l-Tadqiq li-Sharh Ghayat al-Tahqiq, Cairo, n.d., MS Dar al-Kutub 403 *Usul Fiqh*.

4. Cf. al-Ghafur, *al-Taqlid wa'l-Talfiq*, 24–25.

5. Imam Ibn Hanbal, as quoted in al-Ghafur, *al-Taqlid wa'l-Talfiq*, 28, quoting in turn, Yaha b. 'Ali al-Shawkani's *Irshad al-Fuhul min Tahqiq al-Haq ila 'Ilm al-Usul*.

Another example of a twisted *talfiq* is as follows: A Shafi'i follower follows the ruling of the Hanafi school during a land sale by his neighbor in order to take advantage of the right of pre-emption (*shuf'a*) to which adjacent neighbors are entitled in Hanafi law. Then the same person should not be allowed to switch back to the Shafi'i school in order to sell the same piece of land to someone else and deny his neighbor the same right of pre-emption on the premise that Shafi'i law does not take an affirmative position on the right of pre-emption.

Ibn Nujaym al-Misri (d. 970/1536) went on record to say that the negative views toward *talfiq* were only expressed by later scholars (*muta'akhkhirin*), and that earlier authorities did not forbid *talfiq*. Closer to our time, Muhammad 'Abduh (d. 1905) did not shy away from the use of *talfiq*, even in matters of theology. For instance, he not only incorporated some of the positions of Maturidism in the predominantly Ash'ari theology that he expounded in his *Risalat al-Tawhid*, but he also relied on Mu'tazilah positions. Then 'Abduh's disciple, Muhammad Rashid Rida (d. 1935) held that *talfiq* may be used when there is a pressing need for it. Rida looked into the differences of opinion over *talfiq* but sided with its supporters, whose evidence he found more convincing. He went so far as to suggest that *talfiq* is part and parcel of the Hanafi school, which takes positions that sometimes consist of a combination of more than one jurist's opinion.[6]

It may be concluded that the foregoing methods, including *talfiq*, should not be used to conjure up questionable legal stratagems (*hilah*) or to distort the higher objectives (*maqasid* of shariah). They should also not be used in mechanical and questionable ways that seek to realize unlawful and unethical ends. For this reason, we recommend that statutory law and regulatory instruments should be used to facilitate only the beneficial uses of these methods. Questionable uses of *talfiq* that employ lawful means to secure unlawful ends are also likely to invoke the shariah law principle of *sadd al-dhara'i'*, or blocking recourse to lawful means only to obtain unlawful ends.

---

6. Munajjid, *Fatawa al-Imam Muhammad Rashid Rida*, vol. 1, 239.

# 19

# *Legal Maxims of* Fiqh

THIS CHAPTER BRINGS together a selection of the legal maxims of Islamic law (*qawa'id kulliyyah fiqhiyyah*) on the renowned scale of Five Values, namely the halal, the forbidden (*haram*), and that which is recommendable (*mandub*), permissible (*mubah, ja'iz,* halal), and reprehensible (*makruh*). The maxims listed below are presented in bare skeletal forms confined to the actual text in English translation (the present author's own), with their equivalent, Arabic appearing in Appendix 2. The main purpose is to see how the subjects of concern find expression in this genre of the *fiqh* literature. The brevity here is also justified because the relevant details on the various shariah-related themes of halal and *haram* have already been given, or given for the most part, in the preceding chapters of the book. The maxims presented here are self-explanatory for the most part and endorse the information contained in this volume, though they may occasionally add new points. In any case, legal maxims are on the whole educational, usually used as aids to teaching, and do not, as such, bind judges and jurists to comply—unless the maxim in question reiterates a clear directive of Qur'an or hadith. Many of the maxims trace their origins to these sources, either replicating the text of the Qur'an or hadith, or they may consist, as is more often the case, of a rehash in the words of the jurists who compiled them. Legal maxims are epithetic and concise, often not exceeding a single line, and are expressive of the main principles of Islamic law pertaining to a particular subject. Some of these maxims are broad and apply to all aspects of the shariah, whereas others are applicable only to certain areas or aspects thereof. For instance, "harm must be eliminated (*al-dararu yuzal*)" is one of the leading legal maxims, derived in turn from the renowned hadith: "harm may not be inflicted nor reciprocated in [the name of] Islam—*la darar wa-la dirar fi'l-Islam.*" This maxim applies to all aspects of the shariah in all of its parts, but to say that "*ijtihad* is not vitiated by its equivalent—*al-ijtihad la-yunqad bi-mithlihi*," is specific to the subject of *ijtihad*. Another legal maxim of particular import is that "private authority is stronger than public authority—*al-wilayat al-khassah aqwa min al-wilayat al-'ammah*," evidently meaning that the guardianship powers of a parent or guardian over the ward is stronger than that of the public authority, such as a judge or the head of state.[1] Legal maxims tend to be interscholastic, as the leading schools of Islamic law, including the Shia Imamiyyah, do not differ a great deal on them, although some differences of detail do exist among the schools. The selection presented below relates mainly to halal and *haram* in foods and animals, but since halal and *haram* are not confined only to these subjects, the maxims presented describe Islamic law positions on halal and *haram* and also on some of the intervening value points between them; they are conveyed in a language that subsumes eating, drinking, and animal slaughter, as well as a variety of other aspects of human conduct with special reference to Muslims.[2]

- What is indispensable for the completion of an obligation also becomes an obligation.[1]
- The rules [of shariah] proceed on that which is evident. For what is hidden [in the minds and hearts of people] is referred to God Most High.[2]
- The means to all that which is prohibited is also prohibited.[3]
- What is permissible may be subjected to safety requirements.[4]
- When the *haram* and the halal co-exist, the *haram* prevails.[5]
- The effective causes of [shariah] rules indicate the purpose of the Lawgiver and should be upheld whenever they are known.[6]
- Avoidance of the reprehensible is preferred to securing a recommendable.[7]
- The best of every man's conduct is that which is most beneficial to others, most fruitful, and most refined.[8]
- The reprehensible is not committed for [the sake of securing] the recommendable.[9]

---

1. See, for details, Kamali, *Shariah Law*, 141–162.

2. Most of the legal maxims quoted in the list presented here can be found in the 43-volume encyclopedia titled *Mu'allimatu Zayid li'l-Qawa 'id al-Fiqhiyyah wa'l-Usuliyyah*, Abu Dhabi: Mu'assasah Zayid bin Sultan Aal-Nahyan li'l-A 'mal al-Khayriyyah wa'l-Insaniyyah, wa majma' al-Fiqh al-Islami al-Duwali, 1434AH/2013. Legal maxims in this encyclopedia are listed in alphabetical order in Arabic. Volume 37 contains a large number of the legal maxims on halal and *haram*. English translation of the maxims presented here has been supplied by the present writer. Some maxims have also been taken from Zaydan, *al-Wajiz fi-Sharh al-Qawa'id al-Fiqhiyyah*.

- What is indispensable for securing a recommendable is also recommendable.[10]
- The obligatory is not abandoned for the sake of recommendable.[11]
- The Islamic shariah has permitted all that which is pure, and prohibited all that which is unclean.[12]
- No reward and no punishment accrues in the absence of intention[13]
- Custom has no credibility if it contravenes the rules of shariah.[14]
- The norm is that the rules (of shariah) collapse when their effective causes are no longer present.[15]
- Permissibility is the norm in all things unless there be evidence as to its prohibition.
- The norm (of shariah) is freedom from liability.[16]
- *Ijtihad* does not apply to decisive rules.[17]
- *Fatwa* that contravenes the scripture and consensus is invalid.[18]
- Construction of the rules of shariah such that they contravene the higher purposes of God and the shariah is invalid.[19]
- All aspects of *ijtihad* depend on the knowledge of the *maqasid*.[20]
- It is not the Lawgiver's purpose to impose hardship and go to excess in it.[21]
- Repelling prejudice and corruption takes priority over securing benefits.[22]
- The rule stands and falls together with its effective cause.[23]
- The norm is that rules collapse with the collapse of their effective causes.[24]
- The norm [of shariah] in regard to speech is the real/literal meaning.[25]
- No attention is paid to inference in the face of an explicit statement.[26]
- What can be done is not waived due to what cannot be done.[27] (Note: One is advised to do even a part of a duty if one is unable to do the whole of it.)
- Acts of worship are not justiceable.[28]
- Evidence is not turned into proof without the court judgment.[29]
- Certainty overrides probability, and the latter overrides doubt, and suspicion has no credibility in the presence of truth/fact.[30]
- When the direct perpetrator and proximate causer are both present, the ruling falls on the direct perpetrator.[31]
- One who unknowingly drinks alcohol is not liable either to the *hadd* penalty or *ta'zir*.[32]
- One who is certain about doing something but doubts its amount, whether small or large, the smaller is presumed.[33]
- The head of state is not authorized to take away anything from anyone unless it be through a lawfully proven right.[34]
- The head of state may not discontinue that which is indispensable for the Muslims/community.[35]

- All those who have a right remain as they are unless the opposite of it is proven with certainty.[36]
- All dispositions that give rise to harm/corruption or obstruct a benefit are prohibited.[37]
- The norm with regard to clothing/dress is permissibility.[38]
- The norm with regard to [human] actions and customary practices is permissibility and absence of prohibition.[39]
- [The basic norm of] permissibility in human activities is contingent on avoidance of harm to another person.[40]
- The norm [or presumption/with regard to all persons] is [that they possess] integrity [or blamelessness] unless the opposite becomes known.[41]
- The norm [of shariah] is absence of defects.[42]
- The norm in the dispositions of Muslims is validity.[43]
- Hardship begets facility and ease.[44]
- Property that is not guaranteed in respect of a Muslim [such as property temporarily deposited with one for safe keeping] is also not guaranteed in the respect of an unbeliever.[45]
- Muslims, *dhimmis*, and temporary residents are all equal in respect of enacted rights that protect against harm.[46]
- Elimination of injustice as far as possible is an obligation.[47]
- Elimination of harm as far as possible is an obligation.[48]
- The rules [of shariah] are objectively understood regardless of gender specification.[50]
- A woman is like a man in respect of legal capacity.[51]
- All that is forbidden to Muslims in regard to marriage is also forbidden to non-Muslims.[52]
- Whoever owns an object also owns that which is indispensable to it.[53]
- When prohibition and permissibility coexist, prohibition prevails.[54]
- What is forbidden to take is also forbidden to give.[55]
- What is permissible due to an excuse ceases to be permissible with its cessation.[56]
- All that which is permissible to sell can also be mortgaged, and if it cannot be sold may not be mortgaged either.[57]
- The norm [of shariah] in all things is that of permissibility.[58]
- Harm must be eliminated.[59]
- Harm may neither be inflicted nor reciprocated in Islam.[60]
- Necessities make the unlawful lawful.[61]
- Necessity is measured in accordance with its true proportions.[62]
- Harm may not be eliminated by its equivalent.[63]

- Harm to an individual is tolerated if it prevents harm to the general public.[64]
- Prevention of harms [or corruption] takes priority over the attraction of benefits.[65]
- Custom is a [valid] basis of judgment.[66]
- Certainty may not be overruled by doubt.[67]
- Play and games fall under original permissibility unless there be evidence on their prohibition.[68]
- Islam is the religion of [harmony with] human nature.[69]
- When a Muslim takes by force the property of another Muslim he is not entitled to own it.[70]
- The contracts of non-Muslims are held valid even if they oppose Islam but when they convert to Islam they are subject to the rules that apply to Muslims.[71]
- Acts are judged by their intentions.[72] (Hadith-cum-legal maxim.)
- [People's] affairs are determined by reference to their purposes.[73]
- Facilitation is one of the objectives of shariah.[74]
- Building the earth and continuity of its benefits for the good of its inhabitants is a general objective of shariah.[75]
- Primary and explicit prohibitions are indicative of the purposes of the Lawgiver.[76]
- Forbearance and ease are among the purposes of religion.[77]
- Protection of religion is a primary purpose of shariah.[78]
- Protection of life is a primary purpose of shariah.[79]
- Protection of reason is a primary purpose of shariah.[80]
- Protection of lineage is a primary purpose of shariah.[81]
- In the event of conflict among benefits/purposes, that which is certain takes priority over the uncertain and doubtful.[82]

## 20

# *Islam and Science*

## STUNNING, HALAL VACCINES, GMOS, AND MEAT EATING

### *Introductory Remarks*

A few words may be said at the outset on Islam and science, realizing full well, however, that both are too broad and also too important to be treated in a short chapter intended merely to identify what bearings they may have on the halal and *haram* in Islam. However, the first question that arises concerns the basic premise of these concepts. Halal and *haram* are evidently not determined by reference only to human reason or scientific knowledge, but by a combination of these and the guidance mainly of divine revelation (*wahy*). Worship matters (*'ibadat*) are normally determined by the shariah independently of scientific evidence, and this could also be said of a limited number of dietary restrictions Islam has imposed—even though there may be some scientific justification for them.

That said, Islam is on the whole receptive to scientific evidence. If one considers the Islamic prohibition of carrion, spilt blood, alcohol, and pig meat for consumption, most of these, if not all, can perhaps stand the test of scientific knowledge. Scientific rationality essentially confines reality to the data of sense perception, which precludes metaphysical reality and revealed knowledge as well as some of the nonphysical sides of the human existence, such as reducing intelligence to the level of neural chemistry where mental and behavioral phenomena are understood merely as manifestations of physical processes.

Islamic juristic thought recognizes various levels of distinctions with a view to addressing temporal reality within its own parameters. For instance,

*Shariah and The Halal Industry.* Mohammad Hashim Kamali, Oxford University Press. © Oxford University Press 2021. DOI: 10.1093/oso/9780197538616.003.0021

the distinction between shariah and *fiqh* did not exist during the first century of the advent of Islam, and the triple division of the shariah into theology (*kalam*), morality (*akhlaq*), and practical legal rulings (*fiqh*) also developed at a later stage. A certain level of separation was thus recognized between theoretical theology and the practical rules of concern to the daily life and conduct of the individual. In the sphere of the applied sciences and the benefits they can bring to humanity, Islam maintains an open outlook. Thus, it is not only acceptable but may even rank as *maslahah* (public interest) to employ scientific knowledge for the good of the people. Muslims have consequently not seen their faith as a hindrance to scientific knowledge. They have, on the contrary, made significant contributions to the advancement of science in centuries past. The Prophet advocated beneficial knowledge (*al-'ilm al-nafi'*) that responds to people's legitimate needs, and accordingly instructed his followers to seek knowledge "even if it be in China." Thus, it is not difficult to see that Islam accepts beneficial scientific knowledge from any source. China was certainly not known for religious knowledge, let alone Islamic knowledge, but was probably recognized then, as ever since, for its cultural attainments, scientific knowledge, and wisdom.

It is common knowledge that before the advent of Islam, myths, magic, and superstition had profoundly affected people's outlook on reality and reason—so much so that they could totally estrange people from the physical world and were given to mockery and black magic. Islam's strong advocacy of knowledge, rational observation, and development of sense-based observation and intellectual faculties became a major preoccupation of the Qur'an, which is replete with expressions regarding knowledge-seeking Muslims, such as *yanzurun* (they observe), *yatafakkarun* (they think), *ya'qilun* (rationalize), *yatadabbarun* (they ponder), *yatafaqqahun* (they understand with insight), and *ya'lamun* (they know). It is also significant that the Qur'an made itself known to be a collection of *ayat* (signs), from beginning to end, that invite further investigation and truth—or discovery through observation and rational enquiry.

The robust advocacy of *'ilm* in the Qur'an, its open acceptance of knowledge gained through sense perception and observation, and its encouragement of inquiry and investigation of the outer universe and the human earthly habitat, all in all depict a basic alignment and convergence of interests between Islam and science, and not otherwise. Islamic philosophy that mainly studies purposes, as against science, which mainly studies causes, sees objects and events as signs (*ayat*) of the divine presence in the universe. Faith is understood by Muslims not as a limitation on science but as its vista for enrichment and perfection. Thinking Muslims should therefore work to vindicate the symbiotic relation of faith and reason, of knowledge and science, and advance a broader understanding of these and other civilizational objectives of Islam.

The one area where Islam and science part ways is perhaps over the rejection of metaphysical reality and the authority of revealed knowledge. Science is not receptive to these, and Islam will always insist on its own articles of faith. One can, in sum, visualize compatibility in practical concerns of the benefits of science to humanity, without, however, subscribing to its exclusively materialistic vision of reality and existence.

Briefly, Islam's view of reality and knowledge may be divided into three categories: logical, observational, and intuitive.

Logical knowledge is truth obtained through basic assumptions, as in the case of application of deductive logic, or on the most probable result obtained through inductive reasoning. This category of knowledge is *'ilm al-yaqin* (knowledge based on intellectual certainty).

Observational knowledge is obtained through the application of the senses and study and observation of the physical world that yields sense-based knowledge (*'ayn al-yaqin*; Q al-Takathur, 102:7). Scientific knowledge falls, on the whole, under this category, and uses a large variety of tools to study natural phenomena, the signs—or *ayat*—as in their Qur'anic idiom. As for humankind's position of superiority among the rest of God's creatures, the Qur'an declares that "He (God) has subjected to you, as from Him, all that is in the heavens and the earth (al-Jathiyah, 45:13). This being the case, humankind is free to extend the scope of inquiry and observation to any sphere of the created universe, and to benefit by the knowledge that is obtained as a result.

The third category of knowledge is that which is obtained through the inner experiences of the mind and heart, known in its Qur'anic idiom as *haqq al-yaqin* (truth-based certainty—cf. Q al-Waqi'ah, 56:95 and al-Haqqah, 69:51), and may partake in methods known to modern psychology that look into the various levels of the human mind, often described as intuition, inspiration, and revelation. This last category is the prerogative mainly of Prophets and Messengers, who are the conveyors of revelation and its delivery to humankind, and usually supersedes and reaches beyond logic and sense-based observation.[1] What follows next are some halal industry themes that employ

---

1. Cf. Qurashi, *Introduction to Muslim Contributions*, 9–10. See also Shahzad, *Biomedical Ethics*, 134.

science for verification of the outcomes and their compatibility or otherwise with shariah principles.

## Stunning and Halal Slaughtering

There is basically no objection to the use of means and methods, as they are currently employed in modern slaughterhouses, that reduce resistance and pain of the animal, provided in all cases that they do not obliterate consciousness completely prior to slaughter. If the purpose is to reduce pain and suffering, this is acceptable, but this does not extend to hitting the animal with heavy objects or exposing it to high electrical currents that by themselves amount to infliction of torture, which is forbidden.[2] But even so, if the animal is alive and slaughtered through valid slaughter procedures after infliction of suffering, its meat is still lawful for consumption. However, if after the use of procedures that were meant to reduce pain the animal dies prior to a valid slaughter, the meat is non-halal. Furthermore, it is not permissible to draw or drain the blood of an animal with, for example, surgical instruments and then slaughter it without ascertaining that it was still alive before it was slaughtered.

The Malaysian Standard MS 1500-2009 provides in principle that "stunning is not recommended. However, if stunning is to be carried out, the conditions specified under Annex A shall be complied with."[3] Annex A provides details on the permitted methods for electrical stunning, and pneumatic percussive stunning, both to be carried out under the supervision of a trained Muslim and competent authority. Stunning must not kill or cause permanent physical injury to the animal. Electrical stunning is allowed only for certain types of animals. Stunners used for the slaughter of pigs may not be used for stunning halal animals. Stunning used for halal animals shall be "head only stunner," where both electrodes are placed on the head region. Electrical stunning of poultry is allowed using "water bath stunner" only. The strength of electrical current used is to be supervised by a trained Muslim and monitored by the competent authority. MS 1500-2009 also provides guidelines on the strength of currents for various animals in both the "electrical stunning" and "pneumatic percussive stunning" varieties. This latter is only suitable for bovine animals, the air pressure that powers the stunner should be kept below

---

2. al-Zuhayli, *al-Fiqh al-Islami*, vol. 3, 688.

3. MS 1500-2009 (Clause 3.5.2.3).

the specified maximum, and a protective collar is put around the head of the stunner so that it does not protrude more than 3 mm into the skin.[4]

The use of stunning and the thoracic stick procedures, and whether they are acceptable from the shariah viewpoint, has given rise to differences of opinion. Questions have arisen as to how stunning and thoracic stick practices were originally introduced—for reasons of industry convenience, for animal welfare, or both. Although the shariah favors the smooth flow of lawful trade in the marketplace even at the expense of some compromise on other factors, it does not favor measures that would present a threat to its higher values. Any decision that a shariah specialist makes on stunning and thoracic stick issues, without the required scientific input, is bound to be based on externalities and assumptions that would be less than adequate—given the sensitivity of the issues and extensive application of the decisions in question.

This also serves to illustrate the symbiotic relationship that is envisaged, as explained earlier, between *fiqh* and scientific knowledge. Stunning and thoracic stick seem to have gained acceptance on the understanding that they help to make slaughter relatively less painful for the animal. This is also in line with the shariah principles of making the experience less painful for the animal and the whole slaughtering process as smooth as possible. Malaysia's religious authorities have accepted the practice of stunning within a limited range of voltage such that the sense perception of the animal is not completely obliterated. Electric stunning of larger animals like cows and sheep has been accepted in industrial slaughter practices in many Muslim countries. Stunning techniques in Europe, however, are meant to make the animal completely and totally unconscious, which is a main point of difference between the Islamic and European approaches to electric stunning.

Regarding chicken, some Muslim commentators had recorded the concern that, due to their smaller size, chicken may die from the shock that is supposed to only stun them. Yet further investigation conducted in Turkey and by the International Islamic Fiqh Academy seems to favor acceptance of stunning in chicken. Thus, a team of IIFA (International Islamic Fiqh Academy) scholars who visited four plants in Turkey observed that in all the factories, before being slaughtered, chicken were passed through electrified water for up to two seconds. The water, with 40 amps of current, stuns the chicken. The IIFA scholars reported from their observation that the stunned

4. Annex A, MS 1500-2009, 12–13.

chicken regained full consciousness in three minutes—hence the proof that they did not die of the current they were exposed to.[5]

Numerous researchers have responded positively to the use of stunning, just as it has also become a common practice generally on grounds mainly of animal welfare. The slaughter of conscious animals was widely abandoned over the course of twentieth century and is now practically confined only to some Muslim and Jewish communities. A slightly different opinion has been held, however, by Dr. Bert Temple Grandin of Colorado University, a specialist on the subject, who told the BBC at an interview in November 2011 that conventional slaughter with preliminary stunning and religious slaughter without stunning are both acceptable when properly conducted. "There is good and bad stunning, but the research shows very clearly that when you stun an animal properly with a well-maintained captive bolt, unconsciousness is instantaneous. . . . Similarly, when I have seen *shechita* [Jewish kosher slaughter] on a cow done really rightly by a really good *shochet*, the animal seemed to act like it didn't even feel it."[6] A device the size of a hand-held drill is brought to the animal's head, a trigger is pulled, and a four-inch bolt is shot into its brain, causing it to collapse instantly. The unconscious animal is hoisted upside down and slaughtered seconds later with a massive cut to its throat.

Yusuf Altuntas, chairman of the Dutch Muslim umbrella group, said that "it is still unproven that slaughtering with stunning is a better method."[7] The late Al-Hafiz Masri, who founded British Islam's first animal rights movement, argued that there was no Qur'anic prohibition on stunning animals, and added that the main counsel of Islam regarding the slaughter of animals for food is to do it in the least painful manner. Failure to stun animals before slaughter causes them pain and suffering. He also cited the verdict of a special committee appointed by Al-Azhar University in Cairo to decide whether the meat of animals slaughtered after stunning was lawful. The committee

---

5. https://www.upc-online.org/slaughter/poultry_slaughter.pdf .

6. Berg, "Should Animals Be Stunned." Yet a commentator's response to this was as follows: "Have you heard of mad cow disease in humans? It is transferred to humans when they consume meat of a mad cow. The virus that lives in the cow's brain does not reach the meat until the blood-brain barrier is broken by brain trauma—stunning! Stunning causes major brain concussion, allowing virus to enter meat to be consumed. Slaughter without stunning is the way. Scientifically." The commentator, a doctor apparently, is merely identified as "imperialahmed." That said, stunning is a requirement in numerous European countries, but most of them also permit religious slaughtering under certain conditions.

7. Berg, "Should Animals Be Stunned."

decided unanimously that there was no religious objection to modern methods of slaughtering, so long as these methods are swift and clean and do cause bleeding (*museelat al-dam*). If new means of slaughter are more swift and clean, they should be employed.[8] According to the British Halal Food Authority, stunning is permissible. However, there are different forms of stunning; some of which are prohibited, and some are permitted. According to the BHFA, the following are prohibited:

- Captive-bolt stunning
- Percussion stunning
- Gas stunning

There are three types of stunning that the Halal Food Authority approves:

- Water-bath Stun—for poultry only—where birds are dragged through water with an electric stunner within. Stated that sometimes they are not rendered fully paralyzed after the water bath because they lift their bodies up while struggling and do not make full contact with the stunner. Furthermore, the birds come out of the electrified bath paralyzed, but not stunned.
- Electric-Tong Stun—for larger animals, e.g., sheep, cows, camels, goats etc. The tong would have to stay attached to the head when the bovine falls. The neck to neck position must never be used because the current may fail to go through the brain. A headholder that holds the animal's head up when the body falls is strongly recommended.
- Electronarcosis is also often used for larger animals, dulling the animal's senses before the slaughtering and has been agreed upon as licit by the Egyptian Fatwa Committee [a committee that has the authority to declare what is permissible and not in the ritual slaughter techniques of halal].[9]

The Muslim World League (Rabitah al-'Alam al-Islami, or MWL) has also supported the use of stunning by electric shock. In 1955 a MWL delegation of fifty-five Muslim theologians and scientists from all over the world held a joint meeting with World Health Organization and made the following

---

8. As quoted in *VIBE* (a periodical publication of the Halal Development Corporation Malaysia), April 2009, 18. *HDC VIBE*, April 2009.

9. "Dhabihah," *Wikipedia*, https://en.wikipedia.org/wiki/Dhabihah (accessed September 4, 2017).

recommendation about pre-slaughter stunning: "[P]re-slaughter stunning by electric shock is lawful if proven to lessen the animal's suffering, provided that it is carried out with the weakest electric current that directly renders the animal unconscious, and that it neither leads to the animal's death nor renders its meat harmful to the consumer."[10]

The Malaysian National Council of Islamic Affairs' *fatwa* similarly held that electrical stunning was permissible as long as the shock was administered only to the head, the electrical current's strength and duration were controlled within fixed limits, and the process was supervised by accredited Muslim staff.[11]

In a 2012 *fatwa*, Ayatollah Sistani of Iraq stated that it is allowed to stun an animal before slaughtering it, as long as it is still alive after stunning. He added, however, that he thought Ayatollah Khamenei also allowed it, but that he was not sure on this and that he could be wrong. "To my knowledge, there are two types of stunning—'stun to kill' is where the animal is killed by the electricity (this isn't allowed) and 'stun to stun' where the animal is knocked out by the electricity but not dead because the voltage is not high enough to kill it (this is allowed and this is what is used by halal slaughterhouses)."[12] According to available reports, Iran does not make stunning a requirement, yet it has not forbidden it either.

In 2006 the EU commissioned a large committee of religious scholars and scientists to investigate and compare the rules of religious slaughter (mainly halal and kosher) with those of electrical stunning techniques. A series of consultative meetings and events were conducted between 2006 and 2010 and the results were published in 2010, known as the Dialrel research. EU countries adopted the results of many of these reports in their legislation and regulatory instruments. An outline of the Dialrel report is presented under Appendix IV at the end of this volume.

## *Halal Vaccines*

Immunization has curbed many contagious diseases and successfully provided immunity against them among many Muslim communities. It is a process

---

10. *VIBE*, 18.

11. *VIBE*, 18.

12. Rothman, "Halal Slaughter." https://www.vice.com/en/article/d75mea/halal-slaughter-is-more-complicated-than-you-realize 30 October 2014 (accessed February 22, 2021).

where a person is made immune to an infectious disease by the administration of a vaccine. The antigen in vaccine acts to stimulate the immune system to produce antibodies against specific diseases. Immunity is strengthened by priming the body's defense cells to recognize the particular virus or bacteria so that they are ready to fight it in the future. There are many types of immunization that focus on specific groups, such as babies, food handlers, and travelers. However, some people refuse to vaccinate their children, often due to questionable information suggesting that vaccines cause autism.[13]

Developing halal vaccines is the latest instance of market penetration of the halal economy in a new area. Yet unlike the halal food and beverage sectors, halal vaccines, though offering strong commercial prospects, are more challenging insofar as they rely heavily on scientific research and also touch on social sensitivities of its potential users. It takes a significantly more persuasive approach to convince potential users and market participants of the benefits of halal vaccines. This would explain why the newly established halal vaccines industry is facing socio-legal challenges. The industry will need to address three challenging issues: the religio-ethical concerns, safety concerns, and social issues.

First, Islamic legal issues concerning halal vaccines arise from the absence of a standard definition of halal, which has led to differences in the degree of acceptance in different countries. There is suspicion that vaccines include non-halal ingredients. Regarding safety and manufacturing concerns, halal vaccine manufacture involves detailed research and also substantial investment. The social challenges of vaccines generally relate to people's fears over the longer-term effects. There has also been a significant increase in the number of parents rejecting vaccination for their children based on fears that the vaccines are *haram*, as they may contain porcine DNA. In the case of Malaysia, the Ministry of Health has rejected these allegations, calling them baseless. It has made assurances that all medicines and vaccines dispensed to patients in the country are halal and safe.

Media reports by many observers stress that misinformation has been one of the main reasons behind the rejection of vaccination. The Health Ministry director general, Dr. Noor Hisham Abdullah, has been quoted as saying that the spread of fake news and misleading and irresponsible reporting on social media has led to people rejecting vaccines, adding that the World Health Organization identified vaccine rejection "as one of the global health threats

---

13. See, for details, Malek, "Islam and Vaccines," 17. Malek reviews evidence to show that much of the anti-vaccine information lacks scientific credibility.

for 2019."[14] The number of vaccine rejections recorded at government clinics in Malaysia has continued to increase, going from 637 cases in 2013 to 1,603 cases in 2016. Diseases that are preventable by vaccine have also increased in the country; for example, 195 cases of chickenpox were recorded in 2013 but grew to a total of 1,903 cases in 2018. The number of cases of measles due to no immunization similarly increased, from 125 cases in 2013 to 1,467 cases in 2018.[15] This buildup of evidence eventually led to the Ministry of Health announcement in February 2019 to make vaccination compulsory for children. The health minister, Dr. Dzulkifly Ahmad, announced that he would be tabling a proposal to make immunization vaccination compulsory, adding that he would be bringing the matter to the Health Ministry post-cabinet meeting, and if it were supported, it would be brought to the cabinet. He also expected there would be arguments for and against the proposal, and the ministry would consider all views before taking action.[16] The Minister of Health Dr Baba announced, on August 18, 2020, that after much deliberation the decision was made, however, not to make child immunization compulsory in Malaysia.[17]

Ethical considerations on vaccination have also been highlighted pertaining to design and implementation issues, such as the proper role of governments in developing, promoting, and monitoring vaccination programs, conducting research on human subjects, ensuring long-term access to vaccines, and identification of the risks and benefits of vaccines. Ethical concerns also relate to individual choice. The decision made by any individual either to decline or to accept vaccination is not only of concern to his or her own vulnerability to disease, but also affects the community at large. Another ethical objection to vaccination is the "preventive problem," which involves the concern of inequitable distribution of benefit and harm from preventive medicine's focus on population-based interventions. It is suggested that such measures are attributable to several factors, such as (a) whether the preventive measures are practiced on healthy individuals, (b) that such public health

14. As quoted in the *Sun Daily*, January 23, 2019.

15. As quoted in the *Sun* daily, Kuala Lumpur, January 23, 2019, 5.

16. "Health Ministry to propose making immunisation vaccination compulsory." *The Star*, February 24, 2019. https://www.thestar.com.my/news/nation/2019/02/24/health-ministry-to-propose-making-immunisation-vaccination-compulsory/.

17. CodeBlue Health is a Human Right, https://codeblue.galencentre.org/2020/08/18/malaysia-wont-make-childhood-vaccination-compulsory/ (accessed February 22, 2021).

interventions often carries some risk of harmful effects, and (c) that the benefits of such measures are enjoyed by the society at large, whereas the risks of harm fall on the shoulders of individuals.[18]

Malaysia has announced plans to be the main global producer of halal vaccines, as stated by its minister of international trade and industry, Mustapa Mohamed, at the World Halal Forum 2014 in Kuala Lumpur. A Saudi corporation, he added, had already invested US$100 million in the Halal Industry Development Corporation (HDC) of Malaysia to produce halal vaccines for meningitis, hepatitis, and meningococcal disease.[19] Yet it is also reported in the Malaysian press that parental refusal, especially by middle-class parents, to vaccinate their children is primarily due to religious reasons, but is also related to safety concerns. Reports highlighted the risk associated with the lack of vaccination, such as a fatal case involving an unvaccinated four-year-old child due to diphtheria, as the child's parents were doubtful of the safety, as well as the halal status, of vaccines.[20]

According to reports, Malaysia's largest pharmaceutical company, Pharmaniaga, has signed a collaboration agreement with the Malaysian Ministry of Finance's Technology Depository Agency (TDA), and Hilleman Laboratories, a Delhi-based vaccine research organization, to produce various vaccines. Pharmaniaga's managing director, Farshila Emran, explained that the company was in the midst of putting together the laboratory equipment and facilities, and that the company planned to start producing vaccines in "two to three years" time. The vaccine manufacturing facility will conduct clinical trials, manage regulatory measures, and commercialize the products. Emran added that the company will produce vaccines for diphtheria and meningitis, among others, and that halal vaccine is expected to be made available to the public at the latest by 2022.[21]

The March 2017 state visit of King Salman of Saudi Arabia to Malaysia led to the signing of an agreement between the two countries on halal vaccine production and investment. Saudi Arabia agreed to invest a significant sum in Malaysia. A memorandum of understanding was signed between AJ Pharma, a Saudi-based pharmaceutical company under al-Jomaih Group, and

---

18. Abdullah, "Halal Vaccine," 450f.

19. Abdullah, "Challenges Facing Halal Vaccine Industry."

20. Amin et al., "Parental Refusal to Diphtheria Vaccine," 431.

21. Balakrishnan, "Malaysia to Produce and Export the World's First Halal Vaccines."

the Halal Development Corporation of Malaysia for an additional invest-ment of US$300 million (RM1.32 billion) for facilities and infrastructure in Malaysia.[22]

The Malaysian AJ Biologics company is also enhancing its R&D capa-bilities in halal vaccine production, and to this effect it acquired Denmark's Statens Serum Institut (SSI) vaccine production business to develop halal vaccines for hand, foot, and mouth disease (EV71) and meningococcal men-ingitis (MCV4). AJ Biologics is targeting the Middle East and East Asian markets. The MCV4 will be the first ever halal-certified meningococcal vac-cine for all pilgrims traveling to Saudi Arabia. Similar initiatives are being taken by the Chemical Company of Malaysia Berhad (CCM), which has invested in a South Korean company to produce vaccines.[23] Production pla-nning and a number of actual steps to actualize that plan have thus been taken in Malaysia. Time will tell as to how the plans proceed, and when the halal vaccines will be made available to the general public.

## Genetically Modified Organisms

Genetically modified organisms (GMOs) are organism that have been manipulated by molecular genetic engineering techniques to exhibit new traits. It is generally agreed that modern biotechnology differs from classical techniques such as traditional breeding and mutagenesis. Modern biotech-nology involves the selective and deliberate alteration of an organism's DNA through human intervention, by way of introducing, modifying, or eliminat-ing specific genes through recombined DNA techniques.

Genetic modification involves inserting a gene from a bacteria or a virus into an organism where it would normally not be found. The purpose is to alter the genetic code in plants and animals to make them more productive or resistant to pests or farming techniques, like being doused with chemicals that would ordinarily kill them. For example, soybeans that have been genet-ically modified can survive applications of herbicides that would destroy an organic soybean plant.

Genetically modified (GM) crops have been rapidly increasing in pro-duction lines in recent decades. Despite their known benefits, GM crops pose many concerns not only to human and animal health but also to the

22. Abdullah, "Challenges Facing Halal Vaccine Industry."

23. Cochrane, "Overview: How Attractive is Malaysia's Halal Pharmaceutical Sector?"

environment. According to the US Department of Agriculture, only 3 percent of planted acres of corn in 1996 were planted with GMO herbicide-tolerant corn. In 2009, it was 89 percent. Meanwhile, experts estimate that as much as 75 percent of the processed foods sold in the United States contain GMO ingredients.

There are two different positions of note on GMOs: American companies and government organizations allow the use of GMOs, but their European Union counterparts ban cultivation of GMO plants and products altogether.

The Arab Organisation for Agricultural Development held a conference in Sudan (June 15–17, 2003) on "Evaluating the Environmental Impact of Introducing Various Kinds of Genetically Modified Plants and Animals."[24] One of the presenters, 'Awad-Allaah 'Abd al-Mawla, professor of horticulture and genetics at Khartoum University, described GMO products as genetically engineered crops in which a foreign gene has been introduced into their original genetic material. The foreign gene may come from different sources, and is introduced to increase the value and improve the genetic qualities of the plant.

The production of GMOs involves identifying the gene responsible for the desired quality and isolating it, then introducing it to the living being (the receiver). After this new gene has been mixed with the genetic material of the plant, it is possible to increase the number of cells in which the new gene is successfully mixed, then by means of tissue planting it becomes possible to produce complete plants from the cells, and these plants become genetically modified or engineered.[25]

It is a matter of concern that current biotechnology products are mostly focused on the commercialization of biopharmaceuticals through GM crops.[26]

Yet another point of concern is that biotechnology and biomedical issues are often not amenable to clear answers on the lawful and unlawful (halal and *haram*) issues involved, just as they also give rise to profound philosophical, ethical, and religious questions. GMOs thus present a whole series of challenges about which Muslim ethics is as ambivalent and undecided as are other religious traditions. At best, Muslim ethical responses to GMOs can be described as a work in progress. Subject to the relevant principles of shariah, it is permissible, on the whole, to resort to the cloning of microbes, plants, and

---

24. "Ruling on Eating Meat and Plants," Islam Question and Answer.

25. "Ruling on Eating Meat and Plants"

26. Cf. Kamali, *Shari'ah Law*, 189–191.

animals so as to prevent a manifest harm (*darar*) and a fatal disease, or which secures a benefit to humankind, including environmental safety and improvement, or to acquire, for instance, beneficial proteins and hormones to fight hunger and malnourishment.

That said, the Islamic perspective on GMOs is often complex and goes deeper than simply a determination of whether a certain food is halal or non-halal, which is why commentators continue debating these issues. Some Muslim jurists permit the use of GMOs based on the principle of greater good (*maslahah*) of providing a secure food supply to an ever-growing population by improving crop yields and making them more resistant to disease, insects, and a less than ideal growing environment. The opposite view cites risks to both the environment and the human population, as the potential impacts of GMOs often remain largely unknown. Both sides have presented arguments from their readings of the higher purposes of shariah (*maqasid al-shariah*) of protecting life and the natural environment, but also referring to scientific evidence. The Qur'anic position on scientific knowledge is instructive. According to a Qur'anic directive:

> And take not a stand on that over which you have no knowledge (al-Isra', 17:36).

Yet if the purpose of modification is to secure an essentially beneficial result, promote general welfare, or prevent an intolerable harm, then it would be permissible. This is the purport of the divinely ordained nobility of humankind (al-Isra', 17:70), and the grant of permission for us to exploit and utilize the resources of the universe for our benefit:

> And He (God Most High) has subjected to you, as from Him, all that is in the heavens and on earth: behold, herein are signs for those who reflect. (al-Jathiyah, 45:13)

The *fiqh* legal maxim, reviewed earlier, also declares permissibility as the normative position of shariah that deems all things permissible unless proven otherwise. Another principle of shariah is that establishing a *haram* requires decisive evidence, nothing less. According to yet another maxim, "prevention of harm takes precedence over securing a benefit." Altering the genome of plants and (staple) foods for commercial purposes while not knowing the long-term consequences to human safety and environmental health would also stand at odds with the *fiqh* maxim that "certainty may not be overruled by doubt." The state of certainty here is the natural goodness of wholesome food and agricultural produce that should not be overruled in favor of some material gain or doubtful long-term benefits that are, however, not a matter of certainty and definitive knowledge.

A point has also been made that genetic engineering (GE) of animals and plants can give human beings too much power over them, and that it is based on an exploitative view of nature. Many observers have consequently advised greater caution based on the fear that GE technology may disturb the God-ordained balance (*mizan*) in the Creation. Excessive tampering that undermines the fine balance of nature and the universe are clearly proscribed (Q al-Jathiyah, 54:49; al-Rahman, 55:7–9).

In their 2003 conference presentation in Sudan, Lakhdar Khaleefi and Maajidah Khaleefi stated that American law regards GMOs as natural foods that do not pose any danger until proven otherwise, but European law—especially French law—regards GMO foods as unnatural and a possible source of danger until proven otherwise. A Muslim scholar who researches this issue cannot say that it is *haram* to eat GM fruits unless it is proven for certain that they are harmful. Clear Islamic positions can only be established based on definitive research and scientific knowledge about GMOs. [27]

Mohammad Aslam Parvaiz believes that the use of transgenes in food harbors catastrophic consequences. Parvaiz shows how transgenic fish and crops pose serious environmental risks. He also doubts that any scientific grounds can justify altering certain life forms to suit human needs, and adds that such an invasive level of human interference in the ecosystem will produce unforeseen disturbances on the planet. [28]

Following in the footsteps of the Saudi-based Council of Islamic Jurisprudence (CIJ), Muslim religious authorities in Indonesia have approved the use of GMOs in the human food chain. Singapore's Muslim religious authorities have also endorsed the use of GMOs, as have those in Malaysia. Indian Muslim scholars tend to be more conservative compared to their colleagues in the Middle East, but have given a cautionary approval to GMOs. At its October 1997 meeting in Bombay, the Islamic Fiqh Academy of India adopted a resolution approving the cloning of animals and plants, provided this is "beneficial to humans and does not threaten humans from a religious,

---

27. "Ruling on Eating Meat and Plants."

28. Parvaiz, "Scientific Innovation and Al-Mizan," as quoted in Ebrahim Moosa, "Genetically Modified Food," 13–14.

moral and physical perspective."[29] In 2005, Darul Uloom Nadwatul Ulama in Lucknow, India, issued a *fatwa* approving GMOs. Asked whether the consumption of GMOs was permissible, Mufti Masood Hasan Hasni and Mufti Nasir Ali both replied: "To eat such fruit and vegetables is permissible. Unless the harm of a thing is known categorically or by means of a dominant probability, one cannot designate a permissible thing to be prohibited on a mere apprehension of harm. However, if out of precaution one refuses to partake of such foods, then that is the exercise of one's choice."[30]

Shaykh Dr. Hasan 'Ali al-Shadhili of Egypt is positive about biotechnology, yet he is also concerned that it can go in the opposite direction with harmful effects.[31] Iran's Ayatullah Mohammad 'Ali Taskhiri hews close to the scientific debates and invests a great deal of authority in the judgment of science. Ethical and political decisions, Taskhiri points out, cannot be made in advance of the scientific evidence: "There should be no haste in making ethical decisions as long as the scientific results are inconclusive."[32]

The Islamic Food and Nutrition Council of America (IFANCA), the main North American certifying body that designates food as "permissible" (halal) by Islamic standards, is reported to support foods derived from GMOs.[33] However, no explicit statement has been issued in support of GMOs, but one can safely assume, as is also the position under the shariah rules, that all food, including GMO foods, from *haram* sources would be *haram* (prohibited).

Ebrahim Moosa also records reservations and says there are compelling reasons why one should be cautious, adding further that GMO research should not be restricted to science-based decision-making. Religious communities, including Muslims, have generally not been able, however, to go beyond science-based decision making on this issue.[34]

Malaysia ratified the Cartagena Protocol on Biosafety (CPB) in September 2003 and took steps to formulate a regulatory framework for biosafety measures encompassed in the CPB. Malaysia's Biosafety Act (the Act) was approved by Parliament in 2007. The Act is an enabling legislation to ensure the safety of GMO applications, and it came into force on December

---

29. Qasmi, "Jadid Sa'in-si Teknik: Cloning," 75.

30. Moosa, "Genetically Modified Foods and Muslim Ethics," 145.

31. al-Shadhili, "Al-Istinsakh," 204.

32. al-Shadhili, "Al-Istinsakh," 204.

33. Lake, "Current Awareness of Genetically Modified Food Issues," .

34. Moosa, "Genetically Modified Foods," 156.

1, 2009, followed by the Biosafety (Approval and Notification) Regulations 2010 to implement the Act.[35]

The existing law does not contain any provisions, however, dealing with liability for damage that may result from GMOs. Malaysia would probably have to consider available options on this and make appropriate legislative amendments to the Biosafety Act, or else to enact a new law dealing with liability and redress for any damage caused by GMOs to persons and the living environment.[36]

The labeling of GMO products is another issue of concern, especially with the fast developments of GM crops that enter the market. In June 2010 the Malaysian government enacted new regulations on the labeling of GMOs in food, which came into force in July 2014 and requires that consumers are informed through labeling as to whether a package contains GM food or ingredients, and whether the product is derived from the use of GM technology.[37]

## *Meat Eating Then and Now: The Environmental Impact of Meat Eating*

Further to what has been stated in the introductory chapter of this book, scientific research shows that producing one kilogram of protein from kidney beans required approximately eighteen times less land, ten times less water, nine times less fuel, twelve times less fertilizer, and ten times less pesticide than producing one kilogram of protein from beef.[38] In addition, large livestock can provide milk and products such as butter, cheese, and yogurt, which provide greater life-long food yields than if they are slaughtered and consumed as meat.[39]

Over the past forty years or so, world wildlife populations have declined 58 percent, while 20 percent of all species now face the threat of extinction. Livestock farming negatively impacts biodiversity, as well as water quality and availability. It also causes land degradation, and greenhouse gases acidify seas, causing coral reef degeneration. Biodiversity provides essential ecological life

---

35. . Andrew, Ismail, and Djama, Overview of Genetically Modified Crop Governance." Vol. 98, Issue.1, September 2017, 12–17.

36. Ibid.

37. Ibid.

38. Sranacharoenpong et al., "Environmental Cost of Protein Food Choices."

39. Diamond, *Guns, Germs and Steel*, 84.

support for humans. Deteriorating biodiversity affects human well-being and material welfare, community security, resilience of local economies, group relations, and human health. Biodiversity is considered by many to have intrinsic value in which each species has a right to exist, whether or not it is valued by humans.[40]

Research on intensive agriculture confirms that reducing meat consumption is one of the leading challenges of this second millennium: Between 2010 and 2050, as a result of expected increases in population and income levels, the environmental effects of the food system could increase by 50–90 percent in the absence of technological changes and dedicated mitigation measures, reaching levels that are beyond the planetary boundaries that define a safe operating space for humanity.[41] Research further shows that the Western world needs to cut its meat consumption severely by 90 percent to avoid reducing the earth's ability to sustain a forecasted ten billion people by 2050. As a result, scientists have called for a "global shift" toward more plant-based diets.[42]

Furthermore, the livestock sector is responsible for 14.5 percent of all anthropogenic greenhouse gas emissions,[43] which is greater than emissions produced from powering the world's road vehicles, trains, ships, and airplanes combined.[44] Gas emissions derive mainly from belching methane, manure, feed production, land use changes, and fossil fuel and fertilizer use. Livestock also accounts for 70 percent of global agricultural land use.

A major component of global meat consumption is also from pets. Recent research estimates that dogs and cats are responsible for a sizeable 25–30 percent of the total environmental impact of meat consumption in the United States. This meat traditionally comprised offal, but now in developed countries, where pets are being treated less as animals and more like valued family members, it increasingly includes quality cuts of meat.[45]

Currently, the average individual daily meat intake in high-income countries is 200–250 grams, far higher than the UN-recommended 80–90 grams. Oxford Martin School researchers found that switching to the recommended intake, or a vegetarian diet, could save between 5.1 and 7.3 million deaths

---

40. Cresswell and Murphy, *Australia's State of the Environment*, 3.

41. Springmann et al., "Options for Keeping the Food System."

42. "Eat Less Meat to Save the World," *New Straits Times*.

43. Agriculture is the second largest emissions source after the energy sector.

44. Bailey, Froggath, and Wellesley, "Livestock—Climate Change's Forgotten Sector."

45. Okin, "Environmental Impacts."

yearly worldwide. Approximately half of the avoided deaths would be due to a reduction in red meat consumption.[46]

The climate change issue merits individual treatment, which falls, however, beyond our scope. The purpose here is mainly to draw attention to the gravity of the issue and say that in the Islamic context one is faced with a drastic change of conditions compared to what they were in premodern times, and to what humanity is facing in the twenty-first century. The information reviewed earlier showing that Arab communities in the past recommended meat consumption as a favorite food was clearly depicting the prevailing conditions of over a thousand years ago. With sparse populations and a virtual absence of any issues with carbon emissions, abusive industrial practices, and air pollution that are now causing problems, but that this is no longer the case. Climate change is receiving media attention in Muslim countries, yet it is not certain whether Islamic scholars and researchers are paying due attention to these realities. It is time for Islamic scholars and researchers to align their research efforts with scientific findings with a view to revising shariah positions through innovative research and *ijtihad*. The shariah also provides a number of principles, from text interpretation to legal maxims, *usul al-fiqh* principles, and juristic opinion over issues that can, all in all, be used as tools for new research. These are briefly mentioned below.

Some of the relevant Qur'anic passages that provide a scope for interpretation include the verse (al-Baqarah, 2:196) that offers alternative to animal slaughter in haj or Eid al-Adha for those who cannot afford to offer animal sacrifice (such individuals may fast instead for a certain number of days), and the basic Qur'anic principle (al-Nur, 24:55 and passim) that designates human beings as custodian and caretakers of the earth. In addition, many Qur'anic verses (cf. Ghafir, 40:79–80) remind believers of the numerous benefits they can derive from cattle—in addition, that is, to just meat: milk, transport, animals for ploughing, clothing and habitation materials, articles of convenience, and also for religious sacrifice. Although in the developing world all of these may still be relevant, in economically advanced countries there is no longer a demand for cattle to serve for transport, ploughing, or habitation materials.

One may further mention the *usul al-fiqh* position on causation: the rules of shariah stand and fall with their effective causes, and also change with the change of their effective causes—when the effective cause of a ruling no longer obtains, the ruling becomes liable to change through *ijtihad*. Juristic

46. Springmann et al. "Analysis and Valuation," 4146–4151.

opinion has also taken different positions over the question of whether *udhiyah* (animal slaughter during Eid al-Adha, or Eid of Sacrifice) is obligatory (*wajib*), or recommended sunnah (*sunnah mu'akkadah*). The majority (*jumhur*)—excepting the Hanafis—take the position that it is not *wajib* but recommended *sunnah*. The shariah rulings on the elimination of harm (*darar*, as reviewed earlier) occur not only in the clear authority of hadith, but also a number of supportive legal maxims to the effect that harm must be eliminated, minimized, and reduced to the extent possible, especially when it becomes exorbitant. Available evidence suggests that the climate issue has reached a crisis level and threatens human safety and survival on the planet. Many commentators have also observed that the environmental crisis threatens the safety and integrity of almost all of the higher objectives, or *maqasid*, of shariah. The present writer is of the view that environmental protection is one of the higher objectives of shariah that should be pursued through all valid shariah means. Covid-19 also diverted attention form the climate issue.

It is noteworthy also to mention in passing the shariah position regarding scientific and rational issues, which is to consult the experts and carry out fresh *ijtihad* when such is needed in the light of expert opinion and advice. It is relevant, furthermore, to note that eating meat is generally not essential to human well-being, since better and more plentiful alternative protein and nutrient sources exist. Thus, reducing meat consumption is one of the easiest contributions people of all faiths can make to restoring the environment and gain personal well-being and health. Would it not make good sense that the large amounts of funds Muslims spend on animal sacrifice, say in Eid al-Adha, should be donated to disaster-stricken people or war victims facing massive starvation, who are in urgent need of water, food, and medicine for their survival.

# PART II

## Halal Industry in Malaysia

### Introductory Remarks

Malaysia holds a special position in the global halal market. This is partly due to the general perceptions and demands of the Muslims of Malaysia (also of Indonesia), and prevailing consumer behavior among them, that show a keen interest in halal and other aspects of Islamic guidelines on consumption and lifestyle matters. Shafie and Othman reported from their consumer behavior survey that for the Muslim consumers of Malaysia, halal is a key requirement in their choice of food and lifestyle. Muslim expectations have steadily grown stronger, so much so that Muslims today are less prepared to tolerate risk and uncertainty and demand "a near zero halal environment. Furthermore, Muslims are intrinsically motivated to actively boycott brands that are in violation of the teachings of Islam."* Halal products and services in Malaysia have increased over the years and are no longer confined to food, but also cover a wide range of products extending from food and beverage to accommodation, attire, insurance, financial products, medicine, cosmetics, and personal hygiene.

---

* Tieman, "Safeguarding Halal Reputation," 14.

## 21

# *Milestones of Development*

IN 2004, WHEN Malaysia launched its first Malaysia International Halal
Showcase (MIHAS) in Kuala Lumpur, Prime Minister Abdullah Ahmad
Badawi declared that establishing Malaysia as a "global halal hub" was a major
priority of the government, and that MIHAS was the largest halal trade
expo to be held anywhere in the world.[1] According to an industry specialist,
Malaysia is the only country in the Muslim world where the halal industry
development agenda is also backed by the government, which translates into
the existence of a unique ecosystem that allows a synergy between the private and public sectors. In this ecosystem, the private sector players focus on
production, manufacturing, and services, while the public agencies, like the
Halal Industry Development Corporation (HDC) and the Department of
Islamic Development Malaysia (JAKIM), facilitate and coordinate the industry's progress by providing certification and training. "You don't see this kind
of collaboration anywhere else in the world. In most countries private players
dominate their halal industries."[2]

The HDC was established with the purpose of developing the halal industry internationally. HDC commenced operation under the International
Trade and Industry Ministry in 2006. It is also tasked to develop Malaysia's
industrial capacity and bring in foreign direct investment (FDI) into the
country.

Two events are held annually in Malaysia, the Malaysia International
Halal Showcase (MIHAS), as already mentioned, and the World Halal
Forum (WHF), both of which are tasked with spearheading the networking

---

1. Shafie and Othman, "Halal Certification."

2. Ismail, "'Halal' Is Not Just about Food," interview with Jamal Bidin, 12.

*Shariah and The Halal Industry.* Mohammad Hashim Kamali, Oxford University Press. © Oxford University Press 2021.
DOI: 10.1093/oso/9780197538616.003.0022

and internationalization of the halal value chains. Both play pivotal roles in building the country's reputation as the global reference and trade center for the halal industry since 2003. With the government's full support and involvement, Malaysia's credibility and leading role in the halal sector is also recognized by the Organisation of Islamic Cooperation (OIC).[3]

With regard to the financial difficulties that Bumiputera (indigenous Malays) entrepreneurs might face to play active roles in halal industry development, it was said that the government offers assistance through the Rural and Regional Development Ministry and Majlis Amanah Rakyat (Mara) to help them overcome a shortage of funds.[4]

Some rivalry has been noted between Bumiputera and non-Bumiputera companies. The former are seen by their rival non-Bumiputera companies as having too much support from the government, which has led them, in some cases at least, to be too dependent and complacent even at meager levels of achievement. The non-Bumiputera would consequently have to rely on their own creativity and hard work, which eventually proves to work in their favor. Thus, it is advised that the government should not over-lend to the Bumiputera, or even to small and medium-size enterprises (SMEs), and encourage them to be more self-reliant.[5]

The halal pharmaceutical sector has made impressive progress in recent years, taking a prominent place side by side with the food and beverage and cosmetic sectors. Yet for this sector to develop further, it needs to develop its capacity, greater synergy, and economies of scale, such as through halal pharma hubs, bigger market players, and greater reliance on halal ingredients—more so perhaps for the global pharmaceutical sector, which should be more geared toward halal ingredients. It is believed this is gradually happening, with expanded global networking and cooperation with other players like the Department of Standards Malaysia (DOSM) and JAKIM. Much will depend on critical mass when there are enough companies, such as CCM (Chemical Company of Malaysia), manufacturing halal pharmaceuticals, and also a growing consumer demand. There is a certain shortage of halal raw materials for manufacturers to produce ingredients that comply with

---

3. Islamic Tourism. "Malaysia—The world's leading Halal hub." https://itc.gov.my/tourists/discover-the-muslim-friendly-malaysia/malaysia-the-worlds-leading-halal-hub/.

4. Islamic Tourism Centre, "Malaysia—The World's Leading Halal Hub." See also Shah, "Malaysia Accelerating Halal Industry's Growth."

5. Cf. Yusof, Halal Foods, 37–39.

halal and thus help expand the existing production capacities.[6] Currently, halal medicines are estimated to have contributed close to one-third of the total revenue from the global halal market, posing an attractive opportunity for shariah-compliant medicines. This is supported by the fact that demand for halal medicines is growing fast, creating a potential for future economic value added in the industry.[7]

MIHAS is organized annually by Malaysia's External Trade Development Corporation (MALTRADE) under the Ministry of International Trade and Industry, and it provides a value-adding platform that promotes cross-border investments and business partnerships.[8] Malaysia's global halal hub concept aims to create opportunities for small and medium enterprises (SMEs), to penetrate the halal markets in the Middle East, the OIC countries, and elsewhere. The Federal Agricultural Marketing Authority (FAMA) had estimated the market size for frozen food only for the OIC countries to increase to MR193 billion by 2010. Yet actual developments have fallen short of meeting forecasts, owing partly to the limited range of halal products in the market, which are insufficient to cater to the demand. As of 2018, the halal industry in Malaysia was estimated at USD68.4 billion a year, whereas for the global market the figure is estimated at US$3.1 trillion.[9] Food companies such as McDonald's and Nestle have extensively implemented halal food certification in their operations and productions. In announcing this, Deputy Minister of Trade and Industry Mukhriz Mahathir also revealed that Bumiputeras (mainly native Malay Muslims) held only 30 percent of the 4,787 halal certificates issued by JAKIM to companies in the food and beverage industry. He noted that more non-Bumiputera companies were applying for halal certification. "This is despite the fact that being certified halal could be a ticket to growth outside Malaysia," Mahathir said, and added further "that the market potential for halal products is huge, especially in ASEAN, the Middle East and China. . . . In China alone, there are good prospects for halal products, as four provinces there have large Muslim populations with high purchasing

---

6. Cochrane, "Overview: How Attractive is Malaysia's Halal Pharmaceutical Sector?"

7. Salama, "Malaysia: World's First Halal Certification for Prescriptive Medicine issued to CCM." *Halal Focus.* https://halalfocus.net/malaysia-worlds-first-halal-certification-for-prescriptive-medicine-issued-to-ccm/.

8. Since its inauguration, MIHAS has brought together close to 170,000 visitors from 70 countries, 4,000 companies from 48 countries, and generated close to RM10 billion in sales. For details, see Mahmud, "Playing a Leadership Role in Halal Industry."

9. HDC. Halal Industry Master Plan 2030, 2–3.

power."[10] Yet even as of January 2019 it was reported that almost 90 percent of SMEs owned by Bumiputeras operate without a halal certificate. Studies on the attributes of halal certification among food and beverage operators reveal that food products "with halal certification signify trust and safety." So it is vital, it was added, "for the Malaysian SMEs to get halal certificates" to capture the market opportunities that exist.[11]

Four areas where noted developments have taken place in Malaysia's halal industry are halal standards, halal certification, halal parks, and halal pharmaceuticals, which are further discussed in the following pages.

## Halal Standards

Halal food under the Halal Standards currently in force in Malaysia comprises food and drink that are permitted under shariah law and are also clear of any ingredients of non-halal animals or animal products not slaughtered according to shariah. The food must also be clear of impurities, filth, and poisonous and intoxicating contents that are hazardous to health. It is required, furthermore, that no contaminated equipment or parts are used in the preparation of halal food, including its processing, packaging, storage, or transportation, and that it does not contain any human parts or its derivatives not permitted under shariah law.[12]

The first national Halal Standard was released in 2004, effectively making Malaysia the first country to have a documented and systematic halal assurance system, eventually transforming the halal industry from a traditional cottage industry to a vibrant new sector of the economy.

The Department of Standards Malaysia (DOSM), the issuing authority of halal standards in Malaysia, is a department of the Ministry of Science, Technology and Innovation. The establishment of the DOSM marked a milestone of development in the Malaysian halal industry. DOSM was established to formulate uniform halal standards for industry practices in Malaysia. The main function of DOSM is the issuance of halal standards, and also to foster and promote standardization and accreditation as a means of advancing the national economy, industrial efficiency, health and safety of the public, and

10. Mukhriz Mahathir's speech reported by Roziana Hamsawi, "Mukhriz Mahathir's Speech," 5.

11. Omar, "Get Halal Stamp," 19.

12. Department of Standards Malaysia, Malaysian Standards MS 1500-2009 (Clause 2).

consumer protection, as well as facilitating domestic and international trade.[13] It is further added that Malaysian Standards (MS) are developed through consensus by committees comprising a balanced representation of producers, users, consumers, and others with relevant interests. To the extent possible, Malaysian Standards are aligned with or consist of adoption of international standards. Approval of a standard as a Malaysian Standard is governed by the Standards of Malaysia Act 1996 (Act 549).

Malaysian Standards are also reviewed periodically. The use of Malaysian Standards is voluntary except insofar as they are made mandatory by regulatory authorities by means of regulations, local by-laws, or any other similar ways.

An interesting feature of Malaysian halal standards is that they incorporate both Islamic and scientific components, which gives Malaysia a competitive edge in terms of good manufacturing practices that include hazard analysis of critical control points. A Technical Committee on Halal Food and Islamic Consumer Products has been set up that, inter alia, provides seminars and courses to educate the public on halal standards and certification procedures.

Prior to 2004 the country had no national standards for producing halal products and only referred to informal documents and procedures introduced by the Department of Islamic Development Malaysia (JAKIM). MS 1500-2004 was the first documented standard on halal food established by the government of Malaysia to produce coordinated halal guidelines for the country. This business initiative was aimed at boosting Malaysia's exports to other countries and also to capture the global halal food market. The basic purpose was to ensure that there is a set basis for technical agreements to regulate trade with other countries, as well as the halal production activities and businesses within Malaysia.[14] Standards Malaysia has been mandated to develop the local halal standards. The first of these was launched formally in August 2004 by Prime Minister Abdullah Ahmad Badawi. However, in 2009 this standard was replaced by MS 1500-2009—Halal Food, covering the production, preparation, handling and storage of halal food. MS 1500-2009 covers the basic shariah requirements in terms of (a) providing practical guidelines for the food industry and the operation and handling of halal food, including nutrient supplements, and (b) providing basic requirements for halal food products and food trade or business in Malaysia. MS 1500-2009 is not mandatory,

---

13. This statement appears as a Foreword to MS 1500-2009.

14. Yusof, *Halal Foods*, 26.

however, and only serves as a guideline for firms related to food processing and handling. The Malaysian Standards also do not cover all the halal certification requirements and procedures. MS 1500-2009 has, furthermore, been supplemented by additional standards, in particular MS 1480 on food safety according to hazard analysis and critical control points, and MS 1514–2001 on general principles of food hygiene, which highlight key hygiene controls at every level of the food production chain. All of these standards are interconnected and should be used together. Notwithstanding the optional nature of these standards, many firms in Malaysia are keen to adopt them for customer appeal and global market access.[15] The sixteen halal standards that are currently in force not only certify food items but also food premises, cosmetics, halal packaging, personal care, and shariah-compliant quality of management and services. The full list of these standards is as follows:

1. Malaysian Standards (MS) Description—MS 1500 (2009): Halal Food—Production, Preparation, Handling and Storage—General Guidelines (Second Revision).
2. MS 1900 (2005): Quality Management Systems—Requirements from Islamic Perspectives.
3. MS 2300 (2009): Value-based Management System—Requirements from an Islamic Perspective.
4. MS 2424 (2012): Halal Pharmaceuticals—General Guidelines.
5. MS 2400-1 (2010): Halalan-Toyyiban Assurance Pipeline Management System Requirements for Transportation of goods and/or Cargo chain services.
6. MS 2400-2 (2010): Halalan-Toyyiban Assurance Pipeline Management System Requirements for Warehousing and Related Activities.
7. MS 2400-3 (2010): Halalan-Toyyiban Assurance Pipeline Management System Requirements for Retailing.
8. MS 2393 (2010): Islamic and Halal Principles—Definitions and Interpretation on Terminology.
9. MS 2393 (2013): Islamic and Halal Principles—Definitions and Interpretation on Terminology.
10. MS2200-1 (2008): Islamic Consumer Goods, Part 1: Cosmetic and Personal Care—General Guidelines.

---

15. Ibid., 27.

11. MS 2200-2 (2013): Islamic Consumer Goods, Part 2: Usage of Animal Bone, Skin and Hair—General Guidelines.
12. MS 1900 (2014): Shariah-based Quality Management System.
13. MS 2565 (2014): Halal Packaging—General Guidelines.
14. MS 2627 (2017): Detection of Porcine DNA—Test Method—Food and Food Product.
15. MS 2594 (2015): Halal Chemical for Use in Potable Water Treatment—General Guidelines.
16. MS 2610 (2015): Muslim-Friendly Hospitality Services.

Many of these standards have been revised from time to time and the new versions then replace the earlier edition in each case. MS 1500-2009 on Halal Food, as already mentioned, is the revised version of the original that was introduced in 2004. It is provided at the outset that this standard provides the practical and basic guidelines for halal food products and food businesses in Malaysia.[16] Basic guidelines imply that juridical details, scholastic differences, and information on the sources from which the standard might have been taken are not included. MS 1500-2009 consists of eleven pages of text, two appendices, and a short bibliography of the relevant statutes—altogether covering seventeen pages; its prose and style of expression is concise and confined to statute-like declarations that establish positions of validity or otherwise under shariah, Malaysian laws and operational procedures.

The DOSM standards clearly show that the halal industry and halal products have acquired a degree of specialization on sector-by-sector–based developments. Whereas the general principles of halal as a shariah concept are in common and on the whole observed in all sectors, there are variations in technical details, logistic aspects, and implementation. Both the general and sector-based aspects of halal merit attention, especially in areas where common principles of halal apply to all sectors. Both the general and sector-based aspects have been addressed and regulated by the respective authorities via the issuance of regulations, standards, circulars, etc., which are, however, piecemeal and call for further uniformity and consolidation.

---

16. Department of Standards Malaysia, Malaysian Standard MS 1500-2009: Halal Food – Production, Preparation, Handling and Storage—General Guidelines (second edition), Kuala Lumpur, 2009, 1. The thirteen-item bibliography on page 16 of this document only refers to Malaysian laws and other existing standards, but no reference is made to *fiqh* or substantive sources.

Establishing unified standards internationally is a big challenge by common acknowledgment, just as it is also an important target for the future growth of the halal industry generally. There are numerous certification bodies around the world applying standards that are modified to suit their local culture and requirements. These country standards also differ in accordance with their own interpretation of the Islamic principles and any particular school or madhhab of Islamic law they may be following. What it all means is that there is a certain lack of synchrony among Muslim countries and their procedural specifications in the issuance of halal certificates. This also translates into disparities, adding to challenges of uniformity and standardization in the numerous halal stamps or logos issued across regions and globally, affecting in turn consumer confidence regarding which may be seen to be more authentic.

Yet Malaysia seems to be taking a somewhat practical view of the issue. Malaysian officials often say that plurality of standards may not be a huge problem if there is a level of reciprocal acceptance among the various parties. This is how JAKIM approaches the issue, by taking a practical-cum-philosophical view of it. As it is, JAKIM currently recognizes sixty-seven halal certification bodies from forty-one countries, which means that all the products certified by them can be exported to Malaysia, just as Malaysia can also export to those countries. "We cannot say whose standards are right or wrong," says Sirajuddin Suhaimee, the JAKIM Halal Hub director, adding that these differences have not yet been resolved and there are still arguments about whose standards or certificates are preferable or better. Yet it is not really worth arguing about them for yet another reason, which is that "consumers around the world, especially Muslims, do not care whose logo, standards or certification they use."[17] What is more important is industry development. One should focus on developing the industry and services so that they bring returns to one's economy and enhance the range of available choices, rather than arguing about standards and certification procedures.

There is considerable awareness in the industry, however, of the importance of uniformity for the growth of halal industry worldwide. Efforts are consequently underway in Malaysia to unify the numerous standards that currently obtain in the Muslim world. Malaysia's awareness of its own leading role is manifested in an announcement, made in June 2017, on the setting up of an International Halal Authority Board (IHAB), as part of the Malaysian

---

17. Ismail, "Halal Is Not Just about Food," interview with Sirajuddin Suhaimee, 13.

Halal Council's (MHC) 2018-2020 agenda. Malaysia's former deputy prime minister Ahmad Zahid Hamidi, then also chairman of MHC, announced the said agenda and added that MHC would also establish a halal international research academy, the first of its kind in the region. JAKIM's Suhaimee commented, in turn, that this initiative was "aimed at sustaining the country's global halal player leading status." He added that IAHB would be a way for all certification bodies to come under one platform, and it would also be an important step toward the harmonization of halal standards internationally.[18]

One of the principal guidelines on halal foods is MS 1500-2009, which articulates most of the basic positions on halal, *haram*, and *najis* in foodstuffs, as well as the basic requirements of shariah-compliant animal slaughter. A great deal of the rulings provided in this standard tend to feature in relevant places in almost all of the other dozen or so halal standards. MS 1500-2009 begins with a one-page foreword that specifies the main changes made to the first edition. The standard then features the following information on its first page concerning halal food production, preparation, handling, and storage:

Halal food means food and drink and/or their ingredients permitted under the shariah law and must fulfil the following conditions:

(a) the food or its ingredients do not contain any component or product of animals that are non-halal under shariah law, or products of animals which are not slaughtered according to shariah;

(b) the food does not contain any ingredient that is considered as *najis* (filthy, impure) by shariah;

(c) the food is safe for consumption, non-poisonous, non-intoxicating and non-hazardous to health;

(d) the food or its ingredients are not prepared, processed or manufactured using equipment contaminated with *najis* according to shariah;

(e) [the food] does not contain any human parts or its derivatives that are not permitted by shariah law;

(f) during its preparation, processing, packing, storage, or transportation, the food is physically separated from any other food that does not meet the requirements stated in (a), (b), (c), (d) or (e) or anything that is decreed as *najis* by shariah law.

---

18. Ismail, "Halal Is Not Just about Food," 13.

By their express acknowledgement, these standards are developed to safe-guard the life and well-being of consumers and the public at large, and also to promote and facilitate domestic and international trade. It is a means, fur-thermore, of promoting and consolidating international cooperation in food safety and health. When all of these standards are duly observed, a halal cer-tificate may be issued by the authorized agency that establishes the shariah permissibility and halal status of the substances concerned.

Yet in all of the foregoing, "shariah" or "shariah law" are taken for granted to offer standard guidelines that can be readily known and ascertained. This may not be much of an issue for Malaysia internally, as Malaysia is a Shafiʻi jurisdiction and Shafiʻi interpretations of shariah constitute the first recourse for purposes of implementation. But when the halal unification agenda is visualized in its international context, one comes across many scholastic dif-ferences of interpretation over details, which cannot be overlooked. It may then be proposed that ascertaining commonalities over the essentials of halal and *haram*, and identifying and addressing the scholastic differences of in-terpretation among the various *madhhabs*, should be a main agenda of the proposed International Halal Authority Board. They may decide to take a research-oriented approach regarding issues they may consider of merit in their effort to ascertain the prospects of developing common shariah stan-dards. The standards that are so developed need to be consensus-based, and a procedure is visualized for them to be recognized through an authoritative body of scholars and industry experts. This will in some ways be an exten-sion of the DOSM work, albeit from a different angle in some respects. The end result will be an enhancement for all the participants and an important step for the commercial potentials of halal products and services. The stan-dards so developed will hopefully place the global halal agenda and it jurid-ical grounding in shariah on solid foundations that seek to override scholastic differences and aspire to general acceptance throughout the Islamic world.

The global halal market has steadily expanded over the years, and continues to be growing at a remarkable pace: from an approximately US$3.1 trillion in 2018, the halal sector was expected to double to US$5.0 trillion by the end of 2030.[19] The expected expansion stretches to almost all sectors, although food and beverage, followed by cosmetics and personal care, represent the bulk of the growth. According to State of the Global Islamic Economy Report, by the end of 2019, the halal food industry alone was expected to be worth US$2.02

---

19. HDC. Halal Industry Master Plan 2030, 2–3.

trillion, the halal cosmetics would be worth US$66 billion, and the halal pharmaceuticals industry would be worth US$94 billion.[20] It is projected that the halal food and drink sector may be worth as much as US$2.1 trillion by 2030. Furthermore, the halal market is thriving not only in Muslim-majority countries, but also in major non-Muslim-majority economies such as China, Japan, South Korea, Germany, the United States, and the United Kingdom. In the UK, for instance, food production companies are increasingly recognizing the importance of the Muslim market, with around 20 percent of the sheep meat in England being consumed by the Muslim population. More and more companies are, therefore, catering to the Muslim market by producing halal food items. This is also reflected in Malaysia's Department for Halal Industries establishing cooperation with local councils in the Northeast of England to develop a business hub for producing halal meat.[21]

Malaysia's total halal exports in the first half of 2015 were valued at RM19.5 billion (expected to rise to RM40 billion in 2017), which is about 6–7 percent of the country's total exports.[22] Malaysia has also pursued its vision of becoming the global halal hub persistently, and has taken steps to that effect. Malaysia's minister of international trade and industry, Mustafa Mohamed, spoke in March 2016 of "a complete halal ecosystem" that Malaysia offers, calling it a key factor "that sets the country apart as the leader of the global halal industry . . . and one that is capable of delivering impactful socioeconomic enhancement while preserving halal integrity and assuring sustainability of the supply chain."[23] The minister also recounted salient features of the industry developments to say that in 2011, Malaysia introduced the Halal Business Transformation Programme to facilitate the development of local companies to become halal industry players. The objective was to strengthen the halal companies' sale performance, and to increase the number of halal-certified companies year after year. "The landscape is rapidly changing," he said, as there is an intense competition due to the growing interest from other East Asian countries, such as Japan, China, and South Korea. "The capacity building for local producers is our main priority now," he added.[24] There is

20. Dinar Standard, 2020/21 State of the Global Islamic Economy Report, 4.

21. Shah, "Fostering a True Halal Economy," 12.

22. Rasid, "Global Halal Market Growing Bigger," B2.

23. Rasid, "Report on the Minister's Speech," B4.

24. Rasid, "Report on the Minister's Speech," B4.

currently an undersupply situation in the global market, where halal producers can only cater to 20 percent of the demand. The minister also commented on the World Halal Week (WHW) 2016, themed "Beyond the Economy," advancing a perspective that halal transcends its economic value: "We seek to promote halal practices as a modern lifestyle choice for both Muslims and non-Muslims." WHW 2016 comprised the World Halal Conference, Malaysia International Halal Showcase, and Islamic Development Malaysia Department's Certification Bodies Convention. These developments are reflected, the minister added, in Thompson Reuter's evaluation survey that ranked Malaysia as the "Top Country for the Global Islamic Economy Indicator," surpassing the United Arab Emirates, Saudi Arabia, and Qatar.[25]

The Malaysian International Halal Showcase (MIHAS) 2017 provided a platform for companies from across the world to share their experiences in using technology to capture the halal market, such as in the areas of imports and exports, for example, as well as in improvements in halal products packaging. It showed how an exchange of ideas can benefit the halal industry on a global scale. Although the Fourth Industrial Revolution (Industry 4.0) presents challenges to business and industries worldwide, it also presents opportunities to expand and improve, and to strengthen international links.[26]

There is a disconnect, however, between the two logically interrelated sectors of the halal economy: halal industry and Islamic banking and finance. They have remained isolated notwithstanding their many commonalities and the fact that they both share and observe the same shariah requirements of halal. In a survey conducted by Reuters on 250 companies involved in halal production and with a combined market capitalization of US$132 billion, it was found that only 50 percent of them passed the AAOIFI test, which meant that they were not fully shariah-compliant. This was revealed by Rafiza Ghazali, Thompson Reuters' head of Islamic finance (Asia) at a discussion on "Halal Economy" during the Islamic Financial Summit in Kuala Lumpur in 2011.[27] The AAOIFI test was a screening criterion used by Reuters to determine the shariah compliancy of stocks, she said. "Why is that they [companies in halal production] make sure their production can be consumed by Muslims, yet Muslims cannot invest in them?" Rafiza asked. Another panelist, AmIslamic Funds Management Malaysia director Maznah Mahbob, said,

25. Rasid, "Report on the Minister's Speech," B4.

26. Shah, "Fostering a True Halal Economy," 13.

27. Gunasegaram, "Halal Industry Should Work with Islamic Finance," 3.

"There are so many opportunities for these companies to issue *sukuk*, short term papers, and longer term Islamic debt instruments of various tenures for fund managers to invest in." As a fund management firm, AmIslamic invests in both *sukuk* and equities. If they structure their funding requirements in a shariah-compliant way, they can be operating in a shariah-compliant universe.[28]

It seems that the disconnect still continues for the most part. In his well-publicized keynote address at the World Halal Conference 2018, HRH Sultan Nazrin Shah had occasion to stress the importance of the prospects that still await utilization. He said that as the halal industry continues its rapid expansion, halal industry players, together with the Islamic financial institutions, should "aspire to do more to nurture a halal ecosystem through the use of shariah-compliant trade facilities." This would facilitate the growth of Islamic finance, and would also help to promote the sought-after "end-to-end" compliance for the halal industry.[29] The halal ecosystem could greatly benefit from the capital that can be generated via Islamic finance mechanisms, such as *sukuk* and *takaful*. Indeed, some halal companies are already pursuing these funding methods, such that as of 2014, US$5 billion had been raised by forty issuers from the halal industry. In spite of this, according to the MIFC, however, the fuller "potential of *sukuk* financing in support of halal businesses is yet to be realised."[30]

## Halal Certificates

Halal certificates were first introduced in 1974 when the Research Centre for the Islamic Affairs Division in the Prime Minister's Office started to issue halal certification letters for products that met the halal criteria at that time. Halal certification has since played a focal role in the overall development of the halal industry in Malaysia, especially in regard to meeting international market demands for higher standards in the production and management of halal products.

The rapid development of halal certification in Malaysia also prompted the Department of Islamic Development Malaysia (JAKIM) to extend its halal section into a much bigger organization in 2005, officially named

---

28. Gunasegaram, "Halal Industry Should Work with Islamic Finance," 3.

29. Rokshana Shirin, "Effectiveness of The Existing Halal Laws," 144–5.

30. Shah, "Fostering a True Halal Economy," 14.

JAKIM's Halal Hub. JAKIM was the first halal certification body responsible for monitoring the halal industry, leading to the amendment of Malaysia's Trade Description Act in 2011, which gave JAKIM a much stronger mandate to regulate the halal industry.[31]

Halal brands and certification originate in different places, yet some of the local brands appear to have developed their own niche. In general, Muslim consumers in Malaysia look for the authentic halal certification by JAKIM.

Only companies and businesses that have completed the halal certification procedures may use the JAKIM halal logo on their premises and products. General requirements to complete halal certification include the following:

1. Every producer or manufacturer with halal certification must produce only halal products.
2. Every company that applies for the halal certificate must ensure that the source of the ingredients they use is halal and their suppliers and subcontractors supply halal goods and have halal certificates.
3. A company that is listed under the Multinational as well as Small and Medium Industry category is required to establish an Internal Halal Audit Committee and appoint an Islamic Affairs Executive to oversee and ensure compliance with halal certification procedures.
4. It is required also to have a minimum of two permanent Muslim workers of Malaysian nationality in the kitchen/handling/food processing section.
5. Equipment and appliances used on the premise must be clean and free of contamination by impurities based on Islamic law, and not detrimental to health.
6. Transportation used must be specifically for halal products delivery only.
7. Religious worship paraphernalia are not allowed on the premises or in the food processing area.[32]

Many of these requirements derive from the Islamic law rules to the effect that anything which comes into contact with pig and porcine products, non-halal carcass, and blood is also contaminated and therefore non-halal to consume or use. This is the main reason why manufacturers are required to

---

31. Islamic Tourism Centre. "Malaysia—The World's Leading Halal Hub." See also Aznam Shah, "Malaysia Accelerating."

32. For details, see Malaysian Standard. *MS 1900:2014 Shariah-Based Quality Management System*. Cyberjaya: Department of Standards Malaysia, 2014.

produce only halal products at their factory. Requirement 4 above refers to the need for Muslim employees as witnesses to the process of food production in the facilities concerned. This is to avoid doubt as to the halal authenticity of the products produced by non-Muslims. The same can be said regarding requirement 7, as Muslims do not subscribe to belief in religious statues and symbols as objects of worship.

JAKIM, which supervises halal certification procedures, is entrusted with monitoring operations relating to downstream halal production activities such as handling and packaging. Imported products are being certified by certain organizations accredited by JAKIM and government agencies such as the Department of Veterinary Services and the Food Safety and Quality Division of the Ministry of Health, which issue clearances on suspected hazardous food substances. Malaysia's Halal Hub concept, moreover, aims to establish benchmarks for the eventual development of Global Halal Standards not only for food production and processing, but also for pharmaceuticals, cosmetics, and preservatives.[33] Once a halal certification is issued, the companies may print and display the halal logo on their products and advertisements, and on their company premises and outlets.

One of the reasons the Muslim and Bumiputera (Malay Muslim) portion of the halal certificate owners is relatively small is the cost. It costs up to MR2,000 to get a two-year certificate for each product. To get a halal certificate is described as "a very meticulous process. Every single step of the business or manufacturing process will be evaluated and assessed, from the ingredients, process handling of the materials to the logistics."[34] Yet there are shortcomings in enforcement. As of late 2016, of the 5,726 halal-registered companies in Malaysia, only 32 percent were Bumiputera-owned. Commentators have noted that the lack of adequate enforcement by JAKIM personnel in monitoring the use of the halal logo has caused the public to question the authenticity of some of the products or services claimed to be halal.[35]

JAKIM has consequently made efforts to expedite the certification process through enhanced practical training and involvement of the private sector. Mohamad Shukri Abdullah, CEO of Shapers Malaysia, the main organizers of the Malaysian Halal Festival (Halfest) 2016, which featured over five

---

33. For details, see Din, *Trading Halal Commodities*, 20–21.

34. Hamsawi, "Bumis."

35. Shafie and Othman, "Halal Certification," 5.

hundred halal businesses from all over Malaysia, said that by organizing practical training sessions every few months, Bumiputera small and medium-size
entrepreneurs would have a better understanding of what they need to do to
get halal certificates: "Unlike the perception of the majority, halal is not about
the ingredients of the food per se, but also its preparation processes, facilities
and premises."[36]

Effective from January 2012, only Malaysia's halal logo issued by JAKIM
is recognized, in accordance with the Trade Description Act 2011. This means
that halal logos and certificates issued by private companies and entities are
no longer to be exhibited by business premises. The halal certificate is valid for
two years (renewable) and can be cancelled at any time by JAKIM monitors
in the event the organization or company is found to have contravened any of
the halal requirements and procedures.[37]

Yet instances of violation are occasionally noted in the media, partly because of a lack of awareness, but also due to deceptive operations. In January
2019 a violation was found at a popular restaurant in Shah Alam, Section 25,
which had been operating for ten years as a "halal" Muslim establishment,
but which was found by the Selangor Islamic Religious Department (Jabatan
Agama Islam Selangor, or JAIS) to not have a halal certificate, and to be
obtaining meat, such as mutton, from non-halal suppliers. One of the two
owners was a non-Muslim, and so were almost all the employees. The outlet
had also been festooned with displays of Qur'anic verses and messages in Jawi.
It was clearly deceiving patrons by promoting the eatery as a Muslim establishment. JAIS announced that it would take action, under Section 10(A) of
the Selangor Shariah Crimes Enactment 1995, "for insulting Islam or causing
Islam to be undermined."[38]

According to another report, a Vietnamese restaurant owner in Kuantan
was found to have been "duping its Muslim customers by displaying fake
halal logos in its premises on food packages."[39] The Pahang Islamic Religious
Department (JAIP) that conducted the operation also said that the restaurant was fined for committing the same offense in April 2018, and that
this time if convicted the owner might be slapped with a much bigger fine.

---

36. "JAKIM Pushes to Speed Up Halal Certification," 17.

37. Halal Industry Development Corporation, *Best Halal Practices*. See also Yusof, *Halal Foods*, 31.

38. For details, see "JAIS Raids Bogus Halal Restaurant," 58.

39. "Eatery with Fake Halal Logo Raided." *New Straits Times*, January 30, 2019. 66.

The restaurant had violated the Trade Description Act 2011 and the Trade Description (Certification and Marking of Halal) Order 2011.[40]

Further developments of note in Malaysia's halal industry is manifested in its active engagement in developing world halal standards. Known as the Malaysia International Halal Authorities and Bodies System (MyIHAB), the system features a centralized database under JAKIM's Halal Ecosystem Solutions, and is said to be a first of its kind aimed at setting up an International Halal Accreditation Board "in the near future." The then deputy prime minister of Malaysia, Ahmad Zahid Hamidi, spoke of this at the 8th Halal Certification Bodies Convention held in Kuala Lumpur (April 4, 2017), attended by some 1,000 industry players and stakeholder from forty countries. "It has always been our hope and vision that halal certification will have a brighter future," Hamidi said, and the purpose would mainly be to promote halal products to become a premium brand that inspires credibility for its commitment to quality, safety, and good health.[41] JAKIM's office will monitor the applications for International Halal Certification, while recognized Halal certification bodies in Malaysia will act as JAKIM's monitoring agents abroad to assist the government in the process. In the meantime, the government will engage in capacity-building of these recognized certification bodies through coaching and consultation.[42]

## Halal Parks

As part of its global halal hub policy, the Malaysian government has taken measures in both its Second Industrial Master Plan (1996–2005) and the National Agricultural Policy (1998–2010) to support the halal industry through the creation of a number of halal parks located in strategic places in the country. Currently there are several smaller halal parks located in the states of Selangor, Kedah, Melaka, Negeri Sembilan, Perak, and Pahang, while the bigger ones are the Pulau Indah Industrial Park in Selangor, Tanjung Pelepas Free Trade Zone in Johor, and the largest one yet is the Tanjung Manis Halal Hub in Sarawak.[43] Halal parks are an effective instrument in clustering a big part of a halal value chain geographically in a country. Next to clustering

---

40. "Eatery with Fake Halal Logo Raided," 66.

41. Kannan, "Move Towards World Halal Standards," 13.

42. Kannan, "Move Towards World Halal Standards," 13.

43. Kannan, "Move towards World Halal Standards," 13. See also HDC, "Halal Parks."

advantages (like shortening of supply chain, better access, cost reductions, innovations, etc.), it can create a strong base for halal food products and allows enforcement of a common halal standard in a controlled location. Different halal parks offer different infrastructure facilities and benefits, but overall they all encourage green design and accessibility of raw materials and ingredients, energy efficiency, and intercompany linkages. The idea of linkages is also manifested in the development of networks with other countries. Malaysia has formed a working group with several ASEAN countries to look into global issues such as the accreditation of halal food and registration list for halal preservatives. Yet Malaysia faces a certain shortage of raw materials that can be processed into halal products. Shortages have been noted in regard to livestock, especially cows, goats, and poultry, which means that a great deal of the halal ingredients, including meat and food additives, need to be imported for the industry to continue on its growth path.[44]

Iskandar Halal Park, which is located in Johor, started in November 2015 as a joint venture collaboration between United Malayan Land Berhad (UM Land) and Johor State via Johor Biotechnology & Biodiversity Corporation (J-Biotech) to create a 350-acre international halal park, which will be one of the catalyst projects in Eastern Iskandar Malaysia, Johor. J-Biotech is one of the Johor State investment companies chaired by the chief minister of Johor.

Iskandar Halal Park is an integrated industrial park that consists of industrial and commercial facilities, a corporate HQ, scientific laboratories, a data center, foreign worker enclaves, integrated packaging and warehousing logistic facilities (part of a regional marketing and clearing house), a youth park, an all-inclusive and self-contained center, and recreation- related business facilities. All of these are due to be developed in three separate phases. These will eventually make Iskandar Halal Park the first premium bio-halal industrial park in Malaysia.[45]

Another development of interest was the launching of what was announced to be the world's first halal laboratory in Seremban, known as the Malaysia Halal Analysis Centre (MyHAC) by Deputy Prime Minister Hamidi in Seremban in March 2018. Hamidi stated on the occasion that the laboratory would help boost the halal industry in the international arena. A high level of integrity, he added, was essential to ensure that halal-certified products in

---

44. Cf. Yusof, *Halal Foods*, 34–35.

45. "Iskandar Halal Park," UM Land.

Malaysia not only included documents and field research, but also scientific laboratory analysis to confirm the halal status of ingredients in the products. "With MyHAC the halal certification process will be done more efficiently."[46]

On the international front, non-Muslim countries have also shown a strong interest in the development of halal parks. China's Yangling Demonstration Zone in Shaanxi Province is planning to set up a global halal park to lure overseas producers so as to capture a slice of the world's lucrative halal market. It has even offered to set up a Malaysia halal park if there is strong interest from Malaysian companies. In this connection, China has also sought the help of Malaysia's Halal Development Corporation (HDC) to set up a halal certification unit in Yangling, an education town 80 kilometers west of the ancient city of Xian. "We are planning a global halal park for the processing of Muslim food and products. There will be generous incentives and negotiable taxation terms," said the deputy director of the Administrative Committee of Yangling Demonstration Zone, Liu Qing, to a visiting twenty-three-member business delegation from Malaysia led by Lawrence Low, a political secretary in the Prime Minister's Department in May 2016.

Liu said that because Shaanxi had a huge Muslim population and Yangling was situated along the old "Silk Road" trade route with easy access to the Middle East, it was best suited for the setting up of a halal park in order to capture domestic and Central Asian markets. Low said that Malaysia's halal certification was recognized globally due to the stringent conditions that it imposed, and urged Yangling to work closely with Kuala Lumpur on the halal park so that there was closer Malaysia-China cooperation. Low added that many foreign companies wanted to partner with Malaysian firms because of halal certification, and that Japan was also partnering with Malaysia's Lay Hong Group.[47]

Another area of development in Malaysia's halal industry is halal pharmaceuticals, to which we turn next.

## *Halal Pharmaceuticals*

Halal pharmaceuticals (HP) are a natural extension of the traditional manufacture of pharmaceuticals. The existing manufacturing technologies can logically be extended into the halal pharmaceuticals sector. This extension can

---

46. "MyHAC—World's First Halal Laboratory," 4.

47. For details, see Foon, "Shaanix to Set Up Global Halal Hub."

even push outward the boundaries of manufacturing generally. Muslims in Malaysia and elsewhere are becoming increasingly more aware of the medicines and supplements they take, leading to the exponential growth of halal pharmaceutical industry. In 2016 the sector was valued at US$83 billion, a 6 percent growth compared to the previous year. It is expected to grow 8 percent per year to reach US$132 billion by 2022. Malaysia has been increasing its exports of pharmaceuticals, which, according to the Malaysia External Trade Development Corporation (MATRADE), were valued at RM1.31 billion (US$317 million) in 2015, an increase of 15.8 percent over 2014.

Malaysia has fairly well-developed supporting industries, such as halal logistics, including industrial parks, warehousing, and transportation, which augurs well for further development of halal pharmaceuticals. The JAKIM Halal Hub director, Sirajuddin Suhaimee, said in a 2017 interview[48] that Malaysia had been producing halal pharmaceuticals since 2014, as under the halal certification program, a seven scheme development agenda was to be developed, including food, logistics, manufacturing, cosmetics, slaughterhouses, consumer goods (such as toiletries) and pharmaceuticals. For each scheme there is a special team overseeing the certification process, and they normally collaborate with the private sector industries. For cosmetic products, for instance, the team will collaborate with the Cosmetics, Toiletries and Fragrance Association, while for manufacturing the team will collaborate with the Federation of Malaysian Manufacturers. They support and complement one another. When there are issues on pharmaceutical products, for instance, there will be collaboration to solve them. Both sides will seek to facilitate each other's work, especially relating to production of new halal pharmaceuticals. Suhaimee added that the Halal Hub also has a committee that consists of experts and researchers from higher learning institutions that look into all issues faced by the industry in fulfilling the requirements of Malaysian halal standards. Another committee was planned in order to come up with a first of its kind pharmacopeia (an encyclopedia of halal pharmaceuticals), which was expected to be out by 2020. This will not only help inform industry players, but will also guide consumers on how to make better informed purchasing decisions.[49]

Malaysian pharmaceutical companies like Pharmaniaga and AJ Pharma are spearheading innovation in the Halal pharmaceutical sector, investing

48. Ismail, "'Halal' Is Not Just about Food," 13.

49. Ismail, "'Halal' Is Not Just about Food," 13.

substantial amounts in the development of Halal vaccines. The world's first halal vaccine manufacturing center was also planned to be built in Malaysia by 2020, where the vaccines would be produced and exported to other countries.

According to the State of the Global Islamic Economy Report 2021/21, Malaysia has the best-developed Islamic economy for HP and cosmetics, followed by UAE and Singapore. This is based on four criteria—trade, governance, awareness, and social benefit.[50]

Within the halal pharmaceutical sector, halal nutraceuticals have been identified as a major growth segment that can experience rapid growth if supported by strategic investment. Developing new products based on primary research is critical for HPs to develop a viable business model, as well as the ability to market the products to a broader range of consumers. Growth capital will also be critical to investing in research and development, expanding manufacturing capabilities, and broadening focus in new markets. This is where multinational companies can play a significant role by providing halal products and being an important stepping stone to boost investment.

Malaysia has been at the forefront of the global halal pharmaceutical sector. The country's leadership has particularly been accommodating to the needs of this sector, and to the overall Islamic economy, with a view to shifting the former from being primarily food-focused to also include pharmaceuticals and nutraceuticals.

The country's certification body, JAKIM, has been active in publishing the world's first halal pharmaceuticals standard—the MS 2424-2012 Halal Pharmaceuticals General Guidelines. This halal pharmaceutical standard was developed by the DOSM and the Ministry of Science, Technology and Innovation (MOSTI) in collaboration with JAKIM's Halal Hub Division, the National Pharmaceutical Regulatory Agency (NPRA), and subject matter experts from both shariah and science disciplines. Prior to the availability of this halal pharmaceutical standard, the Halal Food Standard MS1900 was being referred to as a stand-in guide by pharmaceutical manufacturers. This was not ideal, as the standard was not tailored to the peculiarities of the pharmaceutical industry. Since the publication of MS 2424, JAKIM's Halal Hub Division has successfully developed a certification system based on this standard that can be used by not just pharmaceutical companies in Malaysia, but also by recognized halal certifying bodies around the world.

---

50. Dinar Standard, 2020/21 State of the Global Islamic Economy Report, 15.

In 2016–2017, the halal pharmaceutical industry saw several key developments in Malaysia. Among these was the world's first halal license for prescription medicine given out by Malaysia's religious authority, JAKIM, to the Chemical Company of Malaysia (CCM) in 2017. Meanwhile, Indonesia has approved for the mandatory halal certification of its products in 2019,[51] and UAE will require all halal imports to be certified as halal.

CCM was the first to get involved in halal certification for pharmaceutical products, around 2000. This milestone of development marked the start of the transition in the sector, from vitamins and health supplements to over-the-counter medicines such as painkillers, analgesics, eye drops, cough mixtures, ointments, and creams.

Among the challenges halal pharmaceuticals must address is the low level of knowledge and awareness of the general public. Although Malaysia has a large Muslim population, demand is not being driven by knowledge. For the halal pharmaceuticals market to expand, it needs to be seen as an aspect of the religious requirements for Muslims globally, and the public needs to be better informed about halal pharmaceuticals—not only medicines, but also vitamins and health supplements.

Another challenge facing HP is a general shortfall of raw materials for the industry, despite the country's biodiversity, which could be tapped into in order to develop resource-based biogeneric drugs. The local industry has to develop further. Although it is not possible to produce everything, investment should be encouraged in APIs (active pharmaceutical ingredients).

Experts have also identified another major challenge: the limited focus on halal as a proposition. There is a critical life-saving role for halal pharmaceuticals that is not well recognized. This has to do with the growing numbers of people, especially children, not being inoculated against diseases over concerns about ingredients in vaccines, including porcine gelatin and non-halal ingredients. The conventional sector has not addressed this challenge either. It may be noted in this connection that AJ Pharma is working on the world's first non-animal-origin vaccine.

Since about 2010, the number of halal pharmaceutical players, excluding traditional medicines and cosmetics manufacturers, has significantly increased. The Chemical Company of Malaysia (CCM) chairman, Normala binti Abdul Samad, commented that in Islam, non-halal medicines are allowed to be consumed only if there is no other alternative, as one of

---

51. Peraturan Menteri Agama Republik Indonesia No. 26, 2019, "Penyelenggaraan Jaminan Produk Halal."

the main tenets of *maqasid* shariah (higher purposes of shariah) is the preservation of life and health. However, the Muslim population worldwide is becoming better informed and discerning in their choices and are looking for, and often demanding, pharmaceutical products that contain only halal ingredients.[52]

"When we got halal certification in 2013, we were the first, and we now see 20 to 30 companies out of around 70 pharma manufacturers in the country, so the sector has grown quite well," Leonard Ariff, group managing director of CCM Berhad, told Salaam Gateway on 28 November 2016.[53] Ariff estimates the overall pharmaceutical sector to be growing by 10 to 12 percent per year, while CCM's exports are growing at close to 15 percent. Demand is driven at the domestic level by the country's 33 million people, around 60 percent of whom are Muslim, although uptake of halal pharmaceuticals is still low overall.

"What sells the most in the halal segment, at 35 percent of the market, is food and beverage, then ingredients, and pharmaceuticals is at about ten percent. Acceptance is still low at the moment," said Dr. Tabassum Khan, managing director of AJ Pharma Holding and chairman of AJ Biologics, an initiative of the Aljomaih Group of Saudi Arabia, which has facilities in Malaysia.[54]

To generate fresh momentum for HP, Anthony Xavier suggests four actions to push HP into a new growth trajectory: (1) The government and the pharmaceutical industry should carry out a "communication blitz" to educate the public and make the adoption of HPs irresistible. (2) There should be greater investment both locally and abroad. Local pharmaceutical companies should venture into partnerships with foreign companies for large scale manufacturing to meet the huge potential demand. (3) Expanded research and development collaboration between manufacturers and universities will ensure that local ingredients can be expeditiously capitalized for the manufacture of HPs. However, lower costs will make HPs even more accessible. (4) To penetrate and conquer the global HP market, the government should foster global collaboration to develop an internationally recognized certification

---

52. Salama. "Malaysia: World's First Halal Certification."

53. CCM is a publicly listed company on the main market of Bursa Malaysia. Established in 1963, it plays a key role in the development of the pharmaceutical and chemical industries while actively championing and developing halal initiatives in the country.

54. Cochrane, "How Attractive Is Malaysia's Halal Pharmaceutical Sector?"

scheme.[55] That said, the halal industry has grown diverse and is now in need of better coordination for greater efficiency, a subject we turn to next.

## Disparity Issues in the Management of the Halal Industry

One of the issues that calls for attention is that the halal sector in Malaysia is governed by piecemeal legislation and regulatory orders under the care of various bodies carrying different jurisdictional mandates. Trade practices in the halal industries sector are governed by the Ministry of Domestic Trade, and Consumer Affairs, while halal certification matters are managed by the Department of Islamic Development Malaysia (JAKIM). The Halal Development Corporation (HDC), on the other hand, is mandated with the internationalization aspects of Malaysia's halal products and services, and the Department of Standards Malaysia (DOSM) is empowered to issue halal standards. Then there is the issue of different jurisdictions in Malaysia and the challenge of consolidation of the federal and state governments spheres of jurisdiction in halal, which falls within the ambit of Islamic religion and the jurisdiction as such of the state authorities.

A perusal of the halal standards issued by DOSM, and the subsequent ministerial announcements over the future direction of the halal industry, is indicative of the concern for developing uniformity and standardization in the halal industry. Significant efforts are being made by relevant bodies to standardize the substantive guidelines on halal and its organizational aspects, with a view to placing the industry under a single umbrella organization. The DOSM has likewise issued a number of standards that seek to standardize the shariah guidelines on halal for application of the halal industry as a whole. The issuance of the standards was a landmark development in the articulation of the substantive shariah into the operational industry guidelines. Yet a point has been made that they are good for regulatory purposes, and especially for certification of halal, but are too epithetic and concise to provide shariah insight and literacy for industry participants and practitioners, and for the general public. It is further said in this connection that the halal standards currently in force fall short of differentiating between the mandatory, permissible, and optional status of the shariah requirements, and determining whether the requirements are

---

55. For details, see Xavier, "New Halal Frontier Products," 16.

shariah or legal and regulatory in nature. In addition, the mandatory or optional status of operational regulations that enhance the halal management features also need to be identified.

Without formulating credible shariah parameters for general and sector-based applications, there is a risk of the gap between the theory and practice of halal getting wider. Failure to provide the suggested elaborations could also lead to confusion among market operators and participants and the general public.

To minimize the risk of disparity in the governance of halal, and of theoretical and practical gaps developing in the halal industry as a whole, the following may be recommended:

1. To centralize the halal sector within the jurisdiction of the federal government. Notwithstanding the establishment of Malaysia Halal Council in 2016 to standardize the halal management system, there will still be jurisdictional issues between the federal and state governments when the parties involved are non-Muslim. However, any progress in this area will depend on the consent and support of their Royal Highnesses, the Malay Rulers. If they are convinced of the merit of consolidation, whether total or partial, for the overall benefit of the halal industry, they may support it, otherwise the project is not likely to succeed.

2. Uniformity of shariah principles on halal should also be included in organizational uniformity and streamlining. Halal standards need to be synchronized and standardized for the whole of Malaysia. The current state of the halal governance framework, jurisdictions, and piecemeal regulations need to be streamlined. The establishment of the Malaysia Halal Council (MHC) in 2016 should be effectively utilized by all parties, including the federal government and the state governments, regulators, and industry players as an important vehicle of standardization in the halal industry generally. This may again be possible through consultation and prior understanding between the federal and state authorities, especially the Malay Rulers. It is encouraging to note, in this connection, the acknowledgment and emphasis that Sultan Nazrin Muizzudin Shah, the Ruler of Perak, placed on the importance of overall consolidation of the halal industry management when he said in his keynote speech at the World Halal Conference 2018 in Kuala Lumpur that "[t]he regulation and governance of the halal industry is going to be key, especially if it requires strategic collaboration across the whole of the halal ecosystem involving numerous government ministries, agencies and business stakeholders." He stressed the need for collaboration among the industry players

nationally and internationally, if they were to benefit by the opportunities offered by the Fourth Industrial Revolution. The learned speaker then added: "The latest initiative by the Government of Malaysia in setting up the Malaysia Halal Council to coordinate this effort is both timely and welcome. In this country where the final authority on matters referring to Islam rests with Their Royal Highnesses the Malay Rulers, I am pleased that the establishment of this council has the consent and support of the Conference of Rulers."[56]

3. The provisions contained in the Malaysian Standards, Halal Manual, and Halal Assurance System should be segregated and identified as to whether they consist of shariah requirements or of legal and industry operational requirements. Shariah provisions also need to be specified as to which are mandatory and which may be only optional with correspondent labeling and indicators. The path undertaken by Bank Negara Malaysia in issuing parameters governing Islamic banking and *takaful* operations could be taken as a model to follow.

For practical purposes, the following may be suggested with regard to cases where clear segregations between the shariah, regulatory, and operational requirements of halal may be less than clear and categorical: Rules that are clearly derived from the shariah sources should not be difficult to identify, as the source information on these are self-explanatory. Identification in this case should also go a step further to signify whether the rule in question is obligatory, recommended, or permissible/optional. Should there be instances where regulatory and operational measures are mixed with the shariah rules merely to facilitate proper implementation of the latter, they should still fall under the shariah requirements. Should the various elements of the mixed rulings in question prove difficult to identify on a clear and decisive basis, however, but the regulatory/operational aspects are not contrary to any principle or injunction of shariah, they may be classified as shariah-compliant. This is because the shariah itself authorizes the ruling authorities (*uli'l-amr*) to take measures that in their best judgment facilitate good governance and desirable market practices. Then there remain rules and guidelines that are decidedly managerial and extra-shariah, in which case they may be earmarked as such in a way that conveys clear positions to inform the general public and the halal industry operators.

---

56. Shah, "Fostering a True Halal Economy," 13.

## 22

# Fatwa *Issuance in Malaysia*

FATWA ISSUANCE ON matters of permitted and prohibited foodstuffs is entrusted in Malaysia to the state religious authorities, namely the state *fatwa* committee and the national *fatwa* committee. *Fatwa* issuance functions in Malaysia are basically a state matter and are regulated, in turn, under state enactments, usually titled Administration of Islamic Law Enactments, in the various states of Malaysia, which authorize the state mufti and the sultan to issue and ratify *fatwas*. The mufti works, in turn, in close cooperation with the State Islamic Religious Council (Majlis Agama Islam), although the mufti is in principle independent of the Majlis. A *fatwa* duly approved by the state *fatwa* committee and mufti, and then duly assented to by the sultan, only needs to be gazetted to acquire a binding force in its relevant state. These enactments have been in force in the various states of Malaysia for several decades, and *fatwas* were generally for guidance but not binding. The issue took a new turn, however, during the 1990s when legislation on *fatwa* went a step further to make a *fatwa* duly issued and gazetted by the state authorities binding, and it was even declared an offense for "any person who gives, propagates, or disseminates an opinion contrary to any *fatwa* in force." Most of the state enactments also provide that anyone who acts against a *fatwa* will be committing an offense that carries a fine of up to RM3,000, or imprisonment for up to two years, or both.[1]

The National Fatwa Committee (NFC) in Kuala Lumpur operates under the authority of the king (Yang Dipertuan Agong) and the Conference of Rulers. There is no Grand Mufti in Malaysia and the NFC consists of state

---

1. *Syariah Criminal Offences (Federal Territories) Act, 1997 (Art. 12)*. http://www2.esyariah. gov.my/esyariah/mal/portalv1/enakmen2011/Eng_act_lib.nsf/858a0729306dc247482576510 00e16c5/bced11b697691518c82568260002aaa20?OpenDocument. Syariah Criminal Offences Enactment of Johor (S.12) and its equivalent provisions in most other states of Malaysia.

*Shariah and The Halal Industry.* Mohammad Hashim Kamali, Oxford University Press. © Oxford University Press 2021. DOI: 10.1093/oso/9780197538616.003.0023

muftis representing all the fourteen states of Malaysia, inclusive of the Federal Territory of Kuala Lumpur and Labuan. The main functions of the NFC are to standardize the various *fatwas* issued by the state muftis, and respond to issues of national concern as and when they may arise.

The Malaysian public has since the 1970s seen *fatwas* being issued by the NFC on a variety of issues, such as beauty pageants, e-cigarettes, vaping, yoga, shishah smoking, and issues of concern to society, youth, and women, but also on food-related matters. A question thus arose, for instance, over the permissibility or otherwise of consuming bird's nest, and the *fatwa* issued by the 79th Conference of the NFC (September 6–8, 2007), was that "consuming bird's nest is allowed (*harus*) in Islam."[2]

On the use, similarly, of prohibited animals parts or organs other than those of dogs and pigs for cosmetic purposes, the NFC issued the following *fatwa* at its 74th session (July 25–27, 2006): Islam emphasizes cleanliness and safety, hence any cosmetic products containing ingredients or elements that are non-halal or harmful to people, it is totally non-halal.[3]

In response to another query on the status of fish fed with non-halal food, the 76th session of NFC (April 4, 2006) issued the following *fatwa*: fish reared in ponds is non-halal for consumption if it is intentionally kept in unclean water, and fed with pork, carrion, or the like.[4]

A question was also addressed to the NFC on the animal DNA (deoxyribonucleic acid) in genetically modified food (GMF). This DNA, which is transferred to the host, is no longer an original copy, since it has undergone several processes, including the cloning of the gene in the bacteria called *E. coli* and gene transfer from the bacteria to plant mediated by *Agrobacterium tumefaciens* or gene gun. It was added, however, that the resulting protein in the genetically modified plant is identical to original protein in donor organism (swine). The GMF does not, in other words, have any physical substance from the swine, but it has the donor's copy of the genetic information. The NFC held that the method of producing genetically modified plants is not similar to conventional crossbreeding of pig with goat and swine hormone injection into cattle; hence the ruling that these methods cannot be used by analogy (*qiyas*) to provide a ruling for the GMF.

---

2. As quoted in Ibrahim, "Fatwa on Halal Related Issues," 92.

3. Ibrahim, "Fatwa on Halal Related Issues," 92.

4. Ibrahim, "Fatwa on Halal Related Issues," 92.

The NFC decided that the DNA copy that is inserted into the host plant cannot be considered as being transformed through substance transformation (*istihalah*). This *fatwa* was based on the consideration that the copy of the gene in the genetically modified plant still has a relation with the original gene in the swine, and therefore the plant is not permissible.[5] Hence the use of swine DNA in the production of GMF is not shariah-compliant. This *fatwa* is based on the principles that "preventing harm takes precedence over securing benefit," and "when the lawful and unlawful substances are mixed up, the unlawful prevails." The NFC also reviewed some of the advantages of GMF, such as overcoming food shortages due to the increasing world population, as well as to alleviate hunger in the Third World, but held that these problems cannot be used as justification to permit the consumption of GMF that contain swine substance. This is because they believe that the root cause of the problem is unfair distribution of food in society. The issued *fatwa* is also based on the fact that there are many other choices of available halal foods and drinks for Muslims, and when that is the case, they are not in the state of *darurah* (necessity).

Twelve years later (in June 2011), the NFC issued a second *fatwa* on GMF, but in a more general context: it is not permissible to use genes from a halal animal that is not properly slaughtered according to shariah-compliant methods. The production of GMF that may bring harm to human health and unknown long-term risks to the environment is also prohibited. The briefing presented to the NFC explained that halal as well as non-halal genes have been used in the production of GMF. The NFC observed that Islam has put utmost importance on eating of halal and *tayyib* food which do not bring harm to human soul and intellect, and that the processing of the food should not involve a bad impact on human health and the environment. Some of the *fiqh* maxims that were considered in the discussion were "preventing harm takes precedence over securing benefit" and "permitting the benefit and prohibiting the harm." The NFC also gave attention to the issue of using genes from a halal animal that was slaughtered using a method that is not compliant with shariah. They decided that GMF which contains this gene is not halal because conformity to slaughtering methods is a big factor that determines the permissibility for consumption of halal animals. This *fatwa* was issued in response to ethical questions that were being raised by the Muslim community on the impact of the potential risks of GMF on its halal status. It

---

5. Izhar Ariff et al., "Istihalah and Its Effects On Food," 759.

was clearly stated that the Islamic teachings promote preservation of the natural environment. Nevertheless, Muslim scholars do not put much emphasis
on causing no harm to the environment as one of the characteristics of halal
food. Malaysia and Brunei Darussalam have adopted rulings, for instance,
that make no reference to the environmental factor: "Foods and drinks containing products of genetically modified organisms (GMOs) or ingredients
made by the use of genetic material of animals that are non-halal by Shariah
law are not halal" (MS1500-2009, 3.5.1.6 and PBD24-2007, 3.1.6 respectively).
The Indonesian equivalent ruling on this, HAS23201, differs in wording, but
its intent is almost the same: "For microbial materials from recombinant
microbes then . . . the microbes should not use gene[s] derived from pigs or
humans" (4.3e). The only difference here is the addition of human genes as
non-halal.[6]

---

6. Munirah et al. "Study on The Formulation of Fatwa On GMO," 150.

# PART III

# *Regional and International Developments*

## *Introductory Remarks*

Malaysia is not alone in its halal development agenda as other countries in Southeast Asia have also seen milestones of development, including the setting up, for instance, of the Halal Science Center in Thailand, the Halal Authority in Indonesia, and its equivalent in Singapore under the umbrella of MUIS (Majlis Ugama Islam Singapura). Indonesia, India, Pakistan, and Bangladesh will likely be the key growth engines for Asia's halal product demand over the coming decades. These four nations account for about 70 percent of the region's one billion Muslims, according to Pew Research Center data.

## 23

# Halal in Indonesia, New Zealand, and Japan

RISING WAGES AND younger, expanding populations in these countries are among the main drivers of growth. With nearly 88 percent of its 265 million population being Muslim, Indonesia has been advancing its halal agenda in a holistic manner and has passed laws to make halal certification a mandatory requirement. Indonesia's Law No. 33/2014 on halal product assurance in October 2014 required all products to be certified halal starting October 2019. This law also created the Halal Certification Agency (BPJPH—Badan Penyelenggara Jaminan Produk Halal), under the Ministry of Religious Affairs, to oversee the process and provide ongoing certification for products. The Halal Certification Agency also works in close cooperation with the Majelis Ulama Indonesia, especially over *fatwa*-related matters and guidance on Islamic issues. The law requires halal certificates and labels for three sectors—food and beverage, cosmetics, and pharmaceuticals—and in addition stipulates that all equipment and raw materials used during the production process to be acceptable under shariah.[1]

ASEAN generally adopted the Halal Food Guidelines in 1998, and in 1999 it endorsed the ASEAN Halal Logo with the objective of facilitating halal trade in the region. The ASEAN Guidelines on the Preparation and Handling of Halal Food also serve as a practical guide in the production and handling of the same.[2]

---

1. Efendi, "Halal Industry Can Help."

2. Ramli, "Legal and Administrative Regulations," 100.

*Shariah and The Halal Industry.* Mohammad Hashim Kamali, Oxford University Press. © Oxford University Press 2021. DOI: 10.1093/oso/9780197538616.003.0024

Beyond ASEAN, and with reference to halal labeling for Asia generally, the Codex Committee on Food Labelling adopted its Codex, and the
General Guidelines for Use of the Term Halal, at its 22nd session in Ottawa
in 1997. While recognizing the differential positions of the various schools
of Islamic law on the matter, the Codex also provided guidelines and recommended measures on the use of halal logos in food labeling, but it falls short
of developing halal standards, which may well be a future agenda item to be
addressed.[3]

For many years, Malaysia has also been a key partner with New Zealand
companies looking to expand their halal offerings to consumers in Southeast
Asia. New Zealand's Trade and Enterprise Department is working with local
companies in New Zealand to build halal compliance into the business models of those companies, especially the new ones. This means that those companies must ensure that their facilities, supply chain processes, and products
are all halal-compliant even before entering the market.[4] The Federation
of Islamic Associations of New Zealand also works closely with Malaysia's
Department of Islamic Development (JAKIM) to ensure that food products coming from New Zealand to Malaysia, and through it to other countries in the region, are equipped with proper certification of halal status.
To date, "more than 90 percent of New Zealand's beef and lamb products
are compliant with Malaysia's halal standards."[5] Furthermore, the growth
of halal e-commerce in Malaysia and the establishment of the Digital Free
Trade Zone enabled New Zealand companies to go through the e-commerce
route and establish new distribution channels that allow them to reach their
consumers directly.

China is also an emerging halal market with a sizeable Muslim population that is showing increased interest in halal foods and products. Of special interest perhaps is the development of a halal park in Yangling, west of
Xian city along the old silk road, and has entered cooperation agreements to
that effect with the Halal Development Corporation of Malaysia. China is
clearly planning to be a major player in the production and commerce of halal
food to cater for its own Muslim population and also to export it to other
Muslim destinations. Similar developments of interest are noted in Japan. For
example, in preparation for the Rugby World Cup in 2019 and Olympics in

---

3. Ramli, "Legal and Administrative Regulations," 99–100.

4. Hearse, "Seizing the Halal Opportunity in Malaysia," 16.

5. Hearse, "Seizing the Halal Opportunity in Malaysia," 16.

2021, Japanese businesses embraced halal opportunities in recognition of this growing market.[6]

Japan is wooing record numbers of Muslim travelers to visit the country. In 2017 nearly 360,000 Muslims visited Japan, up from 80,000 in 2010. The halal hotels in Japan mark the direction of the *qiblah* in each room. All the meals are Japanese-style cuisine prepared in a certified halal kitchen, and the hotel is alcohol free. In Shinjuku, Japan, MHC Company Ltd., a company run by a Malaysian, is authorized to issue Japan halal standard to Japanese restaurants and food manufacturers. "Our aim is to increase the number of halal restaurants in the Tokyo area for the Olympics," said Lori Numata, an official of MHC. In November 2018, Malaysia and Japan also signed a memorandum of cooperation to step up efforts to penetrate the halal market in both countries. The memorandum was signed by the Malaysian Entrepreneur Development Minister, Mohd Redzuan Mohd Yusof, and the Japanese Economy, Trade and Industry Minister, Hiroshige Seko.

Japan's tourist sector is riding on the boom of the global Muslim travel market, which has seen a massive change since 2010. But Japan has also seen a surge in overall foreign tourist arrivals, which hit a record 31 million in 2018, and was expected to reach 40 million in 2020 for the Tokyo Olympics, before these were postponed due to the Covid-19 pandemic.[7] According to the World Tourism Organization, Asia was the second most visited world market in 2017, next to Europe. The main drivers of this were the prevalence of mobile technology and Internet access across Asia, and the millennial cohort. There are also more female Muslims exploring on their own. By far the biggest Muslim spenders come from Saudi Arabia and the UAE, with travelers from these countries having spent more than $40 billion globally in 2017. Indonesia and Malaysia come third and fourth in expenditures by Muslim travelers. The fast-growing segment of younger Muslims from Southeast Asia visit Japan and south Korea in large numbers.[8]

The Dialrel Project/rules that were introduced and authorized by the European Commission in 2010 address issues regarding religious slaughter (mainly halal and Shechita products) and have also gained wider acceptance and are now practiced by many religious communities in Europe. A summary of the Dialrel Project appears in Appendix IV at the end of this volume.

---

6. Hearse, "Seizing the Halal Opportunity in Malaysia," 16.

7. Hamid, "Japan Making a Mark in Muslim Tourism Market," 13.

8. Hamid, "Japan Making a Mark in Muslim Tourism Market," 13.

# 24

# *Imported Meat*

IMPORTED MEAT OF halal animals, such as beef, mutton, and chicken, from countries that follow Christianity or other monotheistic religions is lawful for consumption by Muslims even if the name of Allah has not been cited, provided they have gone through their own slaughter methods, thus precluding killing by other means. Slaughter that involves electrical shock and stunning in slaughterhouses and production lines is also considered part of their slaughter methods, and therefore halal for Muslims. This is not, however, the case with regard to meats imported from countries that do not practice a monotheistic religion and do not fall under the People of Scripture (Ahl al-Kitab), which is why Muslim countries ascertain that they are duly slaughtered and often import live animals, which are then put through halal slaughter methods after safe arrival in the importing country. Slaughter from the top of the neck is still acceptable, and the meat is halal for consumption according to the majority view of the leading schools, but is considered to be reprehensible (*makruh*) nevertheless.[1] The Shia Imamiyyah are more emphatic on the requirement that slaughter must always be in the correct place on the neck, which is where the vital passages are, especially when there is no situation of necessity to dictate otherwise.[2]

It is not a requirement for Muslims to take an unduly inquisitive approach to that which has not been seen or which might have happened in their absence. Questions such as how this or that animal (whether imported

---

1. al-Qaradawi, *al-Halal wa'l-Haram*, 63; al-Zuhayli, *al-Fiqh al-Islami*, vol. 3, 689. The *ahl al-Kitab* status is extended to Magians and Zoroastrians and the rules of *ahl al-Kitab* also apply to them. This status is not recognized for the associators and idolaters among Arabs such as the pagans of Arabia at the time of the advent of Islam.

2. Cf. al-Tabarsi, *Mustadrak al-Wasa'il*, vol. 16, 133.

*Shariah and The Halal Industry.* Mohammad Hashim Kamali, Oxford University Press. © Oxford University Press 2021.
DOI: 10.1093/oso/9780197538616.003.0025

or of local origin) was slaughtered, were all the ritual slaughter procedures observed, or was the name of Allah mentioned or not are uncalled for, but even if one knows that the slaughter person or butcher was an ignorant person, a sinner, or a Christian or Jew, it is halal to take and consume the meat without such inquisitions. This is the purport of a hadith recorded in al-Bukhari and quoted by al-Qaradawi, in which it is stated that a group of people asked the Prophet about this: "Some people bring to us meat we do not know whether God's name was mentioned on it or not, to which the Prophet replied 'mention God's name yourselves and eat it.'" The conclusion drawn from this and similar other rulings in the sources is that the basic norm and presumption of shariah is that of original validity and acceptance (*al-sihhah wa'l-salamah*), unless there is evidence to suggest that invalidity and corruption have prevailed.[3] Al-Ramlawi's analysis goes into greater details on this issue and may be summarized as follows:

If the majority of the population of the country in which the slaughter took place belong to mixed groups of Muslims and People of the Book, their slaughter is halal for Muslims. However, if the population of the country of origin happens to be about equally divided between those whose slaughter is halal for Muslims and those whose slaughter is non-halal, or who predominantly belong to the latter category, then their slaughter will be deemed as non-halal based on the principles of predominance (*taghlib*) and reasonable caution. Thus, if one comes across a slaughtered goat or bull and has no information on who it was slaughtered by, but knows the country of its origin, then the criterion to apply is the principle of predominance (*taghlib*) that looks at the majority of the population of the country of origin. If the majority are Muslims or People of the Book, and only a minority belong to those whose slaughter is non-halal, the goat or bull is halal for Muslims and the presence of a small minority in that country would be ignored.[4] The Shia Imamiyyah position on this is similar, especially with reference to meat offered in a Muslim market. Thus, it is reported that Imam Ja'far al-Sadiq was asked a question regarding meats bought and sold in a Muslim marketplace, where how it was slaughtered, the identity of the butcher, and so forth are not known to purchasers. The Imam's reply was that "there is no objection to

---

3. Al-Qaradawi, *al-Halal wa'l-Haram*, 64, has recorded the hadith and also the conclusion over the presumption of validity. See also on the presumption of validity, Kamali, *Freedom of Expression in Islam*, 57–61.

4. al-Ramlawi, *al-Halal wa'l-Haram*, 356.

that unless the buyer knows that the slaughter was carried in a way contrary to the Sunnah."[5]

The following *fatwas* have also been quoted on the status of imported meat: (1) The Fatwa Committee (Lajnat al-Fatwa) of al-Azhar University of Egypt issued the following *fatwa*: Food imported from the country of the People of the Book is generally held to be halal even if it is unknown whether it was slaughtered in an Islamic way and whether a name other than that of Allah was mentioned, provided it is not known to be forbidden meat, nor does it come from an animal that was suffocated, hit hard and thrown from a height, etc.[6] (2) The Grand Mufti of Saudi Arabia, 'Abd al-'Aziz bin 'Abd Allah, wrote: The food of the People of the Book is permissible for us unless it is known to us that the animal in question was slaughtered in a non-shariah-compliant way, such as slaughter by electric shock, suffocation, or severe blow. If this is known then it is forbidden to us.[7]

---

5. al-Tabarsi, *Mustadrak al-Wasa'il*, vol. 16, 152.

6. As quoted in al-Ramlawi, *al-Halal wa'l-Haram*, 361–362. The signatories of this *fatwa* included the two leading committee figures, Shaykh 'Abd al-Majid Salim and Shaykh Mahmud Shaltut.

7. As quoted in al-Ramlawi, *al-Halal wa'l-Haram*, 363.

## 25

# *Halal Tourism*

## *Introductory Remarks*

Halal tourism, or halal travel, is designed to cater for the needs primarily of millions of Muslims around the globe performing haj or Umrah, visiting the shrines in Mecca and Medina and those in Najaf and Karbala in Iraq. Halal tourism is also open to non-Muslims. The industry has been making impressive progress in recent years, yet it may still be lagging behind in certain respects, such as depth and diversity, or when compared to mainstream international tourism, and it has yet to realize its full potential. As a major component of the halal industry, halal tourism is developing rapidly, mainly because Muslims today are re-engaging with their traditional values for modern times. From halal food to modest fashion, from pharmaceuticals and cosmetics to shariah-compliant finance, the potential market for the core Islamic economy and service categories is enormous.[1] Driven by a growing demand, halal tourism is one sector that is powering the Islamic economy, and it is set to become a major sector of the wider global economy.

Halal tourism is geared mainly toward practicing Muslims and Muslim families who observe their religious obligations. The hotels in the halal sector do not serve alcohol and have separate swimming pools and spa facilities for men and women. Malaysia, the UAE, Turkey, Indonesia, and many more countries are trying to attract Muslim tourists from all over the world, offering them a range of attractive facilities. Halal tourism also provides flights on which no alcohol or pork products are served, prayer timings are announced, and religious programs are broadcast as part of entertainment offered on board. That said, as of this writing, there exists no internationally recognized

---

1. Maniar, "The Growing Popularity of Halal Tourism."

*Shariah and The Halal Industry.* Mohammad Hashim Kamali, Oxford University Press. © Oxford University Press 2021. DOI: 10.1093/oso/9780197538616.003.0026

standards on halal tourism. The sixteen sets of halal standards issued by the Department of Standards Malaysia (DOSM) provide basic guidelines and principles on halal food, slaughter rules, consumer goods, pharmaceuticals, and *halalan-tayyiban*, but only as of 2016 was a standard on halal tourism added. One of the challenges now facing halal tourism professionals is to create a single global halal certification system that will encourage the expansion of halal tourism as a whole.

In response to a question as to who are the halal tourists, it is said that potentially anyone of Muslim faith, followers of other faiths, and anyone who wishes to observe its regulatory regime could be in this category. In terms of nationality, demand for this type of tourism comes primarily from Indonesia (home to the world's largest Muslim population), Malaysia, Saudi Arabia, and the United Arab Emirates. North African travelers also represent a considerable clientele.[2]

Many international hotels serve halal meat that is slaughtered in accordance with the teachings of Islamic shariah and is free of any substances forbidden by the religion. Some hotels have employed people from parts of the Muslim world to provide translation services and other assistance that may be needed by tourists from other countries.

An article on Halal Business published in the *Economist* in May 2013 noted that "[i]t is not just manufactured halal products. Services such as halal holidays are booming too. Crescent Tours, a London-based online travel specialist, book clients into hotels in Turkey that have separate swimming pools for men and women, no-alcohol policies and halal restaurants, and rents out private holiday villas with high walls." Tripfez, which was featured in *Forbes* magazine, offers Muslim-friendly hotels and advice about halal food options, tour availability, and much more.

Based on a report by Thomson Reuters, in 2014 Muslims from around the globe spent US$142 billion on travel (excluding haj and Umrah). In comparison, travelers from China spent $160 billion on travel in 2014, while US travelers spent $143 billion, placing the Muslim travel sector in third place in global travel spending, and accounting for 11 percent of total global expenditures on travel.[3]

With a consumer base of 1.7 billion predominantly young Muslims around the world, and growing at two times the rate of the global population

2. "Halal Tourism Explained," *The Star*.

3. "Halal Tourism," *Wikipedia*.

growth rate, the influence of the fast-growing and young Muslims is increasingly being felt in the marketplace on industries such as finance, entertainment, travel, and healthcare, and in products as varied as cosmetics, food, and fashion.

According to the International Monetary Fund, the global economy is entering "secular stagnation" due to a decline in investments and an aging population; however, the Islamic economy stands in contrast, offering viable solutions to global economic growth and success stories in the twenty-first century.

The fiftyseven mostly Muslim-majority countries of the world represent more than $7US trillion in gross domestic product and some of the fastest-growing global economies that stretch from Malaysia and Indonesia in the east to Turkey in the west, with the Arabian Gulf states at the center. Their influence stretches beyond Muslim-majority countries, as more than 350 million Muslims reside as minorities in many nations, with the relatively more affluent ones living in the West, and large populations residing in the emerging nations of India, China, and Russia. Global trends indicate a prosperous future for this sector, with fast-developing hotel chains acquiring more properties and a range of services. Abu Dhabi and Dubai are currently building hotels faster than many other cities in the world. According to Dinar Standard, Muslim tourists spent $137 billion (excluding the pilgrims in Saudi Arabia) in 2012, and by 2020 this figure was expected to exceed $180 billion. In Britain alone, Muslim tourists spent 21 billion pounds in 2016, and most were inbound tourists from the Middle East.[4]

## *Shifting Patterns in International Tourism*

Although the halal and *haram* (permissible and prohibited) in food and entertainment are not new, halal awareness as a market phenomenon and its implications for international tourism, trade, fashion, and finance are relatively recent, and much of it seems to have emerged, oddly enough, after the 9/11 attacks, which were by no means meant to encourage Islamic values, let alone halal tourism. The 9/11 attacks marked a decidedly dark patch in Muslim-West relations, with enormously damaging consequences. Many Arab tourist destinations suffered massive declines in the tourism sector, while others benefited from a surge in the number of tourist arrivals and holiday makers due

---

4. "Halal Tourism," *Wikipedia*.

to new visa restrictions and security concerns of travelers to Western destinations. The number of visitors to Arab countries from North America, Europe, and Japan declined, and Arab tourists themselves began to spend their holidays in much larger numbers in the Arab and other Muslim countries. Turkey, Malaysia, Indonesia, Bahrain, UAE, and Egypt benefited from these shifts in tourist flows. Shortly after 9/11, these countries made special efforts and were able eventually to stabilize their tourist industries and achieve significant growth. Some GCC (Gulf Cooperation Council) countries, which were traditionally reluctant participants in international tourism, began to expand their tourism sectors with multibillion dollar investments on new facilities.[5]

Beyond economic stabilization and growth, a cultural drift also became noticeable. The "traditional" cultural tourist destinations, which were popular among European and American visitors, were in most cases losing their appeal to the average Arab tourist. This resulted in a still continuing reorganization of tourist facilities in order to adjust to the demands of a growing flow of young Arab and Muslim tourists. These emerging patterns led, in turn, to increased coordination of tourism policies among Arab states and between Arab and Muslim countries. Tourism ministers from these countries met at regular intervals in a quest to increase tourism between Muslim countries, develop new tourist destinations, and strengthen institutional cooperation among them. The cultural and religious dimensions of this cooperation focused on developing Islamic heritage sites to be visited by Muslim tourists. A fresh focus was also noted on the development of halal tourism that took into consideration shariah rules on halal food, entertainment, and gender-segregated and alcohol-free hotels and restaurants, as well as Islamically financed and organized tourism.[6]

While the Arab world was taking steps to increase Arab tourism, it was noted that concerns over halal food and facilities were even more pronounced in Southeast Asian countries such as Malaysia, Indonesia, and Singapore compared to their Middle Eastern counterparts.

Europe, the United States, Canada, and Australia have large and growing Muslim populations and are therefore seen as major emerging markets for halal products, trade, and tourism. These shifting patterns developed further during the first decade of the twenty-first century, and Islamic tourism grew, not only among Muslim countries and populations, but also in non-Muslim

---

5. Dabrowska, "The Rise of Islamic Tourism," 58.

6. Dabrowska, "The Rise of Islamic Tourism," 60.

countries such as Canada, Taiwan, Hong Kong, and Australia, where Islamic tourism was being developed on a large scale. Jeffri Sulaiman, vice president of the Association of Tour and Travel Agents of Malaysia, stated that tourist facilities and hotel rooms in these countries are expected to be offering prayer rooms and halal food menus to lure larger numbers of Muslim tourists.[7] An Australian tourist expert from Brisbane, Daniel Lynn, also observed that "tourism operators will increasingly need to adjust their menus and provide another bid to meet new market needs."[8]

Muslim dietary rules have also assumed new significance due to the effort many Muslims are making to demonstrate how such rules conform to the findings of scientific research on healthy food and dietary practices. Malaysian researchers have shown, for example, that the halal certification procedures ascertain a number of requirements that include attractiveness, quality, cleanliness, market demand, supporting SME producers and Muslim companies, and clean operations in halal food chains and storage facilities.[9] But the halal industry grew even more exponentially as a result of the quest for alternatives to what is seen to be modeled on Western values and lifestyles. Halal among the migrant groups has also served as a focal point of Islamic identity and culture. In the modern food industry, a number of Islamic requirements are being taken into consideration, including avoidance of substances that may be contaminated with porcine residues or alcohol, non-halal gelatin, emulsifiers, enzymes, and flavorings.

## *Values, Places, and Facilities*

For most Muslims, Islam is not only a religion but also a way of life; it is hard or even unthinkable for some to give up their Islamic path for the sake of relaxation. Even though Muslims want to experience different cultures and environments when on holiday, there are circumstances that differ with their values and faith-based traditions.

Not all Muslims are the same though. They differ in the way they practice their religion and there are gradations in how strict they may be with it. Some do not care if others beside them consume alcohol, or if their hotel has no prayer room, or even if the menus contain non-halal food, as long as they still

---

7. "Jeffri Sulaiman Interview."

8. "Jeffri Sulaiman Interview."

9. Nooh et al., "Halal Certification."

have a range of halal food choices. However, even a moderate Muslim with a family will most likely prefer to go somewhere that includes "halal tourism" aspects.[10]

The rapid growth of the halal tourism industry not only results in the appearance of "Muslim-friendly" or halal-friendly hotels, but also of specialized travel agencies as well as DMCs (destination management companies) that offer halal holiday packages. Another phenomenon is the emergence of specialized booking aggregators, the largest of these being HalalBooking.com, which offers specialized search and booking services for online consumers looking to book their halal trip or halal vacation package via a reliable source in multiple languages and with the widest portfolio of properties. Furthermore, a number of consultancy firms have appeared that help companies to adapt to Muslim holidays or halal holidays.

Apart from Britain and France, which traditionally have relations with Muslim countries, one of the rising destinations for halal tourism is Spain. The number of Saudis visiting Spain in 2013 was, for instance, 85 percent higher than in 2012. The number of Algerian tourists increased by 30 percent, Turkish by 57 percent, and Indonesians tripled in 2015–2016. Another important fact recorded by the Spaniards and with variations happening elsewhere, is that Muslim travelers belong to what is called "premium tourism." While in Spain, the average sums spent by a tourist amounted to 980 euros, for the average Saudi this number was 2,287 euros, for the Egyptian 1,703 euros, for Turks 1,501 euros, and for Algerians 1,340 euros. These development patters ensured, in turn, that menus in Spanish restaurants would soon include halal meat and dish varieties to suit the needs of their Muslims patrons.

## Halal Tourism or Islamic Tourism?

According to the UNWTO definition, "Tourism comprises the activities of persons travelling to and staying in places outside their usual environment for duration of not more than one year for leisure, business and other purposes." According to another definition, tourism is "the temporary movement of people to destinations outside their normal places of work and residence, the activities undertaken during their stay in those destinations, and the facilities created to cater to their needs." Tourism thus includes the movement of

---

10. Battour, Ismail, and Battor, "Impact of Destination Attributes," 537–8.

people, either Muslim or non-Muslim, to other destinations outside their home localities. Some researchers have tried to draw a distinction between Islamic tourism and halal tourism, which are often treated as synonymous. For example, Jafari and Scott define Islamic tourism as "[t]he encouragement of tourists likely to meet the requirements of Sharia law." The definition focuses on shariah law and its requirements to meet the tourists' needs but ignores the religion of tourists (i.e., being a Muslim).[11]

When Muslims travel to another destination for leisure for less than one year, this travel is considered tourism. The question that is often asked is whether the activity is to be referred to as halal tourism or Islamic tourism. In response, it may be said that travel to other destinations can be regarded as halal tourism if all the activities, facilities, actions, and objectives therein are permissible according to Islamic teachings. The same applies in the case of non-Muslim tourists. So a non-Muslim tourist can claim to be engaging in halal tourism if he or she consumes halal food and attends halal entertainment outlets, as long as the activities included in the itinerary are permissible in Islam. However, to describe the traveling activities as being "Islamic tourism" requires another important element: whether the activity is accompanied by *niyyah*, or intention, on the part of the traveler.

If the intention of traveling is to seek the pleasure of God or to strengthen one's faith, then it will be both halal and Islamic. Therefore, the term "Islamic tourism" is more appropriate. However, the place may not necessarily be located in a Muslim country or in a religious location. For example, if a man travels to London to visit the British Museum in order to study the history of British colonization of the Muslim world with the intention to earn God's pleasure, the travel can be classified as *Ibadah* (a religious act) deserving spiritual reward, and can therefore be appropriately referred to as Islamic tourism.

However, if the intention is not in accordance with Islamic teachings, then the travel is not necessarily Islamic. For example, even if a man travels to the holy city of Mecca or Medina during the haj season, but with the evil intention to steal things from *haj* or Umrah travelers, then the action cannot be classified as either Islamic or halal. Thus, the element of *niyyah* needs to be taken into account if one is to draw the distinction, but drawing such a distinction is not a requirement, yet "halal tourism" would seem to preferable.[12]

11. Cited in Battour, "Muslim Travel Behavior in Halal Tourism."

12. Battour, "Muslim Travel Behavior in Halal Tourism."

## Halal Tourism in Malaysia, Turkey, and Indonesia

A little patch of grass sits between international banks and flashy skyscrapers in downtown Kuala Lumpur. There is a big statue of a water jug, and some gold and red *ramadas* (gazebos) meant to recall traditional Moroccan architecture. On the edge of the park are kebab stands and a small mall. The gate at the entrance reads *Ain Arabia*. When it was built in 2005, the "Eye of Arabia" was a small gesture to Middle Eastern and Muslim travelers—that whatever other those from other countries might think of Muslims, they were welcome in Kuala Lumpur.

Twelve years later, that message seems to have paid off. Though it is only about 60 percent Muslim, Malaysia now ranks first on the global list of Muslim-friendly tourist destinations. Malaysia has made special efforts to welcome Muslim travelers by making halal food and prayer rooms readily available and clearly marked. The government's dedicated Islamic Tourism Centre says that from 2015 to 2017 the country of 33 million now receives about 5 million Muslim tourists a year and still rising.[13]

"After 9/11, it became difficult for many Muslims, especially from the Middle East, to travel to many traditional tourist destinations like Europe and the USA," says Fazal Bahardeen, founder of Crescent Rating, the travel company behind the ranking. "Malaysia was one of the first countries to realise the potential of this market."[14]

A common misconception maintains that "Muslim tourism" means people going to do Muslim things. But in reality, they go to do more or less the same things as others—they may want a shopping experience, or a beach experience, or a local cultural experience. They want to see people and places like anyone else, but they just want to know they do not have to worry about their basic faith-based needs, especially food and beverage.

The influx of Muslim tourists has transformed parts of Kuala Lumpur. Ain Arabia now looks almost humble compared to the much larger and more lucrative businesses catering to Muslim tourists. The main strip on Bukit Bintang street in central Kuala Lumpur offers almost entirely Arab and Middle Eastern food, and there are designer fashion boutiques, luxury hotels, and the Pavilion Mall, where families from Saudi Arabia, the United Arab Emirates, and many other countries spend hours shopping.

---

13. Hirschmann, "Total Muslim tourist arrivals to Malaysia."

14. Bevins, "Halal Tourism."

"Out of 57, we (Malaysia) are the only member of the Organisation of Islamic Cooperation with a special Islamic tourism department," said Zulkifly Md Said, director of the country's Islamic Tourism Centre. "We created it in 2009 when we shut down our Commonwealth Tourism Centre."[15] He argues that Malaysia's multiculturalism—the two largest non-Malay groups being the ethnic Chinese and Indian minorities—has accustomed them to being flexible with varying religious interpretations. "It's not so complicated. Our Muslim visitors want something that is comfortable, but at the same time something that is a little different."

The government tries to help by providing advice to local businesses on specific Muslim concerns, such as clearly indicating exactly when daylight begins and ends during Ramadan. He jokes that during the period of fasting, Malaysia can be a nice break—as summer days are shorter than in many Arab countries.

By 2020 more than 160 million Muslim tourists were expected to travel globally and spend more than US$200 billion. Following Malaysia and the UAE, Turkey is among the top three most popular destinations for Muslim travelers around the world. Turkey offers an excellent range of accommodations in its Mediterranean and Aegean resorts, as well as in its historic cities. It also offers a wide selection of halal-friendly beach resorts with separate swimming and sunbathing areas for men and women. Turkey has the largest number of halal-friendly thermal resorts, providing natural health benefits from hot, thermal springs.[16]

According to the Turkish Standards Institution a "halal hotel" must comply with certain standards, including female-friendly swimming and spa areas, no-alcohol bars, proper prayer facilities installed with prayer mats and the direction of prayer indicated, the provision of halal cosmetic and sanitation products in the bathrooms, and the serving of halal food. The hotels that implement these requirements, among others, have the ability to obtain the halal hotel certificate.

The *State of the Global Islamic Economy Report 2016/17* released by Thomson Reuters and Dinar Standard shows that Turkey ranks third among the countries with the best developed ecosystem for halal travel. "Turkey rises four places in this year's ranking, from 7th to 3rd place. While its level of inbound Muslim travel has declined slightly, it has greatly improved its halal

15. Bevins, "Halal Tourism."

16. Halal-friendly holidays worldwide." HalalBooking. https://en.halalbooking.com/halal-holidays (accessed January 5, 2017).

friendly ecosystem scores, while also slightly improving its awareness scores, capitalising on its reputation as a halal friendly destination between East and West," the report stated.

Turkey's natural and historic attractions have long been a magnet drawing tourists from around the world, and in recent years, varied tourism options have attracted tourists from Muslim and Arabic-speaking countries.

Halal cruises are also an offering for Muslim travelers. In the summer, Turkish tourism agencies run ships along the Danube and Rhine Rivers, catering exclusively to Muslims. Everything on board complies with Islamic values: halal food products, separate spas for men and women, female-friendly swimming pools and sports centers, spacious prayer facilities, and separate traditional Turkish *hamams*, or saunas.[17]

Indonesia is a bigger country and also culturally more varied, but Malaysia's comparative wealth has made it more of a draw for well-heeled Arab tourists. While Muslims are a minority of the total number of visitors to Malaysia, they tend to spend more, says Zulkifly Md Said, director of the country's Islamic Tourism Centre.

Yet Indonesia has its own charm, as well as a remarkable depth and diversity that make the country a veritable cultural kaleidoscope, with well-developed resorts that attract tourists from the region and beyond. As the world's largest Muslim country, Indonesia has pinned its hopes on the halal market to expand its US$13 billion tourism industry, which used to lag behind those of its neighbors like Thailand and Singapore. Lombok in West Nusa Tenggara Province is one of three government-designated "priority" halal destinations, along with West Sumatra and Aceh. Jakarta's deputy governor Santiago Uno expressed interest in developing a "sharia tourism zone" in the nation's capital, and then announced that the city would build "sharia-based" hotels. About 2.7 million tourists visited halal destinations in Indonesia in 2016, according to a Tourism Ministry spokesperson, out of about 12 million foreign tourists in total.[18]

A soft launch of halal tourism took place in 2012, which was followed by the introduction of ministerial regulations on shariah hotels in 2014. This included providing guests with halal food, copies of the Qur'an, marking the direction of Mecca in every room, offering access to a halal kitchen, restricting

17. *Daily Sabah*, "Ranking 3rd in Halal Tourism."

18. Varagur, "Indonesia Aims To Attract More Muslim Visitors."

alcohol consumption, and generally developing "halal friendly tourism" in the country.

The government of Indonesia reported that the size of halal tourism in 2018 had reached 3.5 million and there were plans for it to reach 5 million tourists by 2019. As Tourism Minister Arief Yahya explained, "I would like to increase visits for halal tourism to 5 million by 2019." Already, quite early into the implementation of Indonesia's halal tourism strategy, results are becoming apparent. The years 2016 and 2017 saw a 14.7 percent annual increase in Muslim visitors.[19] No further update is given.

International recognition for Indonesia's development of its halal sector is also growing. Sofyan Hotel Betawi (located in Jakarta) won the Best Halal Hotel award during the 2015 World Halal Travel Summit in Abu Dhabi. With only fourteen award categories in total, Indonesia collected three of them. Lombok (one of the twelve nominated Muslim-friendly provinces) was rated Best Halal Tourism Destination and Best Halal Honeymoon Destination.[20] And then, in early December 2016, Indonesia was named the best halal tourism destination in the world for the second year at the World Halal Travel Awards. The country's success at the awards ceremony, which was held in Abu Dhabi, UAE, did not end there, however. Indonesian destinations and companies dominated the awards, winning 12 of 16 total categories, including best airline for halal travelers, best halal beach resort, and best halal honeymoon destination, among others. Hotels, tour operators, airports, and other industry players from the islands of Lombok and Bali, and the Sumateran region of Aceh, performed particularly well, with the majority of Indonesia's awards going to these three regions.[21]

On a different note, however, the halal industry has been negatively impacted by the widening sweep of Islamophobia in recent years, a subject we turn to next.

### Halal Phobia and Halal Reputation Risk

Notwithstanding its impressive pace of development and expansion, the halal industry must also address some significant challenges if this encouraging trend is to continue. One must acknowledge first that halal continues

---

19. Yahya, "Indonesia aims to be top 'halal' destination," *The Jakarta Post*, March 14, 2019.

20. "Halal Tourism in Indonesia," World Folio.

21. Oxford Business Group, "Indonesia Eyes Up Further Growth."

to face some opposition in non-Muslim-majority countries. While many non-Muslims are choosing halal products for their business and personal needs, recent years have also witnessed a rise in what has also been called "halal phobia"[22] in certain countries. In December 2017, for instance, a French supermarket supplying halal products was ordered to close for not selling pork and alcohol. This kind of excessive reaction could well hamper prospective globalization of the halal industry.

In Australia, the 2018 Australian elections also saw the growth of the anti-halal movement led by right-wing parties and various groups opposing halal and halal certification, such as the world "boycott halal" campaign.[23] Those against halal certification argued that such a move imposes costs that are passed on to consumers. Some also alleged that companies selling halal-certified products may channel the proceeds to terrorist organizations. The boycotting of halal-certified food is a move against the perceived encroachment of Islam into the public space of those in this movement.

Singapore is a multiracial and multireligious society and generally tolerant of differences, and the halal food industry has been flourishing there. But the Subway incident in March 2018 created discomfort among some customers. The news of the Subway management decision in Singapore to stop serving pork in its effort to obtain halal certification for all of its outlets in Singapore generated some negative feedback on Subway Singapore's Facebook page. In Singapore, views against halal certification of food outlets and products have largely fallen into two categories. The first of these is spearheaded by those who argue that they would not be able to enjoy non-halal ingredients with the initiation of halal certification. The second is projected by those who have made insensitive statements about Islam. All in all, it appears that the prominence of halal products in today's markets accentuated Islamophobic statements and calls for the boycott of halal-certified products. In the case of Singapore, the trend in going halal in the retail sector is largely a market phenomenon. Companies that go for halal certification do so for their own commercial reasons and as a response to market demand, which in turn widens their reach and market share and ultimately increased profitability. The impetus, it is said, is market driven, not a religiously motivated drive by

---

22. A brief description of halal phobia appears in footnote 1 in the Introduction of the present volume.

23. See Anwar, "Halal Is the Way to Go."

any specific community.[24] The March incident notwithstanding, Subway Singapore went ahead and registered as halal certified in August 2018. The announcement issued to this effect mentioned that the famous pork and bacon sandwiches would be removed from Subway offerings throughout Singapore.

Halal reputation is closely related to halal certification and the performance record of a corporate entity, and plays an exceedingly important role. "Halal reputation" has been defined as a collective representation of a company's past actions and halal performance, as well as that company's future ability to meet halal requirements. The drivers of a company's halal reputation are halal authenticity, the trustworthiness of a halal certification, messages delivered by companies and supply chain partners, and messages by external stakeholders.[25] The Reputation Institute (RI) of ASEAN reported in November 2018 that nearly 84 percent of a company's value is now based on reputational factors. RI estimated that a one-point increase in a company's reputation yields a 2.6 percent increase in its market capitalization. Muslim countries are introducing new halal regulations and existing halal certification bodies are continuously upgrading their halal standards. Evidence supports that halal is going through an evolution from a product approach toward a halal supply chain approach (where, similar to food safety, halal is addressed throughout a supply chain) and halal value chain approach (addressing aspects such as Islamic branding, finance, and insurance).[26] Based on the drivers of halal reputation, companies need to track their halal reputation performance and make this a key performance indicator of their business.

Companies need to beware of halal issues. A halal issue for a corporate entity is a gap between the stakeholders' expected and perceived halal practices of a brand owner. A halal issue can be related to contamination, noncompliance, or perception. Muslim markets today are supplied by global supply networks of multinationals, originating from different production locations with a different halal context. The halal context of a country is linked to the Islamic school of thought it may be following, religious rulings or *fatwas*, and local customs, which are manifested in different halal standards. Although these global supply networks might be efficient, there are also risks in combining different brands from a halal reputation point of view. When one brand is

---

24. Anwar, "Halal Is the Way to Go."

25. For details, see Tieman, "Halal Reputation Management," 118.

26. Tieman, "Safeguarding Halal Reputation," 14.

faced with a halal issue, it easily spreads to other brands of that company and other geographical markets.[27]

Halal scandals involving individual firms may cast an entire industry into disrepute, just as positive publicity may enhance the industry's halal reputation. Therefore, collective halal reputation management, including all activities undertaken by members of a collective to address and alter issues about reputation of that collective, are important in reputation management strategies.[28]

27. Ibid.

28. Cf. Winn, MacDonald, and Zietsma, "Managing Industry Reputation," 35f.

# 26

## Conclusion and Recommendations

THIS CONCLUSION IS presented in three sections, beginning with a roundup of the challenges facing the halal industry generally and what could be done to address them. The second section is on promoting standardization and shariah-based solutions for outstanding issues, whereas the last section makes recommendations on environmental issues relating to meat eating.

### Challenges Facing the Halal Industry

Somewhat like the Islamic banking and finance (IBF) sector some decades earlier, the halal industry started with modest beginnings but then rapidly expanded from the food and beverage sector to pharmaceuticals, cosmetics, halal tourism, halal medicine, halal vaccine, and the like, and it is on an expansive trajectory. The future is likely to be a continuation of the same pattern to see greater expansion and depth, not only within each of these sectors, but also into new areas, products, and services. Once again, like the IBF sector, rapid market-driven developments bring greater and even unexpected challenges, and success in meeting them will depend to a large extent on greater synchrony between religion and science, market know-how, and better cooperation among the major players and resource providers. How shariah scholars and scientists can effectively liaise between themselves and synchronize their endeavors is one of the challenges, and the other concerns the extent to which shariah scholars are able to reduce and minimize scholastic differences that come in the way of standardization. Market know-how and cultural

*Shariah and The Halal Industry.* Moḥammad Hashim Kamali, Oxford University Press. © Oxford University Press 2021.
DOI: 10.1093/oso/9780197538616.003.0027

differentials would also need to be factored into the works of shariah scholars and food science specialists.

Relating to the market know-how and prospects of successful penetration, questions to address could include such issues as finding the best market strategies to address the halal phobia phenomenon discussed in the preceding chapter. The culture-cum-religious resistance that certain sectors of society in Western countries such as France, the United States, and even Singapore have voiced, rightly or wrongly, against halal as another manifestation of radical Islam would also need to be taken into account and addressed through revised marketing strategies. Another question one might raise is whether halal market specialists can create a halal brand of their own, like McDonald's or KFC, or enter into a successful and mutually beneficial liaison with them. An extension of this example may also be relevant, in due course perhaps, to pharmacies and drug stores. One can surmise that scientific innovation in the halal medicine and pharmaceutical sectors has some way to go before one can speak of parity and attainment of a credible market presence to match their conventional counterparts.

One may voice a degree of apprehension over market-driven developments setting the pace rather than industry leaders and planners designing and strategizing market developments before they actually occur. This reminds one of the IBF precedent of overreliance on conventional products to the extent that it became difficult to reverse that pattern, even to this day. In the halal sector, too, halal phobia is already a challenge to be addressed. Market specialists, shariah experts, and industry pundits may take this into consideration and find ways to avoid repeating the IBF weaknesses. Attracting investments and developing new products should not done be at the expense of eroding the credibility of important concepts, or of well-planned and balanced developments that are formulated through a blend of influences and inputs from shariah and science specialists as well as market strategists and others.

A new factor that may be the most challenging to address for all parties concerned, but perhaps more so for shariah scholars, is the environmental factor in the future development of the halal industry. This factor has not effectively entered the halal agenda and has for the most part been untouched. The main challenge is one of finding ways to discourage a heavy reliance on animal slaughter—the lifeline, one might say, of the halal industry, yet at the same time the most crucial for environmental care. It is also in this area where meaningful cooperation among industry experts, shariah scholars, and market specialists would be mostly needed. Our examination earlier of the shariah scriptural sources and sociocultural factors showed that heavy reliance on animal slaughter is entrenched enough to make it difficult to turn the tide and impress Muslim populations to open their eyes to new avenues of innovative *ijtihad*, ones that are undoubtedly most challenging yet also meaningful, inherently meritorious, and humane. The issues are not entirely religious, as environmental protection requires input and action-oriented planning from other disciplines, yet the Islamic religious positions would seem to be fraught with difficult perceptions and receptivity issues, due partly to the fact that animal slaughter is a requirement of the Muslim annual occasion of Eid al-Adha (festival of sacrifice), just as it is also a complementary component of the haj rituals. Two to three million Muslim go to haj annually, and that also translates into the massive scale of animal slaughter on that occasion. Yet there is evidence in the sources that circumstantial developments and exceptional conditions in the lives of Muslims play a role in the giving of charity to advance welfare objectives. There may be possibilities, as mentioned in the previous chapter of this volume, to explore through a fresh interpretation of the scriptural sources and encourage giving charity as a substitute for animal slaughter. Would it not make good sense to convert animal slaughter to its monetary equivalent to be allocated to urgent disaster relief, for instance, of Indonesian earthquake and tsunami victims in Palu, Indonesia, in September 2018, or help for the vast numbers of starving and desperately malnourished victims of the Yemen conflict, or the many desperate refugees of so many ongoing conflicts in Muslim countries. Yet these possibilities and the needed adjustments in *fiqh* positions have remained virtually untouched. The environmental factor is now threatening human survival, especially in underdeveloped countries and communities—the majority of whom happen to be Muslims—and of the other inhabitants of planet earth such that taking urgent preventive strategies now poses a level of unprecedented urgency. The second caliph 'Umar b. al-Khattab's well-known precedent comes to mind, when he asked the people, during the year of the draught in Medina (*'aam al-maja 'ah*), to confine meat consumption to certain days of the week only. This precedent also finds support in the Sunnah of the Prophet, and in the Qur'an itself. Muslim scholars are now called upon to establish a fresh focus not only for individual *ijtihad* over these issues, but also ones that pave the way for collective *ijtihad* (*ijtihad jama'i*) and consensus-based positions to make the desired impact.

## Standardization and Other Shariah Issues

Since the world Muslim community (*ummah*) is a unity in faith, its numerous component parts must remain open to learning from one another and appreciate their respective mores and cultural diversities within the wider crucible of Islamic civilization. Halal food, halal finance, and halal tourism are among the tangible manifestations of the shared values that give the *ummah* its distinctive characteristics. Standardization in the halal industry and its value-based positions is not only desirable but also eminently feasible and resonates well with the higher purposes of Islam and its *maqasid*.

The purpose of standardization would naturally be better served if one aims at the common denominators of values, cultures, and customs that can appeal to greater uniformity in trading practices as well as halal food and finance among Muslim countries and communities across the globe. It is also pragmatic and driven in the meantime by the dynamics of realizing greater commercial gain. Yet there are challenges to be identified and overcome. The larger objectives need to be met by smaller steps along the way. The question may often be what steps these might be and whether they can be taken together, or individually, by the great number of countries and communities that constitute the global *ummah*.

To promote uniformity in halal standards, the following may be proposed:

1. With regard to the halal/*mubah*, and also the *makruh* and the *mandub*, greater uniformity and standardization in the halal industry may be attempted by recourse to the principle of selection (*takhayyur*), which was earlier reviewed in some detail, and by singling out among the various rulings of the leading *madhabs* the ones that may be most suitable for that purpose. As an accepted method of Islamic jurisprudence, *takhayyur* is premised on the recognition that the leading schools of Islamic law have accepted one another as equally valid interpretations of the shariah, which evidently offers potential for greater harmony and unification among them in the pursuit of beneficial purposes. There is a need for better understanding of the shariah with a view of narrowing down the differences among its prevailing interpretations.

2. Another method of selection that may be of use for purposes of standardization is the *fiqh* method of piecing together (*talfiq*), as also reviewed earlier, of certain aspects of the rulings of different schools or jurists with a view to amalgamating them into unified formulas.

*Talfiq* differs from *takhayyur* in that the latter selects the ruling of a different *madhhab* from that of one's own, whereas *talfiq* attempts to combine certain parts of different rulings and interpretations of different *madhhabs*, or indeed of interpretations by individual scholars outside the scholastic framework, into a single formula for the purpose of standardization.[1]

3. Another idea is to set up in every Muslim-majority country and jurisdiction an authoritative halal council (to be followed by the country name—such as Egypt, Pakistan, etc.) that should ideally bring together a group of learned figures of standing from different disciplines, which may include shariah scholars, science experts, community leaders, and market specialists. This should be a representative body and sufficiently diversified that its deliberations, advice, and *fatwas* are informed by the scholastic thought and input of the various schools of Islamic law, as well as the prevailing customs and cultures of countries and cultural zones of the wider *ummah* in the twenty-first century. The proposed council should also include representation from their respective country's Muslim minority in the West, as well as outstanding industry experts and market analysts.

4. A set of procedural guidelines should be formulated to regulate the decision-making process or *fatwa* issuance by the proposed council. Plans should also be drawn up as to how the council decisions could achieve high-level media impact and market penetration in its own jurisdiction but also more widely in other parts of the world.

5. Proactive measures should be taken for standardization of halal practices by governments and industry participants at both the macro and micro levels. One is reminded, in this connection, of an aspect of Islamic jurisprudence that authorizes the ruling authorities (*uli 'l-amr*) to raise what may be a recommended course of action (*mandub*) into an obligatory command (*al-amr*), or a *makruh* into a prohibition (*al-nahy*). The ruling authority may also regulate certain aspects of *mubah* to be adopted into practical requirements in order to secure a valid benefit, just as they may also issue rulings on doubtful matters (*al-mashbuhat*) and provide the needed clarification—if such would be to the manifest benefit and *maslahah* of the people and promote uniformity and standardization in the halal industry. The lawful authorities are thus empowered to introduce

---

1. For details on *takhayyur* and *talfiq*, see also Kamali, "*Shari'ah* and Civil Law."

laws and formulate policies that secure people's best interests in the light of prevailing circumstances. This function may, under the present conditions that obtain in most Muslim countries, be exercised by the elected legislature or a body of experts that works under its supervision. Traditional jurisprudence would subsume most of these under the principle of *siyasah shar'iyah*, which still remains valid—all that is suggested is that parliamentary legislation could now be used as a vehicle of *siyasah* for greater clarity and organization.

6. The above-mentioned halal council should propose ideas and formulas for the needed changes and reforms, as well as suggest practical policies and procedures that promote standardization in the halal industry. These proposals would then be adopted, adjusted if need be, and ratified by the legislative assemblies of the component countries, or by executive order, if need be, to become standard positions. The details of the procedural modalities and how the proposed halal council liaises with the legislative bodies and governments may be proposed by the council itself.

7. Halal is an Islamic value and principle, which might mean that Muslim-majority countries should take the lead in the R&D aspects of the halal industry. Hence it is further proposed that a number of leading Muslim countries with greater halal know-how and experience, such as Malaysia, Indonesia, Turkey, and UAE, should take the lead to create research institutes that bring together researchers in shariah, food sciences, market specialists, and social scientists to look into the prevailing cultural dynamics and customs of the various countries and regions of the Islamic world. One such institute may also be created at the OIC (Organisation of Islamic Cooperation) headquarters. The institute should act as the research arm of the country-based halal councils, and make decisions or recommend action plans to the council over advancing greater levels of standardization of halal internally and with other Muslim countries.

8. Since people's likes and dislikes in food choices and marketing practices are influenced by a variety of factors, including climate, soil characteristics, and even geographical proximity to other cultures, all of this may need to be taken into consideration in the quest for promoting standardization in the halal industry. Cultural proclivities and variations may need to be verified and their shariah-compliance duly scrutinized through research. Hence there is a need to enrich the proposed shariah and scientific research efforts by adequate input into the customary practices of countries and regions. These efforts should be a part of the proposed research institutes.

9. Market researchers have consistently reported ambiguity and malpractice in the issuance and identification of halal logos and their certifying authorities. This may be more extensive even in non-Muslim-majority countries, but the problem is widespread even in Muslim-majority countries. In both cases the use of ambiguous and misleading words, phrases, and signs has become problematic. As mentioned earlier, Malaysian authorities were prompted into action by introducing, as of January 2013, stiff fines for violations, and the amounts of fines also increased for repeated offenders. This is a good approach, but a totally punitive approach may not be the best option. Punitive measures should perhaps be supplemented by educational efforts and incentives for recognition that may envisage conferment of best performance awards to individuals, suppliers, producers, and monitoring agencies of halal products and services.

10. Past experience has also shown that companies and industries that did not adapt to new technology, or upgrade their training efforts on how best to implement such technology, can struggle and even fail. Rapid and unprecedented technological advances are currently transforming economies, jobs, and even culture and civilization. Many of the changes brought by the Fourth Industrial Revolution will be inevitable to negotiate and adopt, however selectively, in order to keep pace with market developments. The halal industry must therefore adapt to new technologies to discover the benefits they offer. The possible rewards of Industry 4.0 can mean enhanced safety and security, the global spread of the halal sector, and greatly increased human capacity building. All this need to be with the full awareness of substantial risks and disruptive ripple effects that such developments can also involve.[2]

11. There is a certain disconnect between the halal industry and Islamic finance. This has been highlighted many times by commentators and industry professionals, yet few have reported on effective steps that have been taken to address it. Halal finance is a natural extension of halal food and lifestyle, as they all subscribe to halal principles. It is therefore proposed that a joint working committee representing both sides should be set up, in each country perhaps, to prepare working plans and an agenda on how the disconnect can be effectively addressed in ways that would add value and actualize profitable cooperation for both sides.

---

2. For details, see Shah, "Fostering a True Halal Economy," 13.

12. International developments of interest concerning halal should aim at strengthening trade expansion and liaison among Muslim countries as a matter of priority, as there are greater commonalities of interest in halal products and services among Muslim countries. Muslim countries may also consider opening regional halal parks, if they have not already done so, as a way of pooling their resources, and also develop levels of specialization in the various components of halal products and services.

13. International cooperation among Muslim countries at regional and international levels should address ways to address and curb halal phobia. As already mentioned, there is a fine line between informative and customer-sensitive labeling and marketization strategies and those that may be considered crude and excessive that can generate negative perceptions and customer resistance.

14. Public awareness of halal, including its theoretical underpinnings and practical manifestations, is on the whole low and superficial even among the Muslim populations. This can only be overcome through concerted public awareness programs over medium and long terms, and careful planning to that effect. If halal products and services are to penetrate new markets in both the Muslim-majority and non-Muslim-majority countries, it will require collective efforts and resources of more than one country to achieve it.

15. Wider penetration of halal products and services into new markets also depends on customer-friendly information and labeling of products and services. Halal products should not only have clear and reliable halal logos but also improved levels of essential information on purity, health and safety aspects of products, and shariah-compliance aspects, for the benefit of discerning customers.

16. New areas of cooperation in which greater investment and scientific know-how may be needed, such as development of halal vaccines, may call for wider scientific cooperation. Projects of this kind with a clear focus and potential should be given priority for international cooperation among Muslim countries. Investment in scientific R&D is generally at a low level among Muslim countries and should be a priority area of greater cooperation.

17. Halal products and services should be made cost-effective and be competitively priced. If they happen to be marginally more expensive compared to their other available counterparts, this should be addressed, minimized, and removed. More effective pooling of resources and

specialization levels across the national boundaries may help to make the prices attractively competitive.

18. There is a shortage of raw materials, livestock, and other items such that existing supplies are not enough to cater to expanding demand levels for halal products worldwide. This would also be a fit subject for regional and international cooperation among Muslim countries. Countries with greater productive potentials in animal husbandry and agricultural produce, such as Sudan, Egypt and Turkey, could play a greater role.

19. "Shariah" and "shariah law" are often used in the relevant halal industry literature and guidelines as if these are self-explanatory and clearly known. This is often not the case, especially in regard to subjects and issues on which the various schools of Islamic law have recorded differences of opinion and interpretation. To develop uniformity and standardization, Muslim countries should identify issues based on their individual needs and characteristics, and develop common research agenda on how to address them together with other counterparts, and also, wherever possible, to unify positions and close ranks over their scholastic differences and interpretations. These efforts should also reflect on their people's customary likes and dislikes on regional and international levels.

20. The halal industry should be seen as a socially responsible area that develops inclusivity from within. New projects can be conceptualized on how poorer and marginalized countries that have good potential to produce healthy livestock and other supplies can be given easier access to market their products, and may also be assisted in terms of easier credit access for investment and productive purposes.

## *Environmental Concerns*

21. Global action to widely disseminate key information is urgently needed to persuade consumers worldwide away from overconsumption of ruminant meat, especially red meat. Action is essential now to persuade rapidly expanding middle-class populations worldwide, expected to exceed five billion by 2030,[3] against adopting red meat consumption and choosing less environmentally damaging options.

---

3. Kharas, *The Unprecedented Expansion of the Global Middle Class.*

22. Livestock farming is a leading cause of environmental destruction world-wide and is the prime culprit in land clearing and deforestation, leading to wildlife extinctions. Richard Eckard at the University of Melbourne concluded that reducing red meat consumption is "the smallest change with the biggest impact of anything people can do" to mitigate greenhouse gas (GHG) emissions.[4]

23. Governments should consider measures to make meat more expensive and fresh vegetables cheaper, so as to encourage people to become healthier and make environmentally-friendly dietary decisions.

24. Research is needed by qualified Muslim scholars, *fiqh* academies, and scientists to determine whether reducing red meat consumption to FAO (Food and Agriculture Organization of the United Nations) healthy dietary guideline levels could be declared a recommended (*mandub*) course of action for Muslims from the shariah viewpoint. In the "Islam and Science" chapter we mentioned a number of other shariah principles and methods that can be utilized to advance fresh shariah positions in an effort to dissuade Muslims from consumption of red meat in favor of alternative food options.

25. Owners and potential owners should consider that having pets, especially cats, puts an added strain on the environment. While cats are carnivorous, dogs are omnivorous and so potentially could derive more of their essential protein from non-animal sources. A veterinarian should be consulted if a dog is to be placed on a vegetarian diet to ensure it still gets essential nutrients. Additional strategies proposed for limiting the impacts of having pets include spaying and neutering pets not intended for breeding. Pet ownership should perhaps be made costlier through raising license fees. Children should be educated about the significant ecological costs of having pets.[5]

International Institute of Advanced Islamic Studies (IAIS) Malaysia
April 2021

---

4. McCormak, "Less Meat, Less Heat."

5. Batchelor, "Islamic Perspectives on Reducing Meat Consumption," 169.

# APPENDIX I

## *Qur'anic Verses in Arabic*

*p.8*

يا أَيُّهَا الَّذِينَ آمَنُوا كُلُوا مِن طَيِّبَاتِ مَا رَزَقْنَاكُم وَاشْكُرُوا لِلَّه إِن كُنتُم إِيَّاه تَعبدون
يا أَيُّهَا النَّاس كُلُوا مِمَّا فِي الارض حَلَالًا طَيِّبًا وَلَا تَتَّبِعُوا خُطُوَاتِ الشَّيطَان ۚ إِنَّه لَكُم عَدُوٌّ مُبِين
كُلُوا مِن طَيِّبَاتِ مَا رَزَقْنَاكُم وَلَا تَطْغَوا فِيه فَيَحِلَّ عَلَيكُم غَضَبِي ۖ وَمَن يَحلِل عَلَيه غَضَبِي
فَقَد هَوَىٰ
فَكُلُوا مِمَّا ذُكِرَ اسْم اللّه عَلَيه إِن كُنتُم بِآيَاتِه مُؤمنِين
الَّذِينَ آتَينَاهُم الْكِتَاب يَتلونَه حَقَّ تِلَاوَتِه أُولَٰئِك يُؤمنونَ بِه ۚ وَمَن يَكفُر بِه فَأُولَٰئِك هُم الخا
سرون

*p.8*

حُرِّمَت عَلَيكُم الْمَيتَةُ وَالدَّم وَلَحم الْخِنزِير وَمَا أُهِلَّ لِغَيرِ اللّه بِه وَالْمُنخَنِقَةُ وَالْمَوقُوذَةُ
وَالْمُتَرَدِّيَةُ وَالنَّطِيحَةُ وَمَا أَكَلَ السَّبُع إِلَّا مَا ذَكَّيتُم وَمَا ذُبِحَ عَلَى النُّصُب وَأَن تَستَقسِموا بِالا
زلام ۚ ذَٰلِكُم فِسقٌ ۗ الْيَومَ يَئِسَ الَّذِينَ كَفَرُوا مِن دِينكُم فَلَا تَخشَوهُم وَاخشَونِ ۚ الْيَومَ أَكمَلتُ
لَكُم دِينكُم وَأَتمَمتُ عَلَيكُم نِعمَتِي وَرَضِيتُ لَكُم الاسلام دِينًا ۚ فَمَن اضطُرَّ فِي مَخمَصَةٍ غَيرَ
مُتَجَانِفٍ لِإِثم ۙ فَإِنَّ الله غَفُورٌ رَحِيمٌ

*p.26*

هُوَ الَّذِي خَلَقَ لَكُم مَا فِي الارض جَمِيعًا ثُمَّ اسْتَوَىٰ إِلَى السَّماء فَسَوَّاهُنَّ سَبعَ سَماوَاتٍ ۚ وَهُوَ
بِكُلِّ شَيء عَلِيمٌ

*p.26*

قُل مَن حَرَّمَ زِينَةَ اللّهِ الَّتِي أَخْرَجَ لِعِبادِهِ وَالطَّيِّباتِ مِنَ الرِّزقِ ۚ قُل هِيَ لِلَّذِينَ آمَنوا فِي الحَياةِ الدُّنيا خالِصَةً يَومَ القِيامَةِ ۗ كَذٰلِكَ نُفَصِّلُ الآياتِ لِقَومٍ يَعلَمونَ

*p.38*

وَيُحِلُّ لَهُمُ الطَّيِّباتِ وَيُحَرِّمُ عَلَيهِمُ الخَبائِثَ وَيَضَعُ عَنهُم إِصرَهُم وَالأَغلالَ الَّتِي كانَت عَلَيهِم

*p.67*

إِن تَجتَنِبوا كَبائِرَ ما تُنهَونَ عَنهُ نُكَفِّر عَنكُم سَيِّئاتِكُم وَنُدخِلكُم مُدخَلًا كَريمًا الَّذِينَ يَجتَنِبونَ كَبائِرَ الإِثمِ وَالفَواحِشَ إِلَّا اللَّمَمَ ۚ إِنَّ رَبَّكَ واسِعُ المَغفِرَةِ

*p.72*

فَمَنِ اضطُرَّ غَيرَ باغٍ وَلا عادٍ فَلا إِثمَ عَلَيهِ ۚ إِنَّ اللّهَ غَفورٌ رَحيمٌ وَما لَكُم أَلّا تَأكُلوا مِمّا ذُكِرَ اسمُ اللّهِ عَلَيهِ وَقَد فَصَّلَ لَكُم ما حَرَّمَ عَلَيكُم إِلّا مَا اضطُرِرتُم إِلَيهِ

*p.74*

وَلا تُلقوا بِأَيديكُم إِلَى التَّهلُكَةِ وَلا تَقتُلوا أَنفُسَكُم ۚ إِنَّ اللّهَ كانَ بِكُم رَحيمًا

*P.110*

لا يُكَلِّفُ اللّهُ نَفسًا إِلّا وُسعَها لا يُكَلِّفُ اللّهُ نَفسًا إِلّا ما آتاها

*P.117*

كُلُّ ذٰلِكَ كانَ سَيِّئُهُ عِندَ رَبِّكَ مَكروهًا يا أَيُّهَا الَّذِينَ آمَنوا أَنفِقوا مِن طَيِّباتِ ما كَسَبتُم وَمِمّا أَخرَجنا لَكُم مِنَ الأَرضِ ۖ وَلا تَيَمَّموا الخَبيثَ مِنهُ تُنفِقونَ وَلَستُم بِآخِذيهِ إِلّا أَن تُغمِضوا فيهِ

*P.127*

وَطَعامُ الَّذِينَ أُوتوا الكِتابَ حِلٌّ لَكُم وَطَعامُكُم حِلٌّ لَهُم

*P.134*

يا أيُّها الَّذينَ آمَنوا لا تَقتُلوا الصَّيدَ وَأنتُم حُرُمٌ

أُحِلَّ لَكُم صَيدُ البَحرِ وَطَعامُهُ مَتاعًا لَكُم وَللسَّيّارَةِ ۖ وَحُرِّمَ عَلَيكُم صَيدُ البَرِّ ما دُمتُم حُرُمًا

*p.170*

هُوَ الَّذي خَلَقَ لَكُم ما فِي الأرضِ جَميعًا

وَقَد فَصَّلَ لَكُم ما حَرَّمَ عَلَيكُم

*p.171*

أُحِلَّت لَكُم بَهيمَةُ الأنعامِ إلّا ما يُتلى عَلَيكُم

اللَّه الَّذي جَعَلَ لَكُم الأنعامَ لِتَركَبوا مِنها وَمِنها تَأكُلونَ

وَلَكُم فيها مَنافِعُ

وَالأنعامَ خَلَقَها ۗ لَكُم فيها دِفءٌ وَمَنافِعُ وَمِنها تَأكُلونَ

وَلَكُم فيها جَمالٌ حينَ تُريحونَ وَحينَ تَسرَحونَ

وَتَحمِلُ أثقالَكُم إلى بَلَدٍ لَم تَكونوا بالِغيهِ إلّا بِشِقِّ الأنفُسِ ۚ إنَّ رَبَّكُم لَرَءوفٌ رَحيمٌ

وَالخَيلَ وَالبِغالَ وَالحَميرَ لِتَركَبوها وَزينَةً ۚ وَيَخلُقُ ما لا تَعلَمونَ

وَما يَستَوي البَحرانِ هذا عَذبٌ فُراتٌ سائِغٌ شَرابُهُ وَهذا مِلحٌ أُجاجٌ ۖ وَمِن كُلٍّ تَأكُلونَ لَحمًا طَريًّا وَتَستَخرِجونَ جِليَةً تَلبَسونَها

*p.174*

وَالخَيلَ وَالبِغالَ وَالحَميرَ لِتَركَبوها وَزينَةً وَيَخلُقُ ما لا تَعلَمونَ

*p.180*

وَما يَستَوي البَحرانِ هذا عَذبٌ فُراتٌ سائِغٌ شَرابُهُ وَهذا مِلحٌ أُجاجٌ ۖ وَمِن كُلٍّ تَأكُلونَ لَحمًا طَريًّا

وَحُرِّمَ عَلَيكُم صَيدُ البَرِّ ما دُمتُم حُرُمًا

*P.186*

وَيَستَفتونَكَ فِي النِّساءِ ۖ قُلِ اللَّه يُفتيكُم فيهِنَّ

يَستَفتونَكَ قُلِ اللَّه يُفتيكُم فِي الكَلالَةِ

*p.191*

يُريدُ اللَّه بِكُمُ اليُسرَ وَلا يُريدُ بِكُمُ العُسرَ

يُريدُ اللَّه أن يُخَفِّفَ عَنكُم ۚ وَخُلِقَ الإنسانُ ضَعيفًا

p.192

وَما جَعَلَ عَلَيكُم فِي الدّينِ مِن حَرَجٍ

p.218

وَلا تَقفُ ما لَيسَ لَكَ بِهِ عِلمٌ

p.223

وَسَخَّرَ لَكُم ما فِي السَّماواتِ وَما فِي الارضِ جَميعًا مِنهُ ۚ إِنَّ في ذٰلِكَ لَآياتٍ لِقَومٍ يَتَفَكَّرونَ

# APPENDIX II

## *Hadith Passages in Arabic*

p.85

قال للرجل السادس: إن القوم لم يدعوك، فاجلس حتى نذكر لهم مكانك ونستأذنهم بك

مَا مِنْ عَمَلٍ أفْضَلُ مِنْ إشباعِ كَبِدٍ جَائِع

إذا كان الماء قُلَّتينِ لم يحمل الخَبَث

p.98

إن الماء لا ينجسه شيء إلا ما غلب على ريحه وطعمه ولونه

p.108

إنَّ اللَّه أنْزَلَ الدَّاءَ والدَّوَاءَ وَجعَلَ لِكُلِّ دَاءٍ دَوَاءً ، فَتَدَاوَوْا وَلَا تَدَاوَوْا بِحَرَام

p.111

إن الله تجاوز لي عن أمتي الخطأ والنسيان وما استكرهوا عليه

p.115

مَنْ أكَلَ ثومًا أو بَصَلًا فَلْيَعْتَزِلْنَا، أو لِيَعْتَزِلْ مَسْجِدَنَا

p.116

كره رسول الله صلّى الله عليه وسلم من الشاة: الذكر، والأنثيين، والقبل، والغدة، والمرارة، والمثانة والدم

p.118

أبغض الحلال إلى الله الطلاق

p.136

إن الله كتب الإحسان على كل شيء ، فإذا قتلتم فأحسنوا القتلة ، وإذا ذبحتم فأحسنوا الذبحة ، وليحد أحدكم شفرته ، وليرح ذبيحته. رواه مسلم لا يورَدُ مُفرِضٌ على مُصِخ

p.140

أيُما إهابٍ ذيغ فقد طهُر

p.144

إنَّ الحلال بيِّن، وإنَّ الحرام بيِّن، وبينهما أمور مُشتبهات لا يعلمهنَّ كثيرٌ من الناس، فمَن اتَّقى الشُّبهات فقد استبرأ لدينه وعرضه، ومَن وقع في الشُّبهات دَغْ مَا يَريبُكَ إلَى مَا لَا يَريبُكَ ، فإنَّ الصّدقَ ظَمأنينةٌ ، وإنَّ الكَذِبَ ريبةٌ

p.151

لا ضرر ولا ضرار في الإسلام

p.173

نهى عن لحوم الحمر الأهلية وأذن في لحوم الخيل

p.177

عَنْ عَائِشَةَ رضي الله عنها: أنَّ رَسولَ الّله صلى الله عليه وسلم قال: خَفْش مِنَ الدَّوَابِّ كُلُّهِنَّ فَاسِقٌ, يُقْتَلْنَ فِي الحَرَمِ: الغُرَابُ وَالحِدَأةُ, وَالعَقْرَبُ, وَالفَأرَةُ, وَالكَلْبُ العَقُورُ,

p.179

هُوَ الطَّهُورُ مَاؤُهُ، الحِلُّ مَيْتَئهُ

p.192

يَسْرَا وَلَا تُعْشِرَا ، وَبَشِّرَا وَلَا تُنَفِّرَا

# APPENDIX III

## *Islamic Legal Maxims in Arabic*

١. مالايتم الواجب إلا به فهو واجب.

٢. الحكم إنما يجري على الظاهر وإن السرائر موكولة إلى الله سبحا نه وتعالى.

٣. كل أمر يتذ رع به إلى محظور فهو محظور.

٤. المباح يتقييد بالسلا مة.

٥. إذا إجتمع الحلال والحرام غلب الحرام.

٦. علل الأحكام تد ل على قصد الشارع فيها فحيثما وجد ت اتبعت.

٧. السلا مة من المكروه أولى من تحصيل المستحب.

٨. أفضل عمل كل رجل ما هو أكثر نفعا لغيره و اجود ثمرة و اتم فا ئدة.

٩. لا يرتكب المكروه لأجل المند وب.

١٠. مالا يتم المندوب إلا به فهو مند وب.

١١. المندوب لايترك له الواجب.

١٢. الشريعة الإسلا مية أباحت كل طيب و حرمت كل خبيث.

١٣. لا ثواب ولا عقاب إلا بنية.

١٤. ألعرف لايعتبر إذا خالف أحكام الشرع.

١٥. الأصل أن تزول الأحكام بزوال عللها.

١٦. الأصل في الأشياء إباحة حتى يد ل الد ليل على التحر يم.

١٧. الأصل براءة الذ مة.

١٨. لا إجتها د في قطعيا ت.

١٩. الفتوى على خلا ف النص أو الإجماع با طلة.

٢٠. التوصل بالأحكا م الشرعية إلى ما يخا لف مرادالله ومقاصده-الشر يعة باطل.

٢١. جميع وجوه الإ جتهاد تحتاج إلى معرفة المقاصد.

٢٢. المباح يتقييد بالسلا مة.

٢٣. د رء المفاسد أولى من جلب المنا فع.

٢٤. الحكم يد ور مع علته وجود ا وعد ما.

٢٥. الأصل أن تزول الأحكا م بزوال علله.

26. الأصل في الكلام حقيقة.
27. لاعبرة با لدلالة في المقابلة التصريح.
28. الميسور لايسقط بالميسور.
29. القضاء لايدخل في العبادات.
30. البينة لاتصير حجة إلا بقضاء القاضي.
31. اليقين مقد م على الظن والظن مقد م على الشك و المظنة لايعتبر مع وجود الحقيقة.
32. إذا اجتمع المباشر و المتسبب يضاف الحكم للمباشر.
33. من شرب خمرا جاهلا به فلا حد و لا تعزير.
34. من تيقن الفعل وشك في القليل أوالكثير, حمل على القليل.
35. ليس للإ ما م أن يخرج شيئا من يد أحد إلا بحق ثابت معروف.
36. ليس للإ ما م أن يقطع ما لاغنى للمسلمين عنه.
37. كل من له حق فهو على حاله حتى يأ تيه اليقين على خلاف ذ لك.
38. كل تصرف جر فسا دا أو د فع صلا حا فهو منهي عنه.
39. اصل اللبا س الإباحة.
40. الاصل في الأفعال والعا دات الاباحة وعد م الحظر.
41. أفعال المباح إنما تجوز بشرط عد م إيزاء أحد.
42. الأصل السلا مه حتى يعلم غيرها.
43. ألأصل السلا مة من العيو ب.
44. الأصل في تصرفا ت المسلمين الصحة.
45. المشقة تجلب التيسير.
46. ما لم يكن مالا مضمونا في حق المسلم لم يكن مالا مضمونا في حق الكافر.
47. الحقوق الموضوعة لد فع الضرر يستوى فيها المسلم والذمي والمستأ من.
48. د فع الظلم واجب بحسب الإمكان
49. د فع الضرر واجب بحسب الإمكا ن.
50. وصف الذ كورة والأنوثة لاتأ ثير له في الوصف المقتضى للحكم.
51. المراءة كا لرجل في الأهلية.
52. يحرم على الكافرين ما يحرم على المسلمين.
53. من ملك شيئا ملك ماهو من ضروراته.
54. إذا إجتمع الحلا ل والحرام غلب الحرام.
55. ما حر م أخذه حر م إعطا ؤه.
56. ما جا ز لعذ ر بطل عند زواله.
57. كل ما جاز بيعه جاز رهنه وما لا يجوز بيعه لا يجوز رهنه.
58. الأصل في الأشياء الإباحة.
59. الضرر يزال.
60. لا ضرر ولا ضرار في الاسلا م.
61. الضرورات تبيح المحظورات.
62. الضرورة تقدر بقدرها.
63. الضرر لايزال بمثله.
64. يتحمل الضرر الخا ص لدفع الضرر العا م.
65. درء المفاسد أولى من جلب المصالح.
66. إذا ضا ق الأمر اتسع.
67. العا دة محكمة.

68. اللهو واللعب أصلهما على الإباحة إلا إن قا م الد ليل على المنع والتحريم.
69. الاسلا م د ين الفطرة.
70. المسلم إذا استولى على مال مسلم آخر لا يصير ملكا له.
71. يحكم لعقود الكفا ر بالصحة وان لم توافق الإسلا م, فإذا أسلموا أجرينا عليهم أحكام المسلمين.
72. إنما الأعمال بالنيا ت.
73. الأمور بمقاصدها.
74. من مقاصد الشريعة التيسير.
75. المقاصد العا م للشريعة هو عمارة الأرض و إستمرار صلا حها بصلاح المستخلفين فيها.
76. د لت النواهي الإبتدائية التصريحية على قصد الشرعي.
77. السماحة واليسر من مقاصد الدين.
78. حفظ الد ين مقصد شرعي كلي.
79. حفظ النفس مقصد شرعي كلي.
80. حفظ العقل مقصد شرعي كلي.
81. حفظ النسل مقصد شرعي كلي.
82. عند تعارض مصلحتين أو مقصود ين يجب تقد يم الا قوى.

# Dialrel Research

**www.dialrel.eu/publications**

The DIALREL project (**www.dialrel.eu**) was undertaken to gather information about religious slaughter practices and aimed at addressing issues by encouraging dialogue between stakeholders and interested parties. The DIALREL project is funded by the European Commission and involves partners from eleven countries. It addresses issues relating to religious slaughter in order to encourage dialogue between stakeholders and interested parties.

EC funded project. No: FP6-2005-FOOD-4-C: From November 1, 2006, until spring 2010

Religious slaughter has always been a controversial and emotive subject, caught between animal welfare considerations and cultural and human rights issues. There is considerable variation in current practices and the rules regarding religious requirements are confusing. Consumer demands and concerns also need to be addressed and the project is collecting and collating information relating to slaughter techniques, product ranges, consumer expectations, market share and socioeconomic issues.

An objective of DIALREL is to evaluate the incidence and the scale of religious slaughter practices (halal and *shechita*) in cattle, small ruminants (sheep and goats), and poultry.

Information on current religious slaughter practices in EU countries (France, Germany, Italy, Spain, the UK, the Netherlands, and Belgium), a candidate country (Turkey), and associate countries (Israel and Australia) was collected through two types of questionnaires during 2007 and 2008. The first questionnaire aimed to collect data from the competent authorities about the number of animals slaughtered for halal and kosher. The second questionnaire was used to collect information on the restraining methods and pre-slaughter and post-cut stunning practices.

The most common stunning method for halal slaughter in the EU member states was penetrating captive bolt, similar to conventional slaughter. In Australia, cattle were stunned with a nonpenetrating captive bolt. Halal-stunned animals were restrained in an upright position in all the abattoirs surveyed in the UK, Australia, and in the majority of Germany and Spain.

### Small Ruminants

Halal slaughter was carried out without stunning in all the abattoirs surveyed in Israel, Turkey, Belgium, the Netherlands, and in most of the Italian, French, and Spanish slaughterhouses. On the other hand, stunning before sticking was the most common practice of the abattoirs surveyed in Germany and the UK.

The main restraining method for halal slaughter without stunning was an upright position in the UK, turning on their side in Belgium, France, Germany, and Italy, and turning on their back in the Netherlands. Small ruminants were partially hoisted before sticking in the majority of the slaughterhouses in Spain and Turkey.

The most common stunning method for halal slaughter in the EU member states and Australia was head-only electrical stunning, similar to conventional slaughter.

### Poultry

Halal slaughter was carried out without stunning in all the abattoirs surveyed in Israel, Italy, and most of the Turkish abattoirs. However, it later emerged that some Turkish poultry plants did not acknowledge the use of stunning, although electrical stunning is commonly used during halal slaughter of poultry in Turkey. On the other hand, stunning before sticking was the most common practice of the abattoirs surveyed in Germany, Spain, and the UK.

The main restraining method for halal slaughter without stunning was shackling before slaughtering in Italy and Spain.

The most common stunning method, outside Italy and Spain, was waterbath electrical stunning, being the same as for conventional slaughter.

Halal stunned poultry were hoisted before stunning in all the abattoirs surveyed in Spain, the UK, and Turkey, and in the majority of the abattoirs in Germany.

# Glossary

*'aam*: general
*'aam al-maja'ah*: year of drought
*'abadat al-awthan*: idol worshippers
*'aqur*: rabby dog
*'asr*: late afternoon prayer
*'ayniyyah/ ayni*: physical
*Adhan*: call for prayer
*Adhiyah*: animal sacrifice
*'afw*: exoneration
*'ajam*: non-Arab
*a'yan*: tangible objects
*ahad*: solitary hadith
*ahkam*: *rulings*
*ahkam al-khamsah*: the five values of shariah
*ahl al-amsar*: urban dwellers
*ahl taba' salimah*: people of sound nature
*akhlaq*: morality. morals
*amr*: command
*aqrab al-maa'*: lobster (lit. water scorpion)
*Athnaam*: idols
*ayat*: signs, Qur'anic verses
*baagh*: rebel
*batil*: null and void
*dabb*: desert lizard
*darar*: harm
*darurah*: dire necessity
*dhabh*: ritual slaughter
*dhimmi*: non-Muslim citizen
*fasid*: voidable, irregular

*fasiq*: sinner
*fatwa*: legal verdict
*fiqh*: Islamic law
*fitrah*: primordial nature
*hadd*: limit
*had'at*: black kite
*hadith*: sayings of the Prophet Muhammad
*hajah*: need
*halal*: permissible
*halalan-tayyiban*: permissible and wholesome
*halqum*: trachea
*haqiqi*: genuine
*haraj*: hardship
*haram*: forbidden
*haram li-dhatih*: haram for its own sake
*haram li-ghayrih*: haram for an extraneous factor
*harbi*: enemy at war
*hayat mustaqirrah*: ascertained life
*hayat tayyibah*: life of purity and excellence
*hilah*: legal stratagem
*hissiyyah*: physical
*hiyal*: ruses
*hud-hud*: woodpeckers
*hukmiyyah*: fictitious
*hukm*: ruling
*hukm taklifi*: obligatory law
*hubub*: pulses
*'ibadat*: devotional practices
*'illah*: effective cause
*ibahah*: permissibility
*'ilal*: effective causes
*idafi*: relative
*iftar*: breaking of the fast
*ihram*: state of sanctity in haj
*ihsan*: beauty and being good to others
*ijma'*: general consensus
*ijtihad*: independent reasoning
*ijtinab*: avoidance
*ikhbar*: conveying/informing
*ikhtilaf*: disagreement
*'ilm*: knowledge
*istibra'*: absolvence

*istihalah*: substance transformation
*istihlak*: extreme dilution
*istihsan*: juristic preference
*istishab*: presumption of continuity
*istislah*: public interest
*jallalah*: animal that feeds on filth
*ja'iz*: permissible
*jumhur*: majority
*al-kaba'ir wa'l-sagha'ir*: *major and minor sins*
*kaffarah*: expiation
*kalam*: theology
*kalb*: dog
*khabith* (pl. *khaba'ith*): revolting, impure
*khalifah*: vicegerent
*khalwah*: illicit retirement
*khamr*: wine
*khinzir al-maa'*: polar bear, lit. water pig
*khubth*: filth
*kufr*: denial of faith
*maal*: valuable object
*madhhab* (pl. *madhahib*): legal schools
*mafsadah*: corruption, harm
*mahzur*: prohibited
*majazi*: metaphorical
*makruh*: reprehensible
*makruh tahrimi*: close to haram
*makruh tanzihi*: reprehensible for the sake of purity
*mamnu'*: forbidden
*mandub*: recommendable
*maqsad*: higher purpose
*maqasid*: higher purposes
*marfu'*: an elevated hadith
*mari'*: oesophagus
*marmahi*: snake fish
*mashbuh*: doubtful
*mashbuhat*: doubtful matters
*mashkuk*: doubtful
*maslahah*: public interest
*maytah*: carcass, carrion
*minfahah*: rennet
*mizan*: balance
*mut'ah*: temporary marriage

*mubah*: permissible

*mufattir*: that which causes inertia

*mughallaz*: intensified

*mujaharah*: openly declaring (one's sinful conduct)

*mujtahid*: scholar competent to conduct ijtihad

*mukhaffaf*: lightened

*mula'amah*: harmony

*munasabah*: appropriate

*muqallid*: imitator

*mushrikun*: associators

*mustahab*: commendable

*mustaheel*: impossible

*mustaqdharat*: filthy objects

*mutawassit*: moderate

*muttafaqun 'alayh*: generally agreed upon

*nabidh*: date wine

*nahlah*: bee

*nahr*: stabbing

*najasah*: filth/impurity

*najasah mughallazah*: intensely unclean

*najasah mukhaffafah*: lightly unclean

*najas/najis*: unclean

*najis haqiqi*: physically dirty

*najis hukumi*: putatively dirty

*nass*: clear text

*nisyan*: forgetfulness

*niyyah*: intention

*qat'i*: definitive

*qisas*: retaliation

*qiyas*: ruling of analogy

*qurbah*: closeness

*raf' al-haraj*: removal of hardship

*riba*: usury

*rijs*: filth

*rukhsah*: concession

*sadd al-dhara'i'*: blocking the means

*sahur*: pre-dawn meal

*salah*: ritual prayer

*salihat*: virtuous conduct

*samak*: fish

*sawm*: fasting

*shirk*: association with God

*shubhat*: doubtful matters

*sihhah*: soundness, validity

*siyasah shar'iyah*: shariah-oriented policy

*sunnah*: exemplary conduct of the Prophet Muhammad

*ta'am (pl. at'imah)*: food of all kind

*tadhkiyah*: valid purification

*taghlib*: predominance

*taharah*: cleanliness

*taharri*: reasonable guessing

*tahir*: clean

*takhayyur*: selection

*takhfif wa'l-taysir*: facilitation and ease

*talfiq*: piecing together

*taqlid*: imitation

*tarsib*: sedimentation

*ta'qim*: sterilisation

*tarjih*: preference

*tas'ir*: price control

*tasmiyah*: short for Bismillah al-Rahman al-Rahim

*tatabbu' al-rukhas*: chasing concessions

*tawaqquf*: suspension

*tawhid*: divine oneness

*tayyib*: pure, wholesome, clean

*uli'l-amr*: ruling authorities

*'urf*: general custom

*usul al-fiqh*: sources of Islamic law

*wadajain*: jugular veins

*wahy*: divine revelation

*wajib*: obligatory

*wali*: guardian

*waqf*: charitable endowment

*yarbu'*: gerbil

*zahir*: manifest text

*zakah*: obligatory alms

*zanni*: speculative

*zina*: adultery

*zuhr*: early afternoon prayer

# Bibliography

Abdullah, Ahmad Badri. "Challenges Facing Halal Vaccine Industry." *New Straits Times*, April 21, 2017.

Abdullah, Ahmad Badri. "Halal Vaccine and the Ethical Dimension of Vaccination Programme." *Islam and Civilisational Renewal* 5, no. 3 (July 2014): 450–453.

Abdullah, Ahmad Badri, Mohd Fariz Zainal Abdullah, and Mohammad Hashim Kamali. "Malay Traditional Customs from the Shariah Perspective." IAIS Malaysia Policy Issue Paper no. 12. Kuala Lumpur: International Institute of Advanced Islamic Studies Malaysia, 2020.

Abidin, Muhammad Amin b. *Hashiyah Radd al-Mukhtar ʿala Durr al-Mukhtar*. Cairo: Dar al-Fikr, 1300AH/1979.

Abu Dawud, Sulaymān ibn al-Ashʿath. Sunan Abu Dawud, *Kitab al-Ashribah, Bab al-Nahy ʿan al-Musakkir*. Translated by Ahmad Hasan. Lahore: Sh. Ashraf, 1984.

Abu Zayd, ʿAbdul Razzaq. *Al-Intifaʿ* (ayn) *biʾl Aʿyan al-Muharramah min al-Atʿimah wa al-Ashribah wa al-Albisah*, Jordan: Dar al-Nafaʾis, 2005.

Ahmed, Pervaiz. "Understanding What Is Permissible." *New Straits Times*, January 11, 2018, 20.

Ali, Abdullah Yusuf. *The Meaning of the Holy Qurʾan: Text, Translation and Commentary*. Kuala Lumpur: Islamic Book Trust, 2011.

Anderson, Norman. *Law Reform in the Muslim World*. London: Athlone Press, 1976.

Andrew, Johnny, Normaz Wana Ismail, and Marcel Djama. "An Overview of Genetically Modified Crop Governance, Issues and Challenges in Malaysia." *Journal of the Science of Food and Agriculture* 98, no. 1 (2018): 12–17.

Anwar, Nur Diyanah. "Halal Is the Way to Go." *New Straits Times*, April 27, 2018.

Al-Ashqar, ʿUmar Sulayman, Muhammad ʿUthman Shabir, et al. *Dirasat Fiqhiyyah fi Qadaya Tibbiyyah al-Muʿasirah*. Amman: Dar al-Nafaʾis, 1421AH/2001.

ʿAshur, Muhammad al-Tahir Ibn. *Maqasid al-Shariʿah al-Islamiyyah*. Edited by Tahir el-Messawi. Amman: Dar al-Basaʾir liʾl Intaj al-ʿIlmi, 1998.

ʿAssaf, Shaykh Ahmad Muhammad. *Al-Halal waʾl-Haram fiʾl-Islam*. 9th ed. Beirut: Dar Ihyaʾ al-ʿUlum, 1411/1991.

Awang, Abdul Rahman. "Istihalah and the Sunnah of the Prophet." In *The Modern Compendium of Halal.* Vol. 1, *The Essence of Halal*, ed. Halal Development Corporation, 58–74. Kuala Lumpur: MDC Publisher, 2011.

Azzam, Salem, ed. *Universal Islamic Declaration of Human Rights.* London: Islamic Council of Europe, 1981.

Bailey, Rob, Antony Froggath, and Laura Wellesley. "Livestock—Climate Change's Forgotten Sector." Research paper. London: Chatham House, 2014. https://www.chathamhouse.org/sites/default/files/field/field_document/20141203LivestockClimateChangeForgottenSectorBaileyFroggattWellesley Final.pdf.

Al-Baji, Abu'l-Walid. *Al-Muntaqa Sharh al-Muwatta'.* 2nd ed. Cairo: Dar al-Kitab al-Islami, n.d.

Balakrishnan, Nandini. "Malaysia to Produce and Export the World's First Halal Vaccines." SAYS News, December 6, 2017. https://says.com/my/news/world-s-first-halal-vaccine-to-be-produced-in-malaysia.

Batchelor, Daud Abdul-Fattah. "Islamic Perspectives on Reducing Meat Consumption to Promote Earth's Sustainability." *Islam and Civilisation Renewal* 10, no. 2 (2019): 161–174.

Battour, Mohamed. "Muslim Travel Behavior in Halal Tourism." In *Mobilities, Tourism and Travel Behavior.* Edited by Lexzek Butowski. IntechOpen, 2018. https://www.intechopen.com/books/mobilities-tourism-and-travel-behavior-contexts-and-boundaries/muslim-travel-behavior-in-halal-tourism.

Battour, Mohamed, Ismail, Mohd Nazari, and Battor Moustafa. "The Impact of Destination Attributes on Muslim Tourist's Choice." *International Journal of Tourism Research* 13 (2011): 527–540.

Al-Bayanuni, Muhammad Abu'l-Fath. *Al-Hukmu al-Taklifi fi al-Shari'ah al-Islamiyah.* Damascus: Dar al-Qalam, 1409/1988.

Al-Bayhaqi, Abu Bakr Ahmad. *Al-Sunan al-Bayhaqi.* Edited by M. 'Abd al-Qadir 'Ata'. Vol. 6. Mecca: Maktabah Dar al-Baz, 1407AH/1987.

BBC Religions. "Animals." July 16, 2009. http://www.bbc.co.uk/religion/religions/judaism/jewishethics/animals_1.shtml.

Berg, Raffi. "Should Animals Be Stunned before Slaughter." BBC News, November 30, 2011. https://www.bbc.com/news/magazine-14779271.

Bevins, Vincent. "Halal Tourism: Kuala Lumpur Welcomes the Muslim Travellers Others Didn't Want." *Guardian*, June 6, 2017. https://www.theguardian.com/cities/2017/jun/06/halal-tourism-kuala-lumpur-muslim-travellers-malaysia.

Al-Bishry, Tariq. "Al-Jama'ah al-Wataniyyah fi Daw' Maqasid al-Shari'ah." In *Taf'il Maqasid al-Shari'ah fi Majal al-Siyasi: Majmu'ah Buhuth*, ed. Muhammad Salim el-Awa. London: Mu'assasah al-Furqan li'l-Turath al-Islami, 1435AH/2014.

Bland, Alastair. "Is the Livestock Industry Destroying the Planet?" *Smithsonian*, August 1, 2012. https://www.smithsonianmag.com/travel/is-the-livestock-industry-destroying-the-planet-11308007/.

Brown, Nathan J. "Shari'a and State in the Modern Muslim Middle East." *International Journal of Middle East Studies* 29, no. 3 (1997): 359–376.

Al-Bukhari, Muhammad bin Isma'il. *Sahih al-Bukhari, Kitab al-Dhaba'ih wa'l-Sayd.* Vol. 7. Edited by Muhammad Zuhair bin Nasir. Beirut: Dar Touq al-Najah, 1422/2000.

Burj, Ahmad Muhammad Isma'il. *Ahkam al-Dhabh wa'l-Mustajidat al- Muta'allaqah bihi fi'l-Fiqh al-Islami.* Cairo: Dar al-Jami'ah al-Jadidah li'l-Nashr, 2004.

Cochrane, Paul. "Overview: How Attractive is Malaysia's Halal Pharmaceutical Sector?" Salaam Gateway, September 29, 2016. https://www.salaamgateway.com/en/story/overviewhow_attractive_is_malaysias_halal_pharmaceutical_sector-SALAAM29092016074936/.

CodeBlue Health is a Human Right. https://codeblue.galencentre.org/2020/08/18/malaysia-wont-make-childhood-vaccination-compulsory/, August 18, 2020.

Consiglio, Flavia di. "Food: The Last Bastion of Faith." BBC Religion and Ethics, September 14, 2015. http://www.bbc.co.uk/religion/0/18591686.

Cresswell, Ian, and Helen Murphy. *Australia's State of the Environment: Biodiversity: 2016.* Canberra: Department of Environment and Energy, 2017. https://soe.environment.gov.au/sites/g/files/net806/soe2016 biodiversity launch version2-24feb17.pdf?v 1488792935.

Dabrowska, Karen. "The Rise of Islamic Tourism: International Conference Discusses the Effects of 9/11 on Arab Tourism." *Islamic Tourism* 13 (September-October 2004): 58–60.

*Daily Sabah*. "Ranking 3rd in Halal Tourism, Turkey Offers Better Hotel Standards for Muslim Travelers." *Daily Sabah*, February 24, 2017. https://www.dailysabah.com/travel/2017/02/24/ranking-3rd-in-halal-tourism-turkey-offers-better-hotel-standards-for-muslim-travelers.

Department of Standards Malaysia. MS 2400-1-2010: *Halalan–Toyyiban Assurance Pipeline–Part 1: Management System Requirements for Transportation of Goods and/or Cargo Chain Services.*

Department of Standards Malaysia. MS 2400-2-2010: *Halal-Toyyiban Assurance Pipeline—Part 2: Management System Requirements for Warehousing and Related Activities*; whereas MS 2400-3-2010 bears the title *Halalan-Toyyiban Assurance Pipeline—Part 3: Management System Requirements for Retailing.*

Diamond, Jared. *Guns, Germs, and Steel: The Fate of Human Societies.* New York: Norton, 2017.

Din, Sabariyah. *Trading Halal Commodities: Opportunities and Challenges for the Muslim World.* Kuala Lumpur: Penerbit Universiti Teknologi Malaysia, 2006.

Dinar Standard, 2020/21 State of the Global Islamic Economy Report. https://www.salaamgateway.com/specialcoverage/SGIE20-21.

Douglas, Susan. "The Fabric of Muslim Daily Life." In *Voices of Islam*, ed. Vincent Cornell. Vol. 3. Westport, CT: Praeger, 2007.

"Eat Less Meat to Save the World, Says Study." *New Straits Times*, October 12, 2018.

Efendi, Rahmat Hidayat. "Halal Industry Can Help Indonesia in International Trade." Halal Focus, May 2, 2018. https://halalfocus.net/halal-industry-can-help-indonesia-in-international-trade/.

"Epilepsy." In *Encyclopaedia Britannica Online*. http://search.eh.com/eb/article-9032798.

Fadlullah, Sayyid Mohammad Hussain. *Fiqh al-At'imah wa'l-Ashribah*. Edited by Al-Shaykh Mohammad Adib al-Qobaysi. Beirut: Dar al-Malak, 1428/2007.

——. *Islamic Lanterns: Conceptual and Jurisprudence Questions for Natives, Emigrants and Expatriates*. English Translation by Adil al-Qadi and S. al-Samara'i. Beirut: Dar al-Malak, 1425/2004.

——. *Islamic Rulings: A Guide of Islamic Practices*. English Translation by A. S. As-Samarra'i. Beirut: Dar al-Malak, 1427/2006.

Fiqh Academy. "Decision on Substance Transformation (*istihalah*)." *Al-Sharq al-Awsat* (London), no. 9173, July 9 2004.

Foltz, Richard C. *Animals in Islamic Tradition and Muslim Countries*. Oxford: Oneworld Publications, 2006.

Foon, Ho Wah. "Shaanix to Set Up Global Halal Hub." *The Star*, May 16, 2016. https://www.thestar.com.my/news/nation/2016/05/16/shaanxi-to-set-up-global-halal-hub-malaysian-help-sought-in-creating-chinese-halal-certification-uni/#OP3RitfWDEEefzue.99.

Furber, Musa. "The Elements of a Fatwa and Other Contributions to Confidence in Its Validity." Taba Analytic Brief no.14. Abu Dhabi: Tabah Foundation, 2013.

Al-Ghafur, Fazl al-Rahman 'Abd. *al-Taqlid wa'l-Talfiq 'Ind al-Usuliyyin*. Unpublished dissertation, International Islamic University Islamabad, n.d.

Al-Ghazali, Abu Hamid Muhammad b. Muhammad. *Ihya' 'Ulum Al-Din*. Beirut: Dar al-Kutub al-Ilmiyya, 1421/2001.

Gunasegaram, P. "Halal Industry Should Work with Islamic Finance." *The Star*, November 16, 2011, 3.

Al-Haaj, Ibn Amir. *Al-Taqrir wa'l-Tahbir 'ala'l-Tahrir*. Cairo: al-Matba'ah al-Amiriyyah al-Kubra, 1316/1899.

Al-Hakim. *Al-Mustadrak 'ala al-Sahihayn, Kitab al-Tafsir*. Vol. 2. Edited by Mustafa 'Abd al-Qadir 'Ata. Beirut: Dar al-Kutub al-'Ilmiyah, 1411/1990.

Halal Development Corporation (HDC) Bhd. Halal Industry Master Plan 2030. Putrajaya: Ministry of Economics Affair, 2018. https://www.hdcglobal.com/wp-content/uploads/2020/02/Halal-Industri-Master-Plan-2030.pdf.

Halal Focus. "Many Still Confused on Accepted Alcohol Content in Food." Halal Focus, March 28, 2012. http://halalfocus.net/malaysia-many-still-confused-on-accepted-alcohol-content-in-food/.

Halal Industry Development Corporation. *Best Halal Practices in the Food Industry: Training Module for Halal Awareness Program in Graduate School of Management*. Selangor: University Putra Malaysia, 2012.

"Halal Tourism." In *Wikipedia*. https://en.wikipedia.org/wiki/Halal_tourism.

"Halal Tourism Explained." *The Star*, October 13, 2014. https://www.thestar.com.my/travel/malaysia/2014/10/13/halal-tourism-explained/#UoujAwUStuv36rrV.99.

"Halal Tourism in Indonesia." World Folio, n.d. http://www.theworldfolio.com/news/halal-tourism-in-indonesia/4169/.

Hamdan, Nurbaiti, and A. Raman. "'Halal' Food Factory Shares Wall with Pig Farm." *The Star*, September 11, 2008, N43.

Hamid, Abdul Jalil. "Japan Making a Mark in Muslim Tourism Market." *New Sunday Times*, December 30, 2018, 13.

Hammad, Nazih. *Al-Mawad al-Muharramah wa'l Najasah fi'l-Ghadha' wa'l-Dawa': Bayn al-Nazariyyah wa'l-Tatbiq*. 3rd ed, Damascus: Dar al-Qalam, 1432/2011.

Hammad, Nazih. "Dieting the Islamic Way." Islam, the Modern Religion, n.d. http://www.themodernreligion.com/health/diet.html.

Hamsawi, Roziana. "Mukhriz Mahathir's Speech 'Bumis Only Hold 30pc of Halal Certs.'" *New Straits Times*, June 29, 2011.

Al-Harithi, Badriyah bint Mash'al. *Al-Nawazil fi'l-At'imah*. Riyadh: Dar Kunuz li'l-Nashr wa'l-Tawzi', 1431AH/2011.

Hasan, Ahmad. *Principles of Islamic Jurisprudence*. Islamabad: Islamic Research Institute, 1993.

HDC (Halal Development Corporation). "Halal Parks." Selangor, Malaysia: HDC, 2012. http://www.hdcglobal.com/publisher/halal_park_location_operation.

Hearse, Simon. "Seizing the Halal Opportunity in Malaysia." *New Straits Times*, December 21, 2018, 16.

Hirschmann, R. "Total Muslim tourist arrivals to Malaysia from 2015-2017, in millions." Statista, https://www.statista.com/statistics/976514/total-muslim-tourist-arrivals-to-malaysia/.

Ibn Biri, Ibrahim bin Husayn. *Al-Kashf wa'l-Tadqiq li-Sharh Ghayat al-Tahqiq*. Cairo, MS Dar al-Kutub, n.d.

Ibn Hanbal, Ahmad. *Musnad Imam Ahmad Ibn Hanbal*. Edited by Shu'aib al-Arnaout. Beirut: Muassasah al-Risalah, 1421/2001.

Al-Haithami, Ahmad bin Muhammad Ibn Hajar. *Tuhfat al-Muhtaj fi Sharh al-Minhaj*. Vol. 9. *Cairo:*Maktabah Tijariyah Kubra, 1983.

Ibn Kathir, Abu'l-Fida' (ayn) Imad al-Din Isma'il. *Tafsir al-Qur'an al-'Azim*. Vol. 2. Beirut: Dar al-Kutub al-Ilmiyah, 2006.

Ibn Majah, Abu 'Abd Allah Muhammad ibn Yazid al-Qazwini. *Sunan Ibn Majah: Kitab al-At' (ayn) imah: Bab al-Lahm*. Cairo: Dar al-Hadith, 1998.

Ibn Qudamah, Muwaffaq al-Din. *Al-Mughni*. Edited by Muhammad Sharaf al-Din Khattab and Sayyid Muhammad al-Sayyid. Cairo: Dar al-Hadith, 1425/2004.

Ibn Taymiyyah, Taqi al-Din Ahmad. *Majmu'ah Fatawa Shaykh al-Islam Ibn Taymiyyah*. Compiled by Abd al-Rahman b. Qasim. Beirut: Mu'assasat al-Risalah, 1398AH/1978.

——. *Al-Qawa' (ayn)id al-Nuraniyyah al-Fiqhiyyah*. Edited by Muhammad Hamid al-Faqi. 2nd ed. Lahore: Idarah Tarjaman al-Sunnah, 1404AH/1983.

——. *Al-Siyasah al-Shariyyah fi-Islah al-Rai wa'l-Raiyyah.* 2nd ed. Cairo: Dar al-Kitab al-Arabi, 1370AH/1951.

Ibrahim, Ahmed Fekry. *Pragmatism in Islamic Law: A Social and Intellectual History.* Syracuse, NY: Syracuse University Press, 2015.

Ibrahim, Mohd Radhi. "Fatwa on Halal Related Issues." In *The Essence of Halal,* ed. Halal Industry Development Corporation. Kuala Lumpur: MDC Publisher, 2011.

Ihsan, Abdul Halim, Azimuddin Ahmad, et al. *The Halal Index, Vol.1: Pig Based Pharmaceuticals.* Kuala Lumpur: Phytorex Press, 2011.

Isa, Noor Munirah, Azizan Baharuddin, Saadan Man and Chang Lee Wei. "Bioethics in The Malay-Muslim Community in Malaysia: A Study On the Formulation of Fatwa on Genetically Modified Food by The National Fatwa Council." *Developing World Bioethics* 15, no. 3 (2014): 143–151.

Ismail, Laili. "'Halal' Is Not Just about Food." Interview with Jamal Bidin, Head of Halal Industry Development Corporation. *New Straits Times,* November 19, 2017, 12.

"Halal Is Not Just about Food." Interview with Sirajuddin Suhaimee. *New Straits Times,* November 19, 2017, 13.

"JAIS Raids Bogus Halal Restaurant." *New Straits Times,* January 9, 2019.

JAKIM (Department of Islamic Development Malaysia). "Halal E-Codes." In *Handbook of Halal Food Additives.* Selangor, Malaysia: JAKIM, 2018. http://www.halalmalaysia.net/HALAL_E-CODES.php.

——. "Local Products with E-code Halal for Muslims," site dated 27 May 2014. https://www.astroawani.com/berita-malaysia/local-products-with-e-code-halal-for-muslims-jakim-36652.

"JAKIM Pushes to Speed Up Halal Certification for Bumi Businesses." *New Straits Times,* September 4, 2016.

Jamaludin, Mohammad Aizat, et al. "Istihalah: Analysis on the Utilization of Gelatin in Food Products." In *2nd Conference on Humanities, Historical and Social Sciences,* 174–178. Singapore: IACSIT Press, 2011.

Al-Jawziyyah, Ibn Qayyim. *Zaad al-Maad fi Huda Khayr al-'Ibad.* 13th ed. Vol. 4. Beirut: Muassasah al-Risalah, 1406/1986.

——. *I'lam al Muwaqqi' in 'an Rabb al' Alamin.* Vol. 2. Cairo: Al Kulliyat al-Azhariyah. 1388/1968.

——. *Al-Jawab al-Kafi li-man Sa' ala 'an al-Dawa' al-Shafi.* Cairo: Dar al-Hadith, 1983.

Al-Jaziri, Abd al-Rahman. *Al-Fiqh 'ala'l-Madhahib al'(ayn)-Arba'ah.* Cairo, Al-Mansurah: Dar al-Ghadd al-Jadid, 1426/2005.

"Jeffri Sulaiman, Vice President of the Association of Tour and Travel Agents Malaysia (MATTA), Interview at Islamic Tourism Media." www.islamictourism.com.

Al-Jurjani, Sayyid al-Sharif. *Kitab al-Ta'rifat.* Istanbul: al-Astanah, 1327/1909.

Al-Juwayni, Abd al-Malik ibn Yusuf. *Ghiyath al-Umam fi Iltiyath al-Zulam.* Edited by Mustafa Hilmi and Fuad Ahmad. Alexandria: Dar al-Da'wa, 1978.

Ibn Juzay, Ahmad bin Muhammad al-Gharnati. *Al-Qawanin al-Fiqhiyah.* Edited by Majid al-Hamawi. Beirut: Dar Ibn Hazm, 1434/2013.

Kamali, Mohammad Hashim. "Actualisation (*Tafil*) of the Higher Purposes of Shariah." *Islam and Civilisational Renewal* 8, no. 3 (July 2017): 295–321.

——. "The Johor Fatwa on Mandatory HIV Testing." *IIUM Law Journal* 9, no. 2 (2001): 99–117.

——. "The Principles of Halal and Haram in Islam." In *The Modern Compendium of Halal*. vol. 1, *The Essence of Halal*, edited by Halal Development Corporation. Kuala Lumpur: MDC Publisher, 2011: 10–56.

——. *Principles of Islamic Jurisprudence*. Rev. ed. Cambridge: Islamic Text Society, 2003.

——. *The Right to Life, Security, Privacy and Ownership in Islam*. Cambridge: Islamic Texts Society, 2008.

——. "*Shari'ah* and Civil Law: Toward a Methodology of Harmonisation." *Islamic Law and Society* 14 (2007): 406–411.

——. *Shar'iah Law: An Introduction*. Oxford: Oneworld Publications, 2008.

——. *Shariah Law: Questions and Answers*. Oxford: Oneworld Publications, 2017.

——. *A Textbook of Hadith Studies*. Leicester, UK: The Islamic Foundation, 2005.

——. "The Parameters of Halal and Haram in Shariah and the Halal Industry." Occasional Paper Series 23. London: International Institute of Islamic Thought, 2013.

Kannan, Hashini Kavishtri. "Move towards World Halal Standards." *New Straits Times*, April 5, 2017.

Al-Kasani, 'Ala' al-Din. *Bada'i' al-Sana'i' fi Tartib al-Shara'i'*. Vol. 5. 2nd ed. Beirut: Dar al-Kutub al-'Ilmiyyah, 1406AH/1986.

Kharas, Homi. *The Unprecedented Expansion of the Global Middle Class: An Update*. Global Economy & Development Working Paper 100. Washington, DC: Brookings Institute, February 2017. https://www.brookings.edu/wp-content/uploads/2017/02/global_20170228_global-middle-class.pdf.

Al-Kurdi, Ahmad al-Hajji. *Buhuth wa Fatawa Fiqhiyyah Mu'asirah*. Beirut: Dar al-Basha'ir al-Islamiyyah, 1427AH/2007.

Lake, Rob. "Current Awareness of Genetically Modified Food Issues Project F 99." Christchurch, New Zealand: Institute of Environmental Science and Research Limited & Christchurch Science Centre, 2001. http://www.moh.govt.nz/notebook/nbbooks.nsf/0/7f6a71cf566315dccc25783600734c95/$FILE/genetically-modified.pdf.

Mahmud, Dzulkifli. "Playing a Leadership Role in Halal Industry." *New Straits Times*, May 10, 2015.

Malek, Muhammad Mushtaq. "Islam and Vaccines." *New Straits Times*, December 21, 2018.

Maniar, Saad. "The Growing Popularity of Halal Tourism." *Khaleej Times*, April 27, 2017. https://www.khaleejtimes.com/business/local/the-growing-popularity-of-halal-tourism.

Al-Maqdisi, Shams al-Din (d. 682/1284, son of Muaffaq al-Din ibn Qudamah). *al-Mughni* (with its commentary *al-Sharh al-Kabir*). Edited by Sharaf al-Din Khattab and al-Sayyid Muhammad al-Sayyid. Cairo: Dar al-Hadith, 1425/2004.

Al-Mawsili, Abu Hafs Umar bin Badr. *Al-Jam'u Bain al-Sahihayn.* Vol. 2. Beirut: al-Maktab al-Islami, 1995.

McCormak, Ange. "'Less Meat, Less Heat': Could Your Diet Save the Planet from Climate Change?" ABC *Triple J Hack,* November 15, 2016. https://www.abc.net.au/triplej/programs/hack/agriculture/8025870.

Moosa, Ebrahim. "Genetically Modified Foods and Muslim Ethics." In *Acceptable Genes: Religious Traditions and Genetically Modified Foods,* ed. Conrad G. Brunk and Harold Coward, 135–159. Albany: State University of New York Press, 2009.

Mohamad, Muhammad Hisyam. "Halal Economy: Ensure Islamic Values Are Adopted." *New Straits Times,* August 29, 2018, 18. https://www.nst.com.my/opinion/letters/2018/08/405955/ensure-islamic-values-are-adopted.

Mohd Kashim, Mohd Izhar Ariff, Muhammad Nazir Alias, Diani Mardiana Mat Zin, Noor Lizza Mohamed Said, Zanmzuri Zakaria, Ahmad Dahlan Salleh, and Ezan Azraai Jamsari. "Istihalah and Its Effects on Food: An Islamic Perspective." *International Journal of Civil Engineering and Technology* 9, no. 1 (2018): 755–762.

*Muallimatu Zayid li'l-Qawaid al-Fiqhiyyah wa'l-Usuliyyah.* Abu Dhabi: Mu'assasah Zayid bin Sultan Aal-Nahyan li'l-A'mal al-Khayriyyah wa'l-Insaniyyah, wa majma al-Fiqh al-Islami al-Duwali, 1434AH/2013. Most of the legal maxims cited in this book were taken from this 43-volume encyclopedia.

Al-Mundhiri, Zakiy al-Din Abd al-'(ayn)Azim. *Mukhtasar Sahih Muslim.* Edited by Muhammad Nasiruddin al-Albani. 6th ed. Beirut: Al-Maktab Al-Islami, 1407/1987.

Munajjid, Salah al-Din, ed. *Muhammad Rashid Rida.* 6 vols. Beirut: Dar al-Kutub al-Jadid, 1970.

Muslim, Abul-Hussain Muslim ibn Hajjaj al-Qushairi. *Mukhtasar Sahih Muslim.* Edited by Muhammad Nasir al-Din al-Albani. Beirut: Dar al-Maktab al-Islami, 1987.

"MyHAC—World's First Halal Laboratory Launched." *New Straits Times,* March 30, 2018.

Al-Nabhan, Muhammad Faruq. *Al-Madkhal li'l-Tashri' al-Islami. Nish'atuh, Adwaruh al-Tarikhiyyah, Mustaqbaluh.* 2nd edn. Beirut: Dar al-Qalam, 1981.

Nafsiyah, Abdul Rahman b. Hasan. *Risalah fi Fiqh as-Siyam,* Cairo: *Majallat al-Buhuth al-Fiqhiyyah al-Mu'asirah,* 2009.

Nooh Mohammad, Norhazian Nawai, Nuradli Ridzwan Shah Mohd Dali, and Shah Bin Mohd Dali. "Halal Certification: What the SME Producers Should Know." https://www.researchgate.net/publication/237318846_Halal_Certification_What_the_SME_Producers_Should_Know.

Okin, Gregory. "Environmental Impacts of Food Consumption by Dogs and Cats." *PLoS ONE* 12, no. 8(2017): 1–14. https://doi.org/10.1371/journal.pone.0181301.

Omar, Nor Asiah. "Get Halal Stamp and Go Global." *New Straits Times,* January 31, 2019.

Organisation of Islamic Cooperation. *Al-Nadwah al-Fiqhiyyah al-Tibiyyah al-Tasi'ah li'l-Munazzamat al-Islami li'l-'Ulum al-Tibiyyah.* Vol. 2. Al-Dar al-Bayda: Organisation of Islamic Cooperation, July 1997.

Oxford Business Group. "Indonesia Eyes Up Further Growth as World Leader in Halal Tourism." In *Indonesia 2018*. https://oxfordbusinessgroup.com/analysis/positive-prospects-country%E2%80%99s-success-halal-destination-indicates-significant-growth-potential.

Parvaiz, Mohammed Aslam. "Scientific Innovation and Al-Mizan." In *Islam and Ecology: A Bestowed Trust*, ed. Richard C. Foltz, Frederick M. Denny, and Azizan Baharuddin, 393–402. Cambridge, MA: Harvard University Press, 2003.

Peraturan Menteri Agama Republik Indonesia No. 26, 2019, "Penyelenggaraan Jaminan Produk Halal." http://www.halalmui.org/images/stories/PMA%20No.%2026%20Tahun%202019%20PENYELENGGARAAN%20JAMINAN%20PRODUK%20HALAL.pdf.

Al-Qaradawi, Yusuf. *Bay' al-Murabahah li'l-Amir bi'l- Shira'*. 2nd ed. Cairo: Maktabah Wahbah, 1407AH/1987.

——. *Dawr al-Qiyam wa'l-Akhlaq fi'l-Iqtisad al-Islami*. 2nd ed. Cairo: Maktabah Wahbah, 1422AH/2001.

——. *Fi Fiqh al-Aqaliyyat al-Muslimah: Hayat al-Muslimin Wasat al-Mujtamaat al-Ukhra*. 2nd ed., Cairo: Dar al-Shurouq, 1406AH/2005.

——. *Al-Halal wa'l-Haram fi'l-Islam*. 15th ed. Beirut: al-Maktab al-Islami, 1415AH/1994.

Al-Qarafi, Shihab al-Din. *Kitab al-Furuq*. Vol. 1. Cairo: Dar al-Kutub al-'(ayn) Arabiyyah, 1346AH/1927.

Qasmi, Qadi Mujahidul Islam. "Jadid Sa'insi Teknik: Cloning" [New scientific technique: Cloning]. New Delhi: Islamic Fiqh Academy, 2000.

Al-Qurtubi, Abu'l Walid Muhammad b. Rushd. *Bidayat al-Mujtahid wa Nihayat al-Muqtasid*. Beirut: Dar al-Qalam, 1988.

Qurashi, Mazhar M. *Introduction to Muslim Contributions to Science and Technology*. Islamabad: International Islamic University, 1998.

Al-Qushairi, Muktasar Sahih Muslim. See Muslim.

Al-Ramlawi, Muhammad Saeed. *Al-Halal wa'l-Haram wa'l Mughallab minhuma fi'l Firqh al-Islamic: Dirasah Tatbiqiyyah Mu'asirah*. Cairo: Dar al-Jami'ah al-Jadidah, 2008.

Ramli, Noriah. "*Food Safety and Quality: A Study of the Existing Legal and Administrative Regulations in Malaysia*." PhD diss., International Islamic University Malaysia, May 2007. https://lib.iium.edu.my/mom/services/mom/document/getFile/NcO3qLscXVQnoqisUpHNrp66iCJrgoqy20080723152609515.

——. "Legal and Administrative Regulation in Halal Production." In *The Essence of Halal*, 93–114. Kuala Lumpur: MDC Publisher, 2011.

Rasid, Amir Hisyam. "Global Halal Market Growing Bigger." *New Straits Times*, February 13, 2016.

——. "Report on the Minister's Speech entitled 'Boosting Malaysia's Halal Initiatives.'" *New Straits Times*, March 30, 2016.

Regenstein, Joe M. "Religious Food Laws and Philosophical Food Choices." In *The Essence of Halal*, 114–130. Kuala Lumpur: MDC Publisher, 2013.

Regenstein, Joe M., Chaudry, Muhammad M., and Regenstein, Carrie E. "Kosher and Halal in the Biotechnology Era." *Applied Biotechnology, Food Science and Policy* 1 no. 2 (2003): 95–107.

http://www.kimia. gov.my/v3/wp-content/uploads/2016/11/Sesi-3.pdf.

Rida, Muhammad Rashid. *Tafsir al-Manar*. Vol. 1. Cairo: Dar al-Manar, 1376AH/1946.

Ripple, William J., Smith, Pete, Haberl, Helmut, Montzka, Stephen A., McAlpine, Clive, and Boucher, Douglas H. "Ruminants, Climate Change and Climate Policy." *Nature Climate Change* 4 (2014): 2–5.

Al-Raisuni, Qutb. *Al-Haram fi'l-Shariah al-Islamiyyah: Fiqhuh wa Dawabituh wa Tatbiqatuh al-Mu'asirah*. Beirut: Dar Ibn Hazm, 1432/2011.

Rokshana Shirin Asa. "Effectiveness of The Existing Halal Laws in Malaysia." *Jurnal Syariah* 26, no. 1 (2018): 14–166.

Rothman, Lauren. "Halal Slaughter is more complicated than you realize." https://www.vice.com/en/article/d75mea/halal-slaughter-is-more-complicated-than-you-realize.

"Ruling on Eating Meat and Plants That Have Been Genetically Modified." Islam Question and Answer. https://islamqa.info/en/119830.

Al-Salam, 'Izz al-Din 'Abd. *Al-Qawa'id al-Ahkam fi Masalih al-Anam*, ed. Nazih Hammad, vol. 1. Damascus: Darul al-Qalam, 1431AH/2010.

Securities Commission Malaysia. *Resolutions of the Shariah Advisory Council*, 2nd ed. Kuala Lumpur: Securities Commission Malaysia, 2007.

Sranacharoenpong, Kitti Soret, Samuel, Harwatt, Helen, Wien, Michelle, and Sabaté, Joan. "The Environmental Cost of Protein Food Choices." *Public Health*. 18, no. 11 (2015): 2067–2073.

Shabbir, Muhammad 'Uthman. *Al-Qawa'id al-Kulliyyah wa'l-Dawabit al-Fiqhiyyah fi'l-Shari'ah al-Islamiyyah*. Amman: Dar al-Nafa'is, 1426AH/2006.

Al-Shadhili, Hasan 'Ali. "Al-Istinsakh: Haqiqatuhu, Anwa'uhu, Hikmatuh Fi Al-Fiqh Al-Islami." *Majallat Majma al-Fiqh al-Islami: ad-Dawra al-'Ashira* 10, no. 3 (1418/1997).

Shafie, Shahidan, and Mohd Nor Othman. "Halal Certification: International Marketing Issues and Challenges." Unpublished conference paper. http://halalrc.org/images/Research%20Material/Report/Halal%20Certification%20an%20international%20marketing%20issues%20and%20challenges.pdf.

Shah, Shaheera Aznam. "Malaysia Accelerating Halal Industry's Growth." *Malaysian Reserve*, September 6 2017.

Shah, Sultan Nazrin Muizzuddin. "Fostering a True Halal Economy: Global Integration and Ethical Practice." Speech delivered at the World Halal Conference, 2018. *New Straits Times*, April 6, 2018.

Shahzad, Qaisar. *Biomedical Ethics: Philosophical and Islamic Perspectives*. Islamabad: Islamic Research Institute, 2009.

Al-Sharbini, Muhammad al-Khatib. *Al-Iqna'*. Vol. 2. Beirut: Dar al-Fikr, 1415AH/ 1995.

Al-Shatibi, Abu Ishaq Ibrahim. *Al-Muwafaqat fi Usul al-Shari'ah*. Vol. 1. 2nd ed. Edited by Abd Allah Darraz. Beirut: Dar al-Ma'rifah, 1975.

———. *Al-I'tisam*. Vol. 2. Cairo: Matbaah al-Manar, 1331AH/1914.

———. Abu Dawud, Sulaymān ibn al-Ash'ath. *Sunan Abu Dawud*. English translation by Nasiruddin al-Khatab. Riyadh: Darussalam 2008.

Springmann, Marco, Clark, Michael, Mason-D'Croz, Daniel et al. "Options for Keeping the Food System within Environmental Limits," *Nature* 562 (2018): 519–525. https://www.nature.com/articles/s41586-018-0594-0.

Springmann, Marco, H. Charles J. Godfray, Mike Rayner, and Peter Scarborough. "Analysis and Valuation of the Health and Climate Change Cobenefits of Dietary Change," *Proceedings of the National Academy of Sciences of the United States of America* 113, no. 15 (2016): 4146–4151. https://www.pnas.org/content/113/15/4146.full.

Al-Suyuti, Jalal al-Din. *Al-Ashbah wa'l-Naza'ir*. Beirut: Dar al-Kitab al-'Ilmiyah, 1994.

Syafinaz Amin, N., I. Faridah, A. H. Rukman, A. S. Fathinul Fakri, O. Malina, G. Fadzillah, and I. Ilina. "Parental Refusal to Diphtheria Vaccine: A Fatal Outcome." *Medical Journal of Malaysia* 68, no. 5 (October 2013): 431.

Al-Tabarsi, Mirza Hossein al-Nuri. *Mustadrak al-Wasa'il wa Mustanbat al-Masa'il*. Qum: Mu'assasah Aal al-Bayt li-Ihya' al-Turath, 1407/1990.

Al-Tabrizi, Muḥammad b. 'Abd Allah al-Khatib. *Mishkat al-Masabih*. Edited by Muhammad Nasir al-Din al-Albani. 2nd ed. Beirut: Dar al-Maktab al-Islami, 1399AH/1979.

Al-Tahanawi, Muhammad 'Ali. *Kashshaf Istilahat al-Funun*. Istanbul: Al-Astanah, 1317/1938.

Al-Tamawi, Sulayman Muhammad. *Al-Sulatat al-Thalath fi Dasatir al 'Arabiyah wa fai'l Fikr al Siyasi al Islami*. Cairo: Dar al Fikr al 'Arabi, 1973.

Tieman, Marco. "Control of Halal Food Chains." *Islam and Civilisational Renewal* 3 no. 3 (July 2011): 538–542.

——— . "Halal Reputation Management: Combining Individual and Collective Reputation Management Strategies." *Islam and Civilisational Renewal* 8, no. 1 (January 2017): 115–119.

——— . "Safeguarding Halal Reputation," Kuala Lumpur: *New Straits Times*, February 23, 2019.

Tyser, C. R., et al., trans. *The Mejelle, Being an English Translation of Majallah el-Ahkam-i Adliya and a Complete Code of Islamic Civil Law*. Kuala Lumpur: The Other Press, 2003.

UM Land. "Iskandar Halal Park." https://www.umland.com.my/portfolio/iskandar-halal-park/.

United Poultry Concerns. https://www.upc-online.org/slaughter/poultry_slaughter.pdf.

Uwais, Abd al-Halim, ed. *Mawsu'ah al-Fiqh al-Islami*. Vol. 1. Cairo: Dar al-Wafa', 1426/2005.

Varagur, Krithika. "Indonesia Aims to Attract More Muslim Visitors in 'Halal' Tourism Push." NPR *Parallels*, November 26, 2017. https://www.npr.org/sections/parallels/2017/11/26/528010256/indonesia-aims-to-attract-more-muslim-visitors-in-halal-tourism-push.

Winn, Monika, Patricia MacDonald, and Charlene Zietsma. "Managing Industry Reputation: The Dynamic Tension between Collective and Competitive Reputation Management Strategies." *Corporate Reputation Review* 11, no. 1 (2008): 35–55.

Wizarat al-Awqaf wa'l-Shu'ūn al-Islamiyyah. *Al-Mawsu'ah al-Fiqhiyyah*. Vol. 18. Wizarat al-Awqaf wa'l-Shu'ūn al-Islamiyyah :Kuwait, 1421AH/2001.

Xavier, John Anthony. "New Halal Frontier Products." *New Straits Times*, August 8, 2017.

Yahya Arief. "Indonesia aims to be top 'halal' destination." *The Jakarta Post*, March 14, 2019, https://www.thejakartapost.com/news/2019/03/14/indonesia-aims-to-be-top-halal-destination.html (accessed February 22, 2021).

Yusof, Raja Nerina Raja. *Halal Foods in the Global Retail Industry*. Serdang: University Putra Malaysia Press, 2013.

Al-Zahiri, Muhammad 'Ali b. Ahmad Ibn Hazm. *Al-Muhalla*. Cairo: Idarat al-Tiba'ah al-Muniriyyah, 1351AH/1932.

Zahrah, Muhammad Abu. *Usul al-fiqh*. Cairo: Dar al-Fikr al-'Arabi, 1377AH/1958.

Zaydan, 'Abd al-Karim. *Al-Wajiz fi Sharh al-Qawa'id al-Fiqhiyyah fi'l-Shari'ah al-Islamiyyah*. Beirut: Mu'assasah al-Risalah, 1425/2004.

Al-Zuhayli, Wahbah. *Al-Fiqh al-Islami wa Adillatuh*. Vol. 5. 3rd ed. Damascus: Dar al-Fikr, 1409AH/1989.

# Index